THE
ANTI-INFLAMMATION
ZONE

THE
ANTI-INFLAMMATION
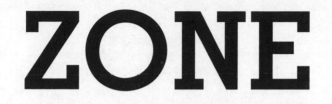

Reversing the Silent Epidemic
That's Destroying
Our Health

Dr. Barry Sears

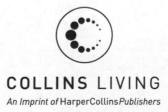

COLLINS LIVING
An Imprint of HarperCollins *Publishers*

This book contains advice and information relating to health care. It is not intended to replace medical advice and should be used to supplement rather than replace regular care by your doctor. It is recommended that you seek your physician's advice before embarking on any medical program or treatment. All efforts have been made to assure the accuracy of the information contained in this book as of the date of publication. The publisher and the author disclaim liability for any medical outcomes that may occur as a result of applying the methods suggested in this book.

A hardcover edition of this book was publishied in 2005 by HarperCollins Publishers.

FIRST PAPERBACK EDITION PUBLISHED 2006.

Designed by Nancy Singer Olaguera

The Library of Congress has cataloged the hardcover edition as follows:

Sears, Barry, 1947–
     The anti-inflammation zone : reversing the silent epidemic that's destroying our health / Barry Sears.—1st ed.
     p. cm.
     ISBN 0-06-059546-9
     1. Inflammation—Alternative treatment. 2. Inflammation—Diet therapy. 3. Fish oils—Therapeutic use. I. Title.

RB131.S43 2005
616'.0473—dc22

                                                                                    2004061350

ISBN 13: 978-0-06-083414-2 (pbk.)
ISBN 10: 0-06-083414-5 (pbk.)

10 ❖/RRD 20 19 18 17 16 15 14 13

Acknowledgments

No book that I write on the Zone is ever done alone. First and foremost is the continuing support of my wife, Lynn, who believed in my mission when no one else would. Equally important has been my brother, Doug, who has been with me through the trials and tribulations of my vision over the past twenty years. Of course, there were my daughters, Kelly and Kristin, who were the first Zone children and had to experience the constant tinkering of my Zone technology at every meal for most of their lives. On this book in particular, I wish to thank Deb Kotz for her excellent advice and Cassie Jones of ReganBooks for her expert editing. Finally, I wish to thank Judith Regan for her continuing faith in the Zone.

Contents

Introduction

The Zone continues to be misunderstood by the vast majority of the population as well as virtually the entire medical profession. It is still perceived as a weight-loss diet, as opposed to the pathway to a new understanding of how hormonal balance determines your state of wellness. The true key to wellness lies in also keeping a certain group of hormones, known as eicosanoids (eye-KAH-sa-noids), within a zone. These little known, almost mystical hormones are the guardians of your future. Keep them in balance, and your future is bright. Allow them to surge out of balance, and your future is bleak.

How I can make such a strong statement? I can because eicosanoids control inflammation, and that is becoming recognized as the underlying cause of many, if not all, chronic disease states that now threaten to destroy our health care system.

The benefits of hormonal control go far beyond weight loss. In fact, hormonal control impacts virtually every aspect of your life. Listed below are some of the powerful benefits beyond weight control that come by following my program to reach the Anti-Inflammation Zone:

- Better health
- Greater longevity
- Reduction of the symptoms of chronic disease
- Improved emotional control

- Greater mental acuity
- Improved physical performance

Diseases such as heart disease, diabetes, cancer, and Alzheimer's consume the vast bulk of our health care resources. Yet they all have a strong inflammatory component. This inflammation is relentlessly driving your body toward chronic disease. Control that inflammation, and you have gone a great distance to minimizing, if not reversing, the symptoms of these chronic diseases, moving you back to a state of wellness.

In fact, everything that is important in your life (health, longevity, physical and mental performance, and emotions) is ultimately controlled by your hormones. Keep these hormones in the appropriate balance and you will obtain the most cherished goal in life—wellness in both mind and body. Wellness is not some elusive state of mind. As I will show you, it can be measured and quantified in your blood. Thus, wellness no longer becomes a philosophical state, but a medical fact. How to get to this zone of wellness by controlling inflammation is the basis of this book.

My previous books on the Zone hormonal control technology over the last ten years have always touched on inflammation control, because the Zone is ultimately based on eicosanoid balance. When I wrote my first book on the Zone in 1995, virtually no one in the medical establishment, let alone the general public, had ever heard of eicosanoids even though the 1982 Nobel Prize in Physiology or Medicine was awarded for understanding their role in human disease. Today, the number of people who understand the power of eicosanoids is still very limited. However, everyone knows enough about inflammation to know that it's probably not a very good thing. What they don't realize is that inflammation is mediated by eicosanoids. Control your eicosanoids, and you control your levels of inflammation and thus your wellness. It's that simple, and in the process you will change your future.

The best tools you have to change that future are the combination of the Zone Diet plus high-dose, ultra-refined fish oil. Two other tools, although not nearly as powerful as diet, are smart exercise and stress reduction to reduce the collateral damage induced by inflammation. All of these approaches combined provide what I call the Zone Lifestyle Program. It will take you only thirty days to begin to master these tools that will change your future. Don't take my word for it—your blood will confirm it loud and clear. But this is only the start, because you have to use these tools on a lifetime basis to keep inflammation under control.

Keep in mind that the day you stop fighting inflammation is the day that you start accelerating the aging process, along with all the chronic diseases that come with it. Yes, losing excess body fat will be a key component in your lifelong struggle against inflammation. This is because it is excess insulin that not only makes you fat and keeps you fat, but also increases inflammation. However, as important as losing excess body fat is, it will not be nearly as important in your battle against inflammation as the use of high-dose, ultra-refined fish oil.

Another goal of this book is to alert you about the new epidemic of a type of inflammation that is below the perception of pain. This is known as silent inflammation. That's what makes it so dangerous; you don't know it's there, although it is constantly eroding your wellness until chronic disease erupts decades later. More important, this book will teach you how to bring the level of silent inflammation in your body under control with the least amount of effort on your part. I emphasize the phrase *with the least amount of effort,* since all change, no matter how positive, induces some stress. I promise you that within a thirty-day period, if not sooner, you will find that your life has dramatically improved. And, when you take the appropriate clinical tests, your blood will validate your movement to a new state of wellness. This is the kind of change that we all welcome.

The continuous control of inflammation is the foundation of the Zone. However, it usually takes at least a year before such habits become ingrained in your lifestyle. So, view this book as a wellness manual that you will refer to constantly to reinforce the necessary dietary and lifestyle skills. More important, you have to have some objective measurement of the benefits these hormonal changes bring. I don't want you to simply take my word for it, even though it is true that you can change your hormonal levels in just one meal, and that you feel, think, and perform better in just a few days once you are in the Zone. That's why I want you to track your changes and ultimately quantify them. Changes in your blood chemistry determine the true extent of your new state of wellness. These blood tests give you a laserlike insight into your future as they are the most precise markers of silent inflammation known to medical science.

If you don't learn how to master your hormones to control inflammation, your future will be much more difficult than it has to be. That's why reaching the Anti-Inflammation Zone gives you the potential to change your future and redirect it into whatever direction you wish. If your future currently looks bleak because of high levels of silent inflammation, don't worry, because you can change it within thirty days. And once you've done so, you're on the pathway to making wellness a permanent state.

Welcome to the Anti-Inflammation Zone—and the return to wellness.

part I

The Epidemic of Silent Inflammation and the Corresponding Loss of Wellness

What Is Wellness?

We assume we have it, and we take it for granted until we're sick. I'm referring to "wellness." Webster's dictionary defines wellness as "the quality or state of being in good health especially as an actively sought goal." This means we have to make an effort if we want to be healthy—something many of us don't do.

You probably think of wellness as simply the absence of chronic disease. If you aren't sick, then you must be well. That definition simply won't cut it because it can take years, if not decades, for diseases like heart disease, diabetes, cancer, and Alzheimer's to finally emerge. The seeds of chronic disease are planted at an early age, sometimes even as early as our childhood. Our genes, body weight, dietary habits, and physical fitness all determine whether we are in a state of wellness, and whether we are already moving toward chronic disease in the years to come. They also determine whether we have a stealth killer: silent inflammation. Having increased levels of silent inflammation means you are not in a state of wellness. In fact, here's my personal definition of wellness:

Wellness\'well-ness\n: the absence of silent inflammation.

You may be asking yourself, What on earth is silent inflammation? Even more perplexing, How can inflammation be silent? Silent inflammation is simply inflammation that falls below the threshold of perceived pain. That's what makes it so dangerous. You don't take any steps to stop it as it smolders for years, if not decades, eventually erupting into what we call chronic disease.

I can't emphasize enough how strong the link is between silent inflammation and life-threatening chronic diseases. If you have high levels of silent inflammation in your body, even if you are not actively sick, it means that you simply cannot be well.

Ironically, inflammation is the life-saving component of your immune system that helps fend off bacteria, viruses, fungi, and other microbial invaders. It also helps damaged tissue repair itself from injury. Without inflammation we would be sitting ducks in a very hostile world, with no way to repair the damage constantly being inflicted on us. But inflammation also has a dark side if it isn't turned off. Study after study points to myriad ways in which chronic inflammation does great harm to the body. It has a damaging effect on arteries, which can lead to heart attacks and strokes. It destroys nerve cells in the brains of Alzheimer's patients. It depresses the immune system and helps promote the formation of cancerous tumors. In essence, silent inflammation is the polar opposite of wellness. It lays the groundwork for chronic disease. What's more, it has become an epidemic in America—and threatens to destroy our health care system as we know it.

The good news is that you can do something to alter your future if you're now on a course to chronic disease. You can achieve a state of wellness when it's still early enough to head off heart disease or diabetes. This, of course, requires you to take action. First you need to find out whether you're in a state of wellness or on the path to disease. If you carry excess body fat, eat poorly, and get little exercise, you're probably heading down the wrong track. That should be fairly obvious, but measuring the extent of silent inflammation in your body will reveal just how bad off you really are. What's amazing, though, is that your state of wellness can now be measured scientifically. Blood tests can reveal your level of silent inflammation. If you have high levels, you need to take the next course of action—to move into the Anti-Inflammation Zone, which is the pathway back to wellness.

THE INSIDIOUS NATURE OF SILENT INFLAMMATION

All pain is ultimately due to inflammation. You generally begin to notice inflammation if you have swelling in your joints and tissues, but you really begin to pay attention when it creates pain. This kind of inflammation manifests itself as what I call *screaming pain*. You know it when you have it, and probably deal with it by reaching for an anti-inflammatory drug like aspirin or ibuprofen. If those over-the-counter drugs don't work, then you may reluctantly go to your physician for more powerful drugs.

If you ask your physician what inflammation actually is, he or she will simply tell you that it's very complex. This is medical shorthand for saying, "I really don't know, but it's probably bad." In fact, the primary focus of medicine since the beginning of time has been the search for compounds that reduce pain. Although pain medications can be very effective at providing temporary relief, they are powerless to stop what's causing the inflammation in the first place.

Let's take this one step further. Let's say you are lucky enough not to have a condition that causes chronic screaming pain. You think you're feeling just fine. You might still be suffering from the dangerous effects of chronic inflammation that is below the threshold of perceived pain. Your body suffers without complaint from this silent inflammation. You might even consider this to be *silent pain*. You don't feel the pain of this type inflammation as it relentlessly takes a toll on your brain, your heart, and your immune system.

MY PROMISE TO YOU

Having silent inflammation means that you are no longer well and are already on your way to chronic disease. You just don't know it yet. I know this can be hard to believe, but the truth is that virtually all chronic diseases work like this. They just don't happen overnight. Most people with cancer are shocked when they get their initial diagnosis. "But I'm feeling just fine. How can I be sick?" is a common question they ask. That's why we call cancer insidious. A tumor can lurk undetected, often for years, in the body before it makes its presence known. Silent inflammation is the same way. It may not announce its presence to you by causing you pain, but that doesn't mean it's not there. And if you have high levels of silent inflammation, you simply aren't well anymore, even if you aren't feeling sick at the moment.

Now imagine you could spot the beginning of silent inflammation years, if not decades, before these chronic diseases develop. Let's say you had the right "wonder drug" that could bring silent inflammation to a halt and greatly slow and possibly eliminate these diseases. Would you take it?

Who wouldn't? Well, I'm handing you this wonder drug in the form of this book, which not only uses the latest research on inflammation but also is designed to show you how to alter the hormonal environment in your body that leads to silent inflammation in the first place. When followed correctly, the dietary and lifestyle prescriptions in this book can reverse silent inflammation, thus preventing it from accelerating into full-blown chronic disease. With this book, you will have a clear pathway back to a state of wellness that can be verified by a simple blood test. That is what you call good medicine.

Achieving wellness means not only altering the pathway to chronic disease but also becomes the pathway to successful aging. Of course, you can't avoid getting older, but can you maintain your quality of life as you age? Can you avoid spending the last years of your life debilitated and dependent on nursing care? If you follow the simple dietary and lifestyle advice in *The Anti-Inflammation Zone,* the answer is an emphatic yes. The longer you maintain yourself in that state of wellness, the better your quality of life will be now and in the future.

In fact, you can start feeling better right now, within days of entering the Zone. This Anti-Inflammation Zone is not science fiction: its concepts have been verified in various studies, including those conducted at Harvard Medical School. Even if you think your quality of life is pretty good at the moment, you'll be amazed at how much better you can feel. Over the years, countless Zone advocates have told me that they never realized how great they could feel until they entered the Zone. Don't take my word for it; try the program for yourself. Get the blood tests. See whether you're in a state of wellness. Then get into the Zone and get your blood tested again. You will see improvements if you follow the plan. And you'll realize what it feels like to be truly well.

THE CONTINUING EVOLUTION OF THE ZONE

When I introduced the Zone a decade ago, I started a revolution about how we think about food. Food is not merely nourishment for the body; it's actually a powerful "drug" that can return you to a state of wellness through better hormonal control. Like a drug, though, food can also make you sick if you use it the wrong way. The Zone is not some mystical place or clever marketing term. It is a real physiological state of your body in which hormones are balanced to maximize wellness and minimize chronic disease. These hormones are controlled largely by your diet. Eat the right kinds of foods in the right amounts and you'll achieve hormonal balance. Eat the wrong foods in the wrong amounts and you'll get increased levels of silent inflammation, which will lead to chronic disease.

My earlier dietary recommendations of balanced protein, carbohydrates, and fats, which I first put forward in *The Zone* more than ten years ago, still remain the best way to control the hormone insulin. Controlling insulin is necessary to help you lose excess body fat and stave off obesity-related diseases like diabetes and heart disease as well as chronic silent inflammation. Taking ultra-refined high-dose fish oil, which I first discussed three years ago in *The Omega Rx Zone,* is the best way to balance your eicosanoids, which ultimately control all inflammation. Following my Zone Diet and taking high-dose fish oil are your keys to maintaining wellness.

There are, however, other steps that can also help you cover all your bases and reduce silent inflammation. These include incorporating smart exercise and simple stress reduction techniques into your daily wellness program. The more you incorporate these additional techniques, the less strict you have to be with the Zone Diet and the less ultra-refined fish oil you have to take.

This book is my most comprehensive Zone program to date. Besides mapping out a personalized dietary prescription, I give you a step-by-step plan to reduce silent inflammation within thirty days. Although you might need to make adjustments in your current lifestyle, you'll see that these changes won't require a radical revamping on your part. My exercise program is designed to be done while watching TV in your home. My relaxation techniques can be done at your office desk or in a comfortable chair. Following the Zone Diet requires nothing more than dividing your plate into three equal sections and then using your palm and eyes to help you get the appropriate portions of protein, fat, and carbohydrates. And you will need no more than fifteen seconds a day to take all the fish oil that you need!

Just a little effort can go a long way toward reducing the ravaging effects of silent inflammation. Here are my guarantees of what will happen during your first week of entering this new Zone of wellness. By reversing silent inflammation, you will:

- Think better
- Perform better
- Look better
- Feel better

All these benefits are the consequence of the rapid reduction of silent inflammation.

Over time, controlling the hormones that cause silent inflammation will:

- Help prevent heart disease and stroke
- Help ward off cancer
- Help reverse type 2 diabetes
- Help prevent neurological disease (Alzheimer's, depression, attention deficit disorder, Parkinson's)
- Help reduce autoimmune disease (rheumatoid arthritis, lupus, multiple sclerosis)
- Help reduce screaming pain (fibromyalgia, migraines, chronic pain, arthritis, and so on)

But most important, you begin to control your own future.

If you want to jump ahead and get started on the program, go immediately to Part II, which begins on page 33. You should notice results in two weeks or less. I don't, though, just want you to believe my promises without scientific data to support them. In the next two chapters, you'll get a brief understanding about what silent inflammation is and why it's so dangerous for your body if it isn't controlled. You'll also understand how the various components of my Zone technology work together to combat silent inflammation. Once you have this knowledge, you'll be convinced that you need to stay in the Anti-Inflammation Zone for life if maintaining wellness is your goal.

Why Is Silent Inflammation So Dangerous?

Inflammation is suddenly big news even though I have been writing about it for the past ten years. It made the cover of *Time* magazine in February 2004 and has been the subject of countless newspaper articles and TV news reports. This attention is certainly warranted. The culmination of decades of research points to one thing: inflammation that you can't feel (silent inflammation) may be the dark force responsible for many of the most feared diseases of middle and old age.

This breakthrough finding has both a downside and an upside. The downside is that average Americans are leading a lifestyle that causes chronic silent inflammation. This may doom them to severe disability in the future, despite all the recent advances in medical technologies. The upside is that instead of needing different treatments for, say, heart disease, cancer, diabetes, and Alzheimer's, a single silent inflammation–reducing remedy could prevent all four of these diseases, as well a number of others. What this means is that you don't need to sit around and wait for some new breakthrough in biotechnology to cure cancer or Alzheimer's that may be decades away (if ever). A simple, effective solution may already be at your fingertips—that is, maintaining yourself in the Anti-Inflammation Zone. Soon you'll understand how it works to fight silent inflammation so effectively while drugs cannot.

INFLAMMATION = PAIN

All pain is caused by inflammation. The primary focus of medicine since the beginning of time has been the search for compounds that reduce pain. Yet your doctor may be at a complete loss to explain what inflammation is and how it triggers pain in the body.

The ancient Greeks described inflammation as an "internal fire." By the first century A.D. ancient Roman physician Celsus elaborated on that definition when he stated that inflammation is "redness (*rubor*) and swelling (*tumor*) with heat (*calor*) and pain (*dolor*)." Two thousand years later, this ancient Roman description of inflammation hasn't changed much. We still think of inflamed areas of injury as swollen, red, and warm to the touch. And, yes, also painful.

Inflammation, however, encompasses much more than meets the eye. As I said in chapter 1, it is our ultimate weapon to fend off alien invaders (such as bacteria, viruses, and parasites) that enter our body and cause infectious diseases. The moment one of these invaders slips into our bloodstream, inflammation coordinates an all-out attack that destroys the enemy and any tissue it may have infected. Inflammation is also the way the body responds to trauma and injury in order to repair itself. Once the healing process begins, inflammation immediately vanishes and the body resumes its normal functioning. Without inflammation, we would be sitting ducks for opportunistic organisms and injuries to our bodies that would never heal.

Sometimes, however, the whole complex process doesn't shut down when it's supposed to. Inflammation becomes chronic rather than transitory, but now it maintains itself below our ability to perceive it as pain. It is this chronic silent inflammation that will ultimately kill you. This constant generation of silent inflammation may be due to a genetic predisposition or a lifestyle factor like obesity, poor diet, or smoking. Whatever the cause, an increased level of silent inflammation becomes a long-term war that decimates healthy blood vessels, tissues, and cells and sets the stage for chronic disease.

Silent inflammation harms the body in a number of ways. Studies have found that it destabilizes cholesterol deposits on coronary arteries, leading to heart attacks and possibly strokes. It also attacks nerve cells in the brains of those predisposed to Alzheimer's and triggers rapid cell division, causing healthy cells to turn into cancerous ones.

The secret to maintaining wellness is controlling silent inflammation the best you can over a lifetime. Yes, your body needs to have a functional inflammatory system to survive, but it also needs to shut down this process once the invader is thwarted or the wound is healed. The foot soldiers of silent inflammation are hormones known as eicosanoids. These hormones work in a coordinated system with your immune cells to win any battle that may arise in the body. They also need to be decommissioned after the battle ends. If they don't, they become the mediators of silent inflammation.

So let's look at your immunological army a little closer.

- **Eicosanoids:** These hormones ultimately control the entire inflammatory process. They allow specialized inflammation cells (neutrophils and macrophages) to mobilize and squeeze between the linings of blood vessels in order to get to the battlefield site. These special cells then destroy the invaders and gobble them up. Eicosanoids also cause the release of more inflammatory proteins, called cytokines, which signal for reinforcements. Soon an army of immune cells descends on the site, destroying the microbes and any damaged tissue. Other eicosanoids are the hormones of repair and rejuvenation. When these opposing eicosanoids are balanced, you are well. When they aren't, you are moving toward chronic disease.

- **Immune cells:** Your body's guardian cells, called mast cells, are always on the lookout for any sign of trouble. At the first sign of a foreign invader, these mast cells release the chemical histamine, which signals to your immune system that it should launch an attack. Histamine circulates through your bloodstream and attaches onto certain cells, causing a cascade of reactions to occur starting with a burst of pro-inflammatory eicosanoids. Blood vessels dilate in response to these eicosanoids, allowing more soldier cells (neutrophils and macrophages) to reach their target as quickly as possible. This dilation of blood vessels is mediated by eicosanoids and causes the trademark signs of inflammation: swelling, heat, and redness.

HOW EXCESS BODY FAT GENERATES SILENT INFLAMMATION

It used to be that fat cells were considered simply to be inert storage sites for excess fat. Unfortunately, research now suggests that fat cells are not as innocent as they seem. They are, in fact, very powerful generators of silent inflammation. This is the smoking gun that links excess body fat to a host of diseases, such as heart disease, cancer, and Alzheimer's.

Fat cells (especially those located in the abdominal region) tend to sequester arachidonic acid (AA), the building block for all pro-inflammatory eicosanoids. This is a protective mechanism to prevent buildup of potentially high levels of AA in your other cells. It's kind of like "out of sight, out of mind" at the molecular level. But as AA keeps piling up in your fat cells, eventually it will start the local production of pro-inflammatory eicosanoids. These locally produced inflammatory eicosanoids generate the production of more pro-inflammatory cytokines in the fat cells, such as interleukin-6 (IL-6) and tumor necrosis factor (TNF). Unlike pro-inflammatory eicosanoids, which cannot enter the bloodstream, the cytokines induced by them can leave the fatty tissue and circulate in the bloodstream, causing a cascade of additional inflammatory responses throughout your body.

The bottom line: the fatter you are, the more inflammation you are generating around the clock. This is why losing excess body fat is your frontline defense in your lifelong struggle against silent inflammation.

How do these immunological soldiers cause pain? Although I will go into more detail later in the book, pro-inflammatory eicosanoids make it easier for immune cells to pass through blood vessel walls to reach the battlefield. The same eicosanoids also trigger an accumulation of excess fluid in the area of the battle. This causes blood vessels to swell even more, which touches off nerve endings, sending a message to your brain that you're in pain. Just to make sure your brain gets the message, eicosanoids increase the sensitivity of the nerve fibers so they send out an even stronger pain signal. Your body wants your brain to know you have an immunological battle going on so you can stop what's causing it and take your body out of harm's way. For instance, if you put your finger into a flame, your body's pain reaction tells you to take it out quickly. After the battle has been won, your body normally recalls the immune system army. It does this by sending out anti-inflammatory agents in the form of the hormones cortisol and anti-inflammatory eicosanoids, which have the opposite effect of pro-inflammatory eicosanoids. These anti-inflammatory agents stop pain and begin to stimulate the healing process.

WHEN INFLAMMATION PERSISTS

Trouble starts when the inflammatory process persists and is transformed into chronic silent inflammation. There is a breakdown in communication so that pro-inflammatory eicosanoids continue to be generated, though at a lower level. These eicosanoids continue to fight an immunological war, but now it's against you. Healthy tissues, cells, and blood vessels come under continuing attack.

If the intensity of the attack is high enough, you'll continue to feel pain. This is the screaming pain that sends you running to the medicine cabinet for anti-inflammatory drugs like aspirin, ibuprofen (Advil, Motrin, Nuprin), or naproxen (Aleve). And yes, you might be able to effectively manage pain with one of these drugs or with new, more expensive prescription drugs, such as COX-2 inhibitors (see page 19), or even more powerful drugs, such as corticosteroids.

That's because virtually all pain medications stop the overproduction of pro-inflammatory eicosanoids.

Unfortunately, like dumb bombs, these same drugs also stop the production of anti-inflammatory eicosanoids, which your body needs not only to repair the damage on the battlefield, but also to maintain a state of wellness. Long-term use of these medications can cause a host of side effects, from stomach ulcers to a digestive lining malfunction called leaky gut syndrome to heart failure or even death. In fact, nearly as many people in America die each year from the recommended use of anti-inflammatory drugs as die from AIDS. For this reason, I don't think these drugs are good ways to control silent inflammation. (I discuss this in more detail in chapter 12.)

At least with screaming pain you're doing something that is proactive. With silent inflammation you do nothing, and that's where the true danger begins. Silent inflammation doesn't trigger the kind of intense inflammation that touches off nerve endings sending pain signals to the brain. You do, though, have enough inflammation to make your body susceptible to long-term damage. It can gradually wear away your blood vessels, immune system, and brain, causing chronic diseases like heart disease, cancer, and Alzheimer's.

Though driven by the same inflammatory eicosanoids as screaming pain, silent inflammation remains hidden for years. You can't feel it, so you do nothing to stop it. And that's why it's so destructive to your health. This gives rise to a terrible trade-off. Do you use anti-inflammatory drugs on a regular basis to keep silent inflammation under control? This would decrease the likelihood of chronic illness like heart disease, but also elevate your risk of gastrointestinal side effects and possibly death. Or is there another alternative? Reaching the *Anti-Inflammation Zone* is that alternative.

The latest research shows that silent inflammation damages your body in a number of ways. What's fascinating is how far the ill effects of silent inflammation seem to extend. Like a poison, it seeps into all the body's systems, wreaking havoc with cell division, the immune system, and major organs like the heart and brain. As a result, much of the conventional wisdom doctors have held about disease is now being challenged. Here are some examples.

HEART DISEASE

Many doctors think of heart disease as mainly a plumbing problem that results from the buildup of fatty deposits on major coronary arteries. These deposits or plaques thicken until they eventually cut off all blood supply to the artery, causing a heart attack. Since plaque is rich in cholesterol, having high levels of cholesterol in the blood should increase heart disease risk. The trouble is, 50 percent of all heart attacks occur in people with normal cholesterol levels, and the best drug that reduces heart attacks (aspirin) doesn't have any effect on cholesterol levels. What's more, doctors have discovered through new imaging tests that the most dangerous deposits often aren't that large, but they are very prone to rupture. These are known as soft plaques.

There must be another contributing factor, but what? The clues actually began in 1848 when Rudolf Virchow, the leading pathologist in Europe, stated that heart disease was an inflammatory condition after observing the heart tissue of individuals who died of heart disease. Virchow's insight was lost, since at that time there was no way to measure inflammation. There was, however, a way to measure cholesterol, which soon became known as the "cause" of heart disease (see chapter 15 for more detail).

Inflammation's link to heart disease wasn't investigated again until the 1970s, when Russell Ross at the University of Washington began to champion the then controversial notion that heart disease was an inflammatory condition. By then, however, the mantra was established that high cholesterol levels are the leading cause of heart disease. Since there was still was no way to measure inflammation, especially silent inflammation, cholesterol reduction remained the Holy Grail of cardiovascular medicine.

Finally, in the late 1990s, the first crude blood marker of silent inflammation was developed. This marker is known as C-reactive protein (CRP), a molecule produced in the liver in response to inflammation. As I will describe later, there is a new, far more sensitive indicator of silent inflammation that detects markers in the blood that rise far earlier in the inflammatory process than does CRP. This new test will tell you at the earliest possible time in your life that silent inflammation is beginning to increase.

DIABETES

Researchers have begun mapping out the complex interplay among inflammation, insulin, and excess body fat. They've learned that fat cells can work like immune cells, releasing pro-inflammatory proteins known as cytokines in greater and greater amounts as you gain weight. In other words, the fatter you are, the more silent inflammation you generate. These cytokines make cells more resistant to insulin, so your body pumps out more and more insulin, which increases the production of still more cytokines. The result is eventually type 2 (adult-onset) diabetes. So which came first, the inflammation or the increased insulin? I believe it's the inflammation, as I will explain later in the book (see chapter 14).

CANCER

Inflammation may work hand-in-hand with genetic mutations to turn normal cells into potentially deadly tumors. Macrophages and other inflammatory cells fire out free radicals, which destroy not only microbes but also the DNA from healthy cells. This is the biological equivalent of the wartime phrase "friendly fire" in which troops get hit by their own artillery. This can lead to genetic mutations that cause a cell to rapidly grow and proliferate. It is known that pro-inflammatory eicosanoids (the ultimate cause of silent inflammation) are not only highly associated with tumor formation, but also facilitate its spread into surrounding tissues (metastasis). Furthermore, these same pro-inflammatory eicosanoids effectively put a barrier between the tumor cell and the body's immune system making the tumor cell all but invisible.

Scientists are now exploring the role of an enzyme called cyclo-oxygenase 2 (COX-2) that makes many of these pro-inflammatory eicosanoids. This enzyme is increased during inflammation—and also in the development of a number of cancers. Several studies have shown that people who take daily doses of aspirin are less likely to develop precancerous growths in the colon called polyps. (Aspirin is known to block the COX-2 enzyme, but it can also cause side effects such as death by internal bleeding, therefore not making it the best possible anticancer drug.)

ALZHEIMER'S DISEASE

In trying to figure out why some Alzheimer's patients develop the disease earlier than others, researchers found an intriguing clue: those patients who were already taking anti-inflammatory drugs for arthritis or other conditions were less likely to develop the disease than those who weren't. Perhaps the immune system wages war against the characteristic plaques that form in the brains of Alzheimer's patients; if so, this inflammatory reaction may actually cause the worsening of the disease.

New research suggests that anything that reduces silent inflammation by reducing pro-inflammatory eicosanoids (like aspirin or eating fish) seems to reduce your risk of Alzheimer's disease. The catch is you have to take these measures to reduce silent inflammation decades before Alzheimer's starts. It's very difficult to reverse dementia in those who already have it, but its likelihood can be significantly reduced if you start early enough (like thirty years earlier).

AUTOIMMUNE DISEASES

These diseases, which include rheumatoid arthritis, multiple sclerosis, and lupus, are the most clear-cut examples of out-of-control inflammation. The body is literally at war with itself as the immune system launches a sophisticated attack on healthy cells and tissues, with no sign of any microbial invader to trigger such a reaction. New, powerful, and very expensive anti-inflammatory drugs introduced in the past few years have given hope to those with severe rheumatoid arthritis. These drugs inhibit the action-specific inflammatory cytokines to help reduce screaming pain. The trouble is, they also have side effects, and like all anti-inflammatory drugs they can't repair the damage that's already been done to the tissue. The only way to do that is to break the constant generation of silent inflammation and allow the body's natural anti-inflammatory machinery to begin the healing process.

Let's say you could find out if you had silent inflammation years, or possibly decades, before you developed one of these diseases. Would you take a blood test to get the diagnosis? Now, let's say you were told you did have high levels of silent inflammation, making it much more likely that you will develop any one of the above-mentioned diseases. Would you do something to stop it?

I suppose the only answer to this question is: How could you not? I came to this conclusion many years ago and have embarked on a mission to reduce silent inflammation in millions of Americans who assume they're healthy. I want them to be truly well and to maintain that wellness as they age. My personal journey to define wellness medically and lay out a simple pathway to reach it is the purpose of this book.

I know I'm well. That's not my perception. I have proof based on the blood tests that I will describe in chapter 4, which give you a complete spectrum of your true state of wellness. You get into this Anti-Inflammation Zone and stay there by following the Zone Diet, supplementing the diet with high-dose ultra-refined fish oil concentrates, and maintaining a moderate activity level.

I want to give this gift of wellness to you. You'll see in the next chapter how reducing silent inflammation will bring you into a state of wellness in less than thirty days and protect you against chronic disease in the future.

The Cause and the Cure for Silent Inflammation

Silent inflammation is the first sign that your body is out of balance and you are no longer well. You can't feel it, but it is grinding down your heart, your brain, and your immune system. Actually, there are three underlying hormonal changes that are linked to silent inflammation. These conditions all set the stage for chronic disease. They involve the overproduction of three distinct types of hormones:

- Pro-inflammatory eicosanoids
- Insulin
- Cortisol

Each of these three hormones contributes to silent inflammation when overproduced by the body. Fortunately, each can be brought back into balance by following the diet and lifestyle prescriptions laid out in *The Anti-Inflammation Zone*.

PRO-INFLAMMATORY EICOSANOIDS

If you've read my previous Zone books, you're probably heard about these hormones time and time again. As I will explain in more detail later in the book, eicosanoids were the first hormones developed by living organisms and are produced by every cell in your body. Although they might be considered primitive hormones, they control everything from your immune system to your brain to your heart. There are two kinds of eicosanoids, those that promote inflammation (pro-inflammatory) and tissue destruction and those that stop inflammation (anti-inflammatory) and promote healing. You need to have both kinds in the proper balance in order to be in a state of wellness. Unfortunately, most of us produce too many pro-inflammatory eicosanoids, which leads to increasing levels of silent inflammation and eventually to chronic disease. The Zone Diet was developed primarily to put these hormones back in proper balance.

Eicosanoids form the command center of your immune system. Knock them out completely, and the immune system goes with them. This occurs in those who have immune-deficiency diseases, such as AIDS. More common, however, is when eicosanoids stage a military coup of the immune system. Like rogue soldiers, if the pro-inflammatory eicosanoids aren't called back to the barracks, inflammation runs amok and your immune system starts attacking your body. Autoimmune diseases like rheumatoid arthritis, multiple sclerosis, lupus, and Crohn's disease can occur when there's too much "friendly fire" from the immune system. In fact, an imbalance of eicosanoids is at the foundation of chronic diseases like heart disease, cancer, and Alzheimer's. It is the imbalance of these eicosanoids that causes silent inflammation.

You can tip the balance back toward anti-inflammatory eicosanoids in a number of ways. First and foremost, you have to modify what you eat. Anti-inflammatory eicosanoids—which I refer to as the "good" ones—come from eating a diet rich in long-chain omega-3 fatty acids (found in fish oil) and spare in omega-6 fatty acids (found in vegetable oils like corn, soybean, sunflower, and safflower). This is because long-chain omega-3 fatty acids reduce pro-inflammatory eicosanoids, whereas omega-6 fatty acids increase the production of pro-inflammatory eicosanoids. Until about eighty years ago, our population ate a 2:1 ratio of omega-6 to omega-3 fats. We ate a lot more fish back then, and many of our grandparents took a daily dose of omega-3-rich cod liver oil. (Yes, it was disgusting, but it was anti-inflammatory, too.) Furthermore, refined vegetable oils were a very small part of our diet. Now all of that has changed. We're eating a lot more omega-6 fats and far fewer long-chain omega-3 fats, with the ratio of these two groups of fatty acids being closer to 20:1. With that dramatic increase in omega-6 fatty acids in our diet, the amount of silent inflammation in our society has correspondingly increased. Heart disease, diabetes, and cancer are all on the rise because they are initiated by silent inflammation, which comes from the overproduction of the pro-inflammatory eicosanoids.

How can the type of fat you eat cause silent inflammation? As a lipid (i.e., fat) researcher, I have been intrigued by this question for more than twenty-five years. It turns out that certain pro-inflammatory eicosanoids (primarily consisting of prostaglandins and leukotrienes) are derived from arachidonic acid (AA), a long-chain omega-6 fatty acid. Prostaglandins and leukotrienes are the usual suspects when you have screaming pain, and they are also the cause of silent inflammation. This is why every anti-inflammatory drug works to stop the overproduction of these particular eicosanoids. (As an added benefit, reducing the levels of pro-inflammatory eicosanoids also reduces the release of pro-inflammatory cytokines.)

The classic symptoms of inflammation are due in large part to those eicosanoids. Prostaglandins cause the pain, and leukotrienes cause the swelling and redness associated with inflammation.

To call off these storm troopers in your inflammatory army that are derived from AA, you need to increase the "good" anti-inflammatory eicosanoids. These are derived from long-chain omega-3 fatty acids, such as eicosapentaenoic acid (EPA). Ultimately, the balance of AA to EPA in your blood determines the levels of silent inflammation in your body. That's why I call this ratio of these two fatty acids your Silent Inflammation Profile (SIP). The higher the SIP, the less well you are and the more likely it is that you are going to develop some type of chronic disease. In other words, the SIP gives you a glimpse into your future. This is why I believe it is the single best test in medicine—because it reveals your state of wellness (or lack of it) with laserlike precision.

Insulin

Simply consuming a lot more fish oil and a lot less vegetable oil will begin to reverse silent inflammation. Changing your dietary habits by following the Zone Diet can also have an immediate impact, because that will reduce the levels of the hormone insulin, which indirectly affects silent inflammation. This is because increased insulin levels increase the production of AA, the building block for all pro-inflammatory eicosanoids. The power of the Zone Diet is that you can see a difference in your insulin levels within seven days. In fact, it has been shown by studies at Harvard Medical School that even one meal can begin to reduce insulin levels and then begin to drive you back to a state of wellness. You'll notice it right away in terms of your energy level and overall well-being. Of course, the opposite is also true: one meal that increases insulin levels can begin to drive you out of the Anti-Inflammation Zone.

You may hear a lot about insulin today, but still may not know exactly why it is important. To start with, insulin is the storage hormone that drives nutrients into cells. It is vital for your survival, since it allows cells to either store nutrients or immediately use them for energy. Without adequate levels of insulin, your cells would literally starve to death. This is exactly what happens in type 1 (childhood-onset) diabetes, in which the person is producing no insulin. (In fact, only a small percentage of diabetics have this type of diabetes.) Without daily injections of insulin, death is the inevitable outcome. But most of us are much more likely to have the opposite problem: we make way too much insulin. This is bad news, since it is excess insulin that makes you fat and keeps you fat. And it is also excess insulin that increases silent inflammation. This is the smoking gun that links excess fat to a wide range of chronic diseases such as heart disease, type 2 diabetes (more than 90 percent of all diabetics have this type), cancer, and Alzheimer's.

As you age, your cells become less responsive to insulin, and your pancreas needs to continually churn out more and more insulin to get the message through to the cells in the liver and the muscles that incoming dietary nutrients (primarily sugar and amino acids) need to be taken up by the cells. This is called insulin resistance. In general, the more excess body fat you have, the more insulin resistance you have, and the more insulin your body needs to produce in order to overcome this resistance. This means an increase in the levels of silent inflammation and a much higher risk for the development of chronic disease.

Excess insulin's link to silent inflammation stems from the fact that it increases the production of AA. And if that isn't bad enough, recent research shows that insulin induces inflammation by increasing the production of Interleukin-6 (IL-6), a pro-inflammatory cytokine that causes the formation of CRP, another marker for silent inflammation. The bottom line: controlling insulin is essential if you want to reverse silent inflammation and move toward a state of wellness.

A quick and easy way to tell if you're making too much insulin is to stand naked in front of your mirror and ask yourself two questions. First, are you overweight? Second, is much of the excess fat located around your abdomen (i.e., are you apple-shaped)? If the answer to both questions is yes, then it's a pretty good bet that you have insulin resistance. Insulin resistance is a precursor to type 2 diabetes and heart disease. In type 2 diabetes, the pancreas eventually begins to fail since it can no longer continue to pump out the megadoses of insulin (hyperinsulinemia) needed to push glucose into the cells. Without this excessive output of insulin to keep blood glucose levels under control, they now rise to dangerous levels. In heart disease, the increased production of insulin leads to increased silent inflammation that is the underlying cause of its development. These are two very different manifestations of long-term insulin resistance. The Zone Diet was developed specifically to reduce excess insulin production, and as a result the Zone Diet also reduces silent inflammation. You'll get all the added benefits that go along with this, including a loss of excess body fat, a reduced risk of heart disease, diabetes, and other insulin-related illnesses, and an increased life span. Not a bad deal.

The hormonal systems of both eicosanoids and insulin are intricately linked. They both trigger silent inflammation if they're out of balance. They both reduce silent inflammation when they're brought back into balance. Neither operates in a vacuum, since they are interrelated. The bad news is most of us have both systems out of balance at the same time, and it only gets worse as we age. The good news is the Zone Diet can normalize both systems, which is why it's the ultimate antidote to silent inflammation.

Cortisol

When your body is in a constant state of silent inflammation, it reacts by having your adrenal glands pump out high amounts of cortisol, the primary anti-inflammatory hormone you have to shut down excess inflammation. We tend to think of cortisol as a stress hormone, but in reality it is an anti-stress hormone. At the cellular level, all stress creates an inflammatory state caused by an overproduction of pro-inflammatory eicosanoids. Cortisol is sent out to lower the levels of these eicosanoids, which is fine over the short run when stress is temporary. But having a high level of constant silent inflammation means you are going to have high levels of cortisol on a permanent basis, causing a number of nasty consequences such as increasing insulin resistance (which makes you fatter), killing nerve cells (which makes you dumber), and depressing your entire immune system (which makes you sicker). This is the collateral damage that comes from increased silent inflammation. The diet and lifestyle prescriptions of *The Anti-Inflammation Zone* allow you to decrease silent inflammation and prevent the need for your body to increase cortisol levels. In fact, the more successful you are, the more control you'll have over cortisol. You might even be able to reduce your levels to what you'd normally produce if you were on a relaxing vacation at some tropical paradise.

IS SILENT INFLAMMATION IN YOUR GENES?

Why do we have this growing epidemic of silent inflammation? Blame it on your genes. Evolution tends to favor those biological characteristics in a particular species that make them better equipped to pass their genes on to the next generation. These are the genes that give the next generation an unfair advantage over others. Over the last 150,000 years, evolution has been working hard to favor the lucky few of our ancestors who had a higher chance for survival after birth, a survival long enough to be able to procreate. In those days, lack of food was a real problem, not to mention the constant hazard of alien bacteria, parasites, fungi, and viruses.

Nature dealt with these hurdles in a number of ways. It favored those individuals who were more efficient at storing fat, which would enable them to survive during lean times. Body fat is vital for survival. It's compact, high energy, and travels with you wherever you go. For example, it would take a 100-pound liver to store as much energy (in the form of carbohydrates) as 10 pounds of body fat. Who wouldn't rather tote around the 10 pounds of body fat instead of the 100-pound liver? Insulin is the hormone that allows us to easily store away fat for a rainy day. Thus, our early ancestors needed to develop the genetic propensity for producing large amounts of insulin whenever they ate excess calories during the times of feasting. Our genes evolved to increase insulin in two ways: eating too many carbohydrates or eating too many calories.

Now fast-forward to present-day America. We have no more famines, and we're constantly feasting on unlimited amounts of inexpensive food that is rich in carbohydrates. But our DNA still lives in the Stone Age, even if we don't. Our genes haven't had time to adapt to the Krispy Kreme doughnut generation. So if we eat too much on a regular basis, our cells pump out more and more insulin. As a result, we sock away more and more fat, and voila! We now have an obesity epidemic on our hands and that means a corresponding epidemic of silent inflammation. The very genes that saved us tens of thousands of years ago are now our biggest liability.

The same is true of our ability to generate a strong inflammatory response. This was the only way to survive microbial or parasitic invasions. As recently as seventy years ago, we had very few weapons against infectious diseases except a strong inflammatory response to kill such organisms. All we could do was hope and pray that our immune system would protect us against these ravages. Picture the Norman Rockwell painting of the physician wringing his hands over the patient, hoping the fever would break. That's the way medicine was practiced seventy years ago.

Those of us with overactive immune systems had a better chance of survival than those with weaker immune defenses. Thus, we've inherited a genetic predisposition for an intense inflammatory response from our ancestors who were the only ones to survive these constant microbial attacks. Today, we are faced with far fewer infectious disease threats. Vaccinations, clean water, and increased sanitation have banished many of these microbes. What's more, we have a whole arsenal of drugs to take against microbial infections.

Unfortunately, we no longer need our genetic propensity for mounting an excessive inflammatory response. Yet, again, we are stuck with this propensity since our genes haven't had time to evolve. This sets the stage for increased silent inflammation, which gets activated by our diet and lifestyle. Our dramatically increased intake of vegetable oils (rich in the building blocks for pro-inflammatory eicosanoids) and our decreased consumption of fish oil (rich in the building blocks for anti-inflammatory eicosanoids) is one dietary habit that has activated this inflammation. It's like adding kerosene to the already burning fire of silent inflammation that's fueled by the obesity epidemic.

While it's true that you can't replace your genes, you can change their expression by altering your diet and lifestyle. Reaching the Anti-Inflammation Zone will alter the functioning of these genes and reverse the course of silent inflammation throughout your lifetime.

CONTROLLING YOUR GENES

If the genes that increased our chances for survival also increase the likelihood of silent inflammation, then how did we get as far as we have? The answer lies with diet and lifestyle. For much of our time on earth, humans followed an anti-inflammatory diet that worked in concert with our pro-inflammatory genes. Ten thousand years ago, this was a diet rich in fruits and vegetables, lean protein, and long-chain omega-3 fats (coming primarily from fish) and was simultaneously poor in omega-6 fats. This Paleolithic diet had virtually no grains or starches. It was the diet of hunters and gatherers and acted as a way to manage our increased genetic propensity to generate inflammation and excess insulin. As a result, silent inflammation was kept under control.

With the advent of agriculture, things started to change, but it has only been in the last two generations that our diet has gotten completely out of harmony with our genes. Of course, we can't go back to the hunter/gatherer caveman days. Who'd want to give up supermarkets? But we can alter our current eating habits to better reflect the anti-inflammatory actions of a Paleolithic diet. This diet was able to keep the immune system at full alert without causing chronic silent inflammation. It's the diet we should all be following now if we truly want to keep silent inflammation under control and reach the zone of wellness.

As long as our diet can counterbalance our increased insulin and inflammation responses honed by evolution, then life is good. It's only when things get out of balance that chronic silent inflammation begins to emerge. The modern-day version of this Paleolithic diet is the Zone Diet that I have been writing about for the past ten years. This is the key to returning to a state of wellness and keeping yourself there for a lifetime. In the Anti-Inflammation Zone, silent inflammation is no longer elevated, as you are in a new physiological state in which your inflammatory genes are balanced by an anti-inflammatory diet to keep silent inflammation under control. This is the molecular definition of wellness.

Reaching the Anti-Inflammation Zone also incorporates a host of new strategies against silent inflammation in addition to the Zone Diet. Certain anti-inflammation foods like extra-virgin olive oil, wine, sesame oil, turmeric, and ginger are featured prominently in the recipes to fight against silent inflammation. A comprehensive (but simple-to-follow) exercise plan is needed to help keep insulin levels in check. Cortisol reduction strategies such as meditation will boost these hormonal benefits even further.

Think of these lifestyle changes as if they are "drugs" that you have to take on a daily basis to control silent inflammation. The power of reaching the Anti-Inflammation Zone lies in keeping the hormones you can control (eicosanoids, insulin, and cortisol) in their appropriate zones (not too high and not too low) so that you can live a longer and healthier life—in essence, maintain a state of wellness. Or you can choose to do nothing—but then you'll have to face the ravages of aging, a consequence of increasing levels of silent inflammation. The choice is in your hands.

part II

Entering the Anti-Inflammation Zone: How to Combat Silent Inflammation on a Lifetime Basis

Testing for Silent Inflammation

Wellness is ultimately dependent on the levels of inflammation and especially silent inflammation in your body. If you have screaming pain or an existing chronic disease, you know, of course, that you aren't well. Having type 2 diabetes, heart disease, cancer, or Alzheimer's means you have inflammation. Having an autoimmune condition such as multiple sclerosis or lupus also indicates that inflammation is present. Any chronic pain condition—those that end with "itis"—means you have inflammation in the area that is causing you pain. But silent inflammation is different. It is ongoing inflammation that is below the perception of pain. Until recently there was no way to test for it. Now that there is, you can find out if you have it and begin to mount a lifelong anti-inflammatory program to keep it at bay. You can also have periodic clinical testing to determine whether your efforts have been successful.

The first step you need to take to reach the Anti-Inflammation Zone is to determine whether you have silent inflammation and, if so, the extent of it. Silent inflammation is hard to detect, and it's impossible to determine by sight alone. You might have it if you're obese, or you might not. In fact, you can be overweight and still be in a state of wellness if your insulin levels are in the healthy range (good news for millions of Americans). On the flip side, you might have significant silent inflammation if you're at your ideal weight.

So how can you figure all this out? A clinical assessment of your blood to determine your degree of silent inflammation is the only definitive answer. However, there are subjective ways to help give you a clue. Many years ago, I developed what I call a Silent Inflammation Report to help both heart disease patients and world-class athletes make the necessary dietary changes to combat this type of inflammation. The questionnaire is purely based on observations, but it is an easy way to give you a general indication of whether you're likely to have silent inflammation.

SILENT INFLAMMATION REPORT

Parameter	Yes	No
Are you overweight?	_____	_____
Are you always craving carbohydrates?	_____	_____
Are you constantly hungry?	_____	_____
Are you tired, especially after exercise?	_____	_____
Are your fingernails brittle?	_____	_____
Is your hair limp with little texture?	_____	_____
Are you constipated?	_____	_____
Do you sleep excessively?	_____	_____
Are you groggy upon waking?	_____	_____
Do you have a lack of mental concentration?	_____	_____
Do you lack a sense of well-being?	_____	_____
Do you have headaches?	_____	_____
Are you constantly fatigued?	_____	_____
Do you have dry skin?	_____	_____

If you answer yes to more than three questions, you probably have elevated levels of silent inflammation. Admittedly, this is not a very scientific way of determining the levels of silent inflammation in your body, but it does tell you whether you're a likely candidate. If you are, your next step should be to test your blood to determine the true extent of the inflammation, and thus your current state of wellness.

PRIMARY BIOMARKERS FOR THE ANTI-INFLAMMATION ZONE

It is only within the past few years that blood tests have been developed to measure silent inflammation. These tests look for specific biomarkers of silent inflammation and the levels that indicate that significant inflammation is already under way. These biomarkers are the best indication that you need to start taking immediate action because real trouble is brewing. Think of silent inflammation as kindling. Try to light a log with a match, and nothing happens. On the other hand, light the kindling with a match, and the log is soon engulfed by flames. Now consider the log to be your body, the flames are screaming pain or chronic disease. Those are the symptoms that you see, but the first step was the lighting of the kindling.

Silent Inflammation Profile

This is the gold standard test for silent inflammation. It measures the balance of pro-inflammatory eicosanoids and anti-inflammatory eicosanoids by measuring the key fatty acid building blocks in the bloodstream for eicosanoids. These are also the hormones that ultimately control inflammation. Since eicosanoids don't circulate in the blood, there is no direct test for them. This is why they are little understood by today's medical community. Eicosanoids exist only momentarily to carry information from one cell to another, and then they are deactivated in a matter of seconds. They are, however, synthesized from fatty acid building blocks that circulate in the blood. Measuring the ratio of fatty acid building blocks for pro-inflammatory "bad" eicosanoids (arachidonic acid or AA) and the building blocks for anti-inflammatory "good" eicosanoids (eicosapentaenoic acid or EPA) can tell us the balance of "bad" to "good" eicosanoids, and provides a reasonably precise indicator of the levels of the same fatty acids in the rest of the 60 trillion cells in the body.

It is the ratio of AA to EPA in the blood that provides the most precise marker of silent inflammation, and this is why I call this test your Silent Inflammation Profile (SIP). Your SIP can alert you years, if not decades, in advance of real trouble. The higher the SIP, the greater your likelihood of having a heart attack, getting cancer, or developing Alzheimer's disease. These diseases don't happen overnight and take decades to develop. The more advance warning you have, the easier it will be to make the necessary changes to bring silent inflammation under control and to dramatically reduce your likelihood of developing chronic disease in your future.

I cannot emphasize enough the importance of the SIP. Science backs me up. Consider the landmark Lyon Diet Heart Study that demonstrated the most striking reduction in cardiovascular mortality known to medical science. In this study, two randomized groups of patients who survived recent heart attacks were put on different diets. One followed the standard American Heart Association diet, which is rich in grains and starches and low in fat but high in pro-inflammatory omega-6 fatty acids (found in vegetable oils). The other group followed a diet rich in fruits and vegetables but low in pro-inflammatory omega-6 fatty acids. After four years, the group that had dramatically reduced their intake of omega-6 fatty acids experienced a 70 percent reduction in the number of fatal heart attacks compared to the other group, who did not reduce their intake. They also experienced *no* sudden cardiovascular deaths. This is vitally important, since sudden death normally accounts for more than 50 percent of all cardiovascular mortality. More important, the divergence in mortality between the two groups began to appear as early as three months into the study. There is no drug that has such a striking impact on reducing the likelihood of heart attacks. So what was the cause of this miracle?

Researchers were amazed to find no differences in cholesterol, triglycerides, glucose, or blood pressure levels between the groups. (So much for cholesterol causing heart disease, but more on that later.) The only difference was that the group that avoided omega-6 fatty acids had a 30 percent drop in their SIP, compared to the control group. It appeared that for each 1 percent reduction in the SIP, the risk of dying from heart attack was reduced by 2 percent. I'd say that's a pretty strong case for SIP as a diagnostic test for your future.

Decreasing the SIP has also been associated with the reversal of multiple sclerosis, an autoimmune condition that causes inflammation in the brain and nervous system. At this point, no medication can reverse multiple sclerosis; drugs only slow the relentless progress of this disease. Yet preliminary research from Norway indicates that reducing the SIP can actually reverse nerve damage caused by multiple sclerosis in some patients. Other published studies have indicated that those who have a high SIP seem to have an increased risk of developing dementia, depression, and attention deficit disorder. Such published research, coupled with the thousands of SIP tests that I have done in the past three years, is why I consider the SIP to be the most powerful blood test you can take. I firmly believe that it predicts your likelihood of developing cancer, Alzheimer's, and heart disease decades before these diseases manifest themselves. The higher your SIP, the more silent inflammation you have and the further you are from a state of wellness. Before you get too depressed, the good news is that you can dramatically reduce your SIP within thirty days using my dietary prescription, which I describe later in this book.

WHERE CAN YOU GET THE SILENT INFLAMMATION PROFILE?

Until recently the Silent Inflammation Profile (SIP) had been done only in specialized university research laboratories. But now a handful of commercial laboratories are offering the test. You can ask your physician to order a blood test to measure your ratio of AA to EPA. The laboratory with which I have had the greatest success is Nutrasource Diagnostics in Canada, which is associated with the University of Guelph. They measure the ratio of AA to EPA in the plasma phospholipids, which yields a far more reliable (and consistent) result than measuring the ratio from the red blood cells. It's a complicated test and not covered by most insurance, but the results are well worth it. Here's how you or your doctor can contact Nutrasource Diagnostics, Inc:

130 Research Lane, University of Guelph Research Park
Guelph, Ontario, Canada N1G 5G3

U.S. physicians: 519-824-4120 x58817
U.S. consumers: 800-404-8171
Canadian physicians and consumers: 866-MDS-TEST (866-637-8378)

Fasting Insulin Levels

Although the SIP remains the gold standard of quantifying the levels of silent inflammation, measuring your degree of insulin resistance is the next best biomarker. As I will discuss later, insulin resistance is the underlying cause of obesity and type 2 diabetes and is characterized by excess levels of insulin in the bloodstream. The best clinical blood test for determining the extent of insulin resistance is your fasting insulin level. The higher your insulin levels, the more inflammation your body is producing, because insulin stimulates the production of AA from omega-6 fatty acids. What's more, it increases the amount of stored body fat, which generates an increased amount of silent inflammation, as I will explain in chapter 14.

Unlike the SIP, fasting insulin blood tests are relatively routine and are often covered by medical insurance. They are used to screen for not only diabetes but also heart disease. (Fasting insulin levels are a far better predictor of future risk of heart disease than cholesterol tests.) Unfortunately, they are also expensive, so some physicians are reluctant to order them, as HMOs may be reluctant to cover the cost of the fasting insulin test. But if you make a strong case for why you need it, you'll probably get coverage.

If you really want to be considered well, then both your SIP and fasting insulin should fall within the parameters shown below that define the Anti-Inflammation Zone, and hence your state of wellness.

PRIMARY CLINICAL BIOMARKERS OF THE ANTI-INFLAMMATION ZONE

Parameter	Good	Ideal
Silent Inflammation Profile	3	1.5
Fasting Insulin (uIU/mL)	10	5

Where did these numbers come from? The SIP numbers are based on studies of the Japanese who have the longest life span, the longest health span (longevity minus years of disability), the lowest rates of heart disease, and the lowest rates of depression in the world. They also have an average SIP of about 1.5. In comparison, the SIP of the average American is about 12. Not only are Americans the fattest people in the world, but we probably also have the most inflammation. This helps explain why we spend so much on health care and have so little to show for it. Once silent inflammation gets a foothold in the body, it can be difficult to stop.

If a high SIP is bad, then shouldn't you aim for the lowest possible SIP (say, below 1)? Not necessarily. If your SIP is too low, you won't be making enough pro-inflammatory eicosanoids and will have a difficult time mounting an appropriate response against infection. This was found to be the case in epidemiological studies of the Greenland Eskimos in the 1970s. These Eskimos had very low rates of heart disease, depression, multiple sclerosis, and diabetes but tended to die more readily of infectious disease. Their average SIP was about 0.7. Those who had an SIP of 0.5 had a much higher risk of hemorrhagic strokes. Again, you are looking for maintenance of your inflammatory reserves within a balanced Zone. Once your SIP is beyond 15, you definitely have significant levels of silent inflammation. In fact, I tested some patients with SIP levels as high as 50 (and in some children as high as 100), but these people usually also have severe chronic pain or neurological problems. The higher your SIP is above 15, the greater your risk of facing real trouble in a relatively short period of time. Shown below is the relationship of the SIP to chronic disease risk.

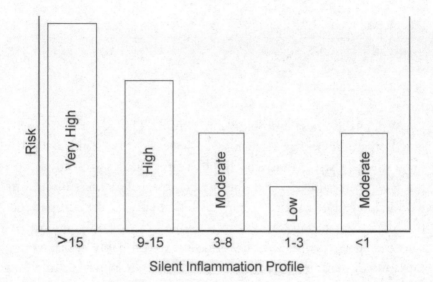

Silent Inflammation Profile

If your level of fasting insulin is greater than 10 uIU/mL, then your likelihood of developing heart disease increases more than five-fold. Keep in mind that if you have high cholesterol, your likelihood of developing heart disease is increased only by a factor of two. Although we have a national war against cholesterol, we never hear of the war against excess insulin. This is why I strongly advise you to get an insulin blood test as opposed to a general cholesterol screening.

If your fasting insulin levels are greater than 15, then you know that you are generating a lot of silent inflammation and fast-tracking yourself to an early heart attack and premature mortality. By the time you reach this level of insulin you are already probably overweight, insulin resistant, and also well on your way to becoming a type 2 diabetic.

SECONDARY BIOMARKERS FOR THE ANTI-INFLAMMATION ZONE

The SIP is not a routine test, although it can be ordered from specialized clinical laboratories. Likewise, doctors are reluctant to perform a fasting insulin test since it's more expensive than standard blood tests. What else will give you a clue to your future? Fortunately, there are some secondary blood tests for wellness that are cheaper and more routinely performed. They will give you a general indication of wellness, though they're not nearly as precise as the SIP or fasting insulin tests.

TG/HDL Ratio

You can get this ratio by getting a standard fasting blood lipid test, which is generally done to get your total cholesterol levels broken down into their individual components. The important numbers are not total cholesterol or even the "bad" (LDL) cholesterol. Rather, you want to look at the level of triglycerides (TG) and the level of "the good" (HDL) cholesterol. The TG/HDL ratio will tell you if you have what is called metabolic syndrome, which is caused by insulin resistance. Metabolic syndrome is a cluster of chronic conditions (obesity, type 2 diabetes, heart disease, and hypertension) that are related to high insulin levels (hyperinsulinemia) caused by insulin resistance. Therefore, the TG/HDL ratio becomes a surrogate marker of insulin. The higher the TG/HDL ratio, the higher your insulin levels and the more silent inflammation you may be generating. (Note: You can have a normal fasting insulin or TG/HDL ratio and still have a high SIP, so this test won't catch all silent inflammation. A ratio greater than 2, however, does indicate that you have increased silent inflammation.)

The TG/HDL cholesterol ratio can also give you information

on your heart disease risk. The lower your TG/HDL ratio is, the greater your protection against heart disease. This protection comes from having a high percentage of nonatherogenic (i.e., friendly) LDL particles in the bloodstream.

In recent years, the cholesterol picture has become more complicated; we now know there is *good* "bad" cholesterol and *bad* "bad" cholesterol. The good "bad" cholesterol is fluffy "beach-ball-like" LDL particles, which are relatively harmless to your arteries. On the other hand, the bad "bad" cholesterol is small, dense LDL particles, which can be deadly. They oxidize more readily and accumulate in cells that line the blood vessels, eventually leading to the development of atherosclerotic plaques that protrude into the bloodstream and occlude the arteries. These baseball-like particles can do a lot of damage to your arteries and dramatically increase your risk of heart disease. How can you tell which kind of LDL particles you have? The higher your TG/HDL ratio, the more of the dangerous "baseball" particles you have and the fewer the harmless "beach balls."

If you doubt that this TG/HDL ratio really predicts future development of heart disease, consider this: A 2001 study found that those who had a low TG/HDL ratio—even if they smoked, were sedentary, or had high LDL cholesterol or hypertension—had half the risk of developing heart disease than those with a high TG/HDL ratio who had no other risk factors for heart disease. This isn't to say you should take up smoking, become a sloth, drive up your LDL cholesterol levels, or develop high blood pressure. But if you have a low TG/HDL ratio, then you are far better protected against future heart disease than those who are doing all the right things but have a high TG/HDL ratio.

What's more, studies from Harvard Medical School indicate that patients with a high TG/HDL ratio can be up to sixteen times more likely to suffer a heart attack than those with a low TG/HDL ratio. For comparison, the average American has a TG/HDL ratio of 3.3; those who have a ratio of 4 or more are either pre-diabetic or have type 2 diabetes. I'm not telling you this to let you off the hook for engaging in heart-damaging behaviors like smoking. You should definitely do what it takes to avoid smoking, to get active, and to keep your blood pressure down. However, your primary focus should be on getting your TG/HDL ratio into the ranges that define the Anti-Inflammation Zone.

C-Reactive Protein

Currently, the most popular way to test for inflammation is a blood test that measures a marker called C-reactive protein (CRP). But is it as good as it appears? Synthesized in the liver in response to acute inflammation, CRP was first discovered about fifty years ago when researchers found that it's extremely elevated during times of infection by bacteria, viruses, or other microbes. Not much followed that discovery, since it wasn't very useful. By the time you could measure CRP levels, the patient was obviously very ill. A few years ago, researchers developed a more sensitive test for CRP, called high-sensitivity CRP (hs-CRP), that could detect much lower levels of this protein. They discovered that when CRP is only slightly elevated, it might indicate silent inflammation rather than an acute infection. Initial studies indicated that mildly elevated CRP levels may be a far better predictor than cholesterol levels of heart disease risk. Unfortunately, more recent studies have not confirmed this. In fact, a lot of things, like being overweight or having hypertension or type 2 diabetes, also elevate CRP. When you take all of these nonlipid factors into account, the predictive value of CRP for future heart disease is virtually eliminated.

With the information we now have, CRP appears to be a nonspecific marker of inflammation. It's present during inflammation, but lowering CRP levels may not help alleviate inflammation. Aspirin, for instance, is an excellent anti-inflammatory drug, but it doesn't significantly lower CRP levels. Likewise, vitamin E lowers CRP levels but doesn't decrease inflammation or prevent cardiovascular mortality. So at this point CRP simply appears to signal that inflammation is already present without being the actual culprit of inflammation. An interesting aside to this point comes from a lecture I gave at Harvard Medical School a few years ago on the SIP. After the lecture, one of the professors came over to tell me that my lecture scared him. He said his lab had just begun studying the SIPs of their graduate students, and he found that their levels were very elevated, whereas their CRP levels were perfectly normal. The scary part, he said, was that Harvard had been using such students as the control groups for a number of years, and now he was wondering if they had to reexamine all their data because the "normal" controls might have already been highly inflamed.

Even though the high-sensitivity CRP test is being heralded in the media, I consider it the poor man's marker for silent inflammation. Nonetheless, something is better than nothing. Your risk of heart disease goes up dramatically once you get above 3 mg/L, even if you have normal LDL cholesterol levels. Ideally, you want to keep this marker under 1 mg/L, but at the very least, it should be under 2 mg/L. The ranges for the secondary biomarkers for the Anti-Inflammation Zone are shown below.

SECONDARY BIOMARKERS FOR THE ANTI-INFLAMMATION ZONE

Parameter	Good	Ideal
TG/HDL	2	Less than 1
High-sensitivity CRP (mg/L)	2	Less than 1

Finally, if you are reluctant to have a blood test, you can always measure your percentage of body fat or simply measure your waist at your belly button, since both are surrogate markers for insulin levels. (However, it is quite possible to be overweight and still be well if your markers of inflammation are in the appropriate zones.)

Although I consider these relatively weaker markers of silent inflammation, you need only a tape measurement and pencil to calculate either of them as shown in Appendix E. You can also log on to my website at www.drsears.com and use the online calculator once you have your measurements. Here are the ranges you want to strive for:

WEAK BIOMARKERS FOR THE ANTI-INFLAMMATION ZONE

Parameter	Good	Ideal
Percent Body Fat		
Males	15	12
Females	22	20
Waist measurement (measured at the belly button)		
Males	Less than 40 inches	Less than 35 inches
Females	Less than 35 inches	Less than 30 inches

The reason I call these tests weak markers for silent inflammation is that they don't cast as wide a net as the primary biomarkers for silent inflammation, the SIP or fasting insulin, does. Yes, if your insulin levels are high, you are going to have high levels of silent inflammation. But you may also have silent inflammation even if your insulin levels and body fat fall within the healthy range. A great number of world-class athletes have high levels of silent inflammation induced by their intensive training. They are physically fit, but often not well. This eventually leads to a weakened immune system, which is why these athletes get more frequent colds, are often in a state of chronic pain and fatigue, and constantly keep breaking down.

SUMMARY

Knowledge is power when it comes to silent inflammation. Silent inflammation is insidious and the greatest threat to your wellness. Keep in mind that wellness is not a multiple choice test: you have to keep both insulin and eicosanoids within their appropriate ranges that define the Anti-Inflammation Zone. Only then can you be assured of being in a state of wellness. Don't make wellness a guessing game. Take the time to invest in the medical tests that will determine exactly where you stand. If you find you aren't quite there, keep making the adjustments to your diet and lifestyle until your blood says for sure that you're moving toward the Anti-Inflammation Zone, which indicates your state of wellness.

Your First Line of Defense Against Silent Inflammation: The Zone Diet

To keep inflammation at bay, you need a drug that you can safely take over the course of your lifetime. That "drug" is an anti-inflammation diet—the Zone Diet. The word *diet* comes from the ancient Greek root, which means "way of life." We have corrupted the real meaning of diet to now think of it as simply a short-term period of hunger and deprivation to hopefully get you into a swimsuit. But fighting silent inflammation is a lifelong struggle, which means you have to have a lifelong diet to control it. The Zone Diet is exactly that: it gives you your primary "drug" to reverse silent inflammation, slow the aging process, and lower your risk of chronic disease. But like any drug, you have to take it at the right time and the right dosage to get the maximum effect. Go off the Zone Diet, and you may usher in the return of silent inflammation, acceleration of chronic disease, and a decreased life span.

The Zone Diet was designed to reverse inflammation by reducing the production of pro-inflammatory eicosanoids. This is done by both reducing excess body fat (a primary mediator of inflammation) and reducing excess insulin levels (a primary mediator of arachidonic acid [AA] formation). I will explain both in more detail later in the book. Since Americans have become the fattest people on the face of the earth, it also means we have the unfortunate distinction of also having highest rates of silent inflammation.

This linkage of excess body fat and increased silent inflammation is the smoking gun that links obesity to a wide variety of chronic diseases like heart disease, type 2 diabetes, cancer, and Alzheimer's. Increasing levels of silent inflammation accelerate the development of all of these chronic diseases.

Losing excess body fat is hard, but keeping it off is an even greater challenge. The question is: Why has it become so much more of a challenge in recent years? Was there some strange genetic mutation that occurred only in America? Probably not. Up until 1980, the rates of obesity in America remained fairly constant, at about 14 percent of the population. Over the past twenty-five years, however, obesity has surged to a current record-setting 33 percent of Americans. To add more fuel to the fire, more than two-thirds of Americans are now overweight. Why is our collective weight spinning out of control?

Although I will discuss this in greater detail later in the book, the short answer is that we're eating more calories because we're hungrier. The best way to lose excess body fat and reduce silent inflammation is simply to eat fewer calories. This is incredibly difficult to do if you're always hungry.

Here's a strange paradox to consider: the more calories you eat, the hungrier you become. This paradox won't seem so strange once you understand what really makes you hungry: low blood sugar. The brain needs a certain amount of glucose (blood sugar) to fuel itself. It's a glucose hog, using 70 percent of your blood glucose to keep itself functioning, though it accounts for less than 3 percent of your total body weight. When blood glucose levels fall, your brain throws the equivalent of a temper tantrum: you may feel irritated or in a mental fog or may feel increased hunger. Whatever the symptom, you learn to self-medicate this drop in blood glucose levels by eating more carbohydrates, especially candy bars, sugar-laden soft drinks, cookies, corn chips, and so on, that quickly enter the bloodstream as glucose. Once you do, you feel better. Your brain is rewarding you for giving it the glucose it desperately needs. The faster the brain gets fed, the quicker you feel better. You may not even realize it, but you're setting yourself up for another bout of low blood glucose (hypoglycemia), because the same carbohydrates that rapidly increased your blood glucose have also caused a rapid increase in the secretion of excess insulin, which will dramatically reduce your blood glucose levels within one to two hours. Do this self-medication on a constant basis, and excess body fat piles on because it is excess insulin that makes you fat and keeps you fat.

You might assume that if your brain relies on a constant supply of blood sugar to function, then you should feed it by eating primarily carbohydrates all day long. But that would only upset the delicate balance of insulin and glucagon. These two hormones work in concert to keep hunger at bay and keep your brain feeling happy. Insulin drives blood glucose into your liver cells to use at a later time, and glucagon releases this stored glucose when your brain needs it. Carbohydrates stimulate insulin secretion; protein stimulates glucagon secretion. When these two hormones are in balance from a properly proportioned diet, such as the Zone Diet, you keep hunger at bay and lose excess body fat because of lack of hunger between meals. Unfortunately, the hormonal partnership that was built over millions of years of evolution can be easily destroyed by a high-carbohydrate diet.

For a decade, nutritionists espoused the mantra that a calorie is calorie. Since, gram for gram, carbohydrates contain fewer calories than fat, they stated we would lose excess weight by eating more carbohydrates and less fat. Many Americans took this advice, and guess what? We gained weight and became a fat nation with an obesity crisis, even though we are eating less fat than we were twenty years ago. On the other hand, we are eating a lot more fat-free carbohydrates to self-medicate our constant hypoglycemia.

No one ever asked what the hormonal effect would be of making the dietary recommendations to replace fats with fat-free carbohydrates. This ignorance of the effects of carbohydrates on insulin, protein on glucagon, and fats on eicosanoids has driven up the costs of our health care system as we deal with more diabetes, heart disease, and other obesity-related problems.

High-carbohydrate diets lead to an overproduction of insulin. The more insulin you have, the more blood sugar is driven down, and the hungrier you are as you try to maintain adequate blood glucose levels for the brain. So, following dietary recommendations to reduce fat and increase carbohydrate intake has led us to eat an excess of calories but has not kept our hunger at bay. It's no wonder our nation has gotten fatter.

When produced at healthy levels, insulin has an extremely important job: it drives all nutrients, carbohydrates, protein, and fat into cells for either immediate usage or long-term storage. Insulin is, of course, necessary for your survival. But excess insulin can do a number on your body, primarily by increasing the levels of silent inflammation. The biochemistry behind why that happens is complex and will be explained later, but the end result is the acceleration of chronic disease and a corresponding loss of wellness.

There are only two fuels the body can readily use for energy: glucose and fat. When your body is at rest, more than 70 percent of your energy needs comes from circulating fat. Your brain, however, can use only glucose for energy. This works fine if there are adequate amounts of both glucose and fat circulating in the bloodstream. The brain gets what it wants (glucose) and the rest of the body's cells get what they want: a high-octane fuel (fat). Excess insulin, however, can upset this balance by blocking the release of stored fat into the bloodstream. This forces your body and brain to compete for a relatively limited amount of glucose in the blood. You feel hungrier as a result and will seek out more calories to consume, probably in the form of carbohydrates, to replenish blood glucose levels. This causes another rise in insulin, feeding a vicious cycle that eventually leads to weight gain and increased silent inflammation.

UNDERSTANDING CARBOHYDRATES

Here's a riddle: why do five grams of carbohydrate from a potato cause a bigger insulin spike than five grams of carbohydrate from a sugar cube? To understand the science, you have to think like a biochemist.

Nutrition used to be so simple in the old days. There were only two types of carbohydrates: simple ones (such as table sugar), and complex ones (such as bread, pasta, potatoes, and rice). Simple carbohydrates were bad for blood sugar levels, and complex carbohydrates were good. Then a perfectly good theory was totally destroyed by actual studies. This research found that some simple carbohydrates enter the bloodstream as glucose at a much slower rate than many complex carbohydrates. More than twenty years later, the nutritional establishment is still, for the most part, in a state of denial.

This flip-flop on carbohydrates is due to biochemistry. All carbohydrates have to be broken down into simple sugars, such as glucose and fructose, to be absorbed. (Milk and dairy products contain another simple sugar, called lactose, which many people cannot digest.)

Grains and starches (bread, pasta, rice, corn, potatoes, and so on) are composed of long strings of glucose held together by very weak chemical bonds that are rapidly broken down during digestion. As the glucose is rapidly released, it flows into your bloodstream, causing an increase in the secretion of insulin. The more rapidly glucose enters the bloodstream, the more insulin is secreted. On the other hand, fructose is rapidly absorbed but is very slowly converted into glucose in the liver. As a result, the simple sugar fructose will actually enter the bloodstream as glucose at a much slower rate than the glucose coming from a complex carbohydrate. Less glucose in the bloodstream means less insulin is secreted.

Vegetables are about 30 percent fructose, fruits are about 70 percent fructose, and grains and starches are 100 percent glucose. This should help you see why eating more complex carbohydrates, such as grains and starches, has a stronger impact on increasing insulin levels. Add soluble fiber (found primarily in fruits and vegetables) to the mix and you reduce the rate of entry of glucose into the bloodstream even more, producing a smaller increase in insulin. (Note: the insoluble fiber found in grains and starches has little impact on slowing down glucose entry into the bloodstream, which is another strike against grains and starches.) Now that your head is spinning from this quick biochemistry course, just remember this: eating carbohydrates primarily in the form of vegetables and fruits is a great way to control insulin levels, whereas eating grains and starches is not.

Each carbohydrate-containing food enters your bloodstream at a particular rate. The rate at which a particular food enters your bloodstream is called the glycemic index of that carbohydrate. The higher the glycemic index of a food, the faster that particular food raises your blood glucose levels and the quicker the rise in insulin secretion. For example, a sugar cube is composed of one-half glucose and one-half fructose, whereas a potato is 100 percent glucose. This is why an equivalent amount of carbohydrate in the form of a sugar cube enters the bloodstream as glucose at a slower rate than the same amount of carbohydrate in a potato. No wonder the nutritional establishment hates the concept of the glycemic index.

Although there has been a lot of hype about the glycemic index, it has significant limitations in the real world. It is based on eating 50 grams of carbohydrate of one particular food at a single sitting. Since you don't normally eat that much of any one food, it doesn't tell you how much a real serving of that food raises your blood sugar levels and also doesn't take into account your total carbohydrate intake in a given meal or snack. This means it doesn't give you the big picture, that is, how much your blood levels are going to rise from a particular meal or snack. Instead, you have to rely on a relatively new term called the *glycemic load* to get that information.

Glycemic Load

The glycemic load takes into account not only the rate of entry of a carbohydrate into the bloodstream (the glycemic index) but also the total amount of carbohydrates that you eat in one sitting. The glycemic load predicts how much insulin your body will produce in response to carbohydrates actually consumed. In fact, studies at

Harvard Medical School show that the higher the glycemic load of your diet, the more likely you are to become obese, develop diabetes, and suffer a heart attack. Why? Harvard researchers also found that the higher the glycemic load of your diet, the greater your levels of silent inflammation.

How the Glycemic Load Explains the Differences Among Various Popular Diets

Every year another 1,000 diet books are published. In fact, there are more than 15,000 different diet books in print today. Yet despite the abundance of this dietary advice, there are only four main types of diets known to medical science, and they can be described on the basis of their glycemic load. This is why understanding the glycemic load begins to take all the mystery out of the various diets on the market today. In essence, the concept of the glycemic load is a universal translator to characterize any diet. Shown below are typical diets that can be broken down by their actual glycemic load.

Dietary Glycemic Load	Popular Diet Name
Very low	Atkins
Low	Zone
High	USDA Food Pyramid, Weight Watchers, American Heart Association, American Diabetes Association, and so on
Very high	Typical American

Note: Some popular dietary plans try to hedge their bets. A good example is the South Beach diet. For the first two to three weeks, it is the Atkins diet, falling into the very low glycemic-load category. Thereafter it is the Zone Diet, falling into the low glycemic-load category.

Once you grasp the concept of the glycemic load, such terms as *high-protein, high-carbohydrate, low-fat,* or *low-carbohydrate* become meaningless to describe diets. The key to finding a lifelong anti-inflammatory diet lies in finding a diet with the appropriate glycemic load for your biochemistry. If the glycemic load of your diet is higher than what you can genetically handle, you will increase the levels of silent inflammation in your body due to increasing insulin production. On the other hand, if the glycemic load of the diet is too low, a complex series of hormonal events begins to occur that leads to increased secretion of cortisol (the hormone that makes you fat, dumb, and sick). Neither is optimal if your long-term goal is wellness.

CALCULATING THE GLYCEMIC LOAD

Once you find your optimal glycemic load, all you need to do is stick with it for a lifetime to keep silent inflammation at bay. The glycemic load has very little to do with the actual amount of carbohydrates consumed. This means that food labels are not going to be much help. That's because glycemic load takes into account the dynamics of the blood-glucose-raising effects of any carbohydrate and its impact on insulin secretion.

The power of the glycemic load is calculated by taking the glycemic index (GI) of a particular carbohydrate multiplied by the total amount of that carbohydrate (g) in a meal and then dividing that by 100 as shown below.

$$\text{Glycemic Load (g)} = \frac{\text{GI of the carbohydrate} \times \text{grams of carbohydrate per serving}}{100}$$

The glycemic load of a meal or your daily diet strongly correlates with the amount of insulin that will be secreted. Adding up the glycemic load of each meal gives you the total dietary glycemic load during the course of a day. Since grains and starches are composed almost entirely of glucose, they will have a higher glycemic load than fruits and vegetables, which are richer in fructose. Although particular foods may have the same total grams of carbohydrates, their glycemic loads can be wildly different based on their content of fructose and glucose. Thus, a carbohydrate-rich diet based on grains and starches is a high glycemic-load diet that increases insulin and silent inflammation, whereas a carbohydrate-rich diet based on fruits and vegetables—even one with the same amount of carbohydrate grams—is a low glycemic-load diet that will be your best pathway to reducing silent inflammation. The following table shows the dramatic differences in the glycemic loads of typical serving sizes:

Type of Carbohydrate	Glycemic Load (g) of a Typical Serving Size
Nonstarchy vegetables	1–5
Fruits	5–10
Grains and starches (pasta, rice, potatoes)	20–30
Typical junk foods (candy, chips, soda)	20–30

You can see from this table that, in terms of glycemic load, there isn't a lot of difference between grains and starches and typical junk foods. If you want to keep the glycemic load of the diet under control, it is just common sense to eat more fruits and vegetables and fewer grains and starches (and, of course, less junk food). This explains why switching to a fruit- and vegetable-based diet lowers rates of heart disease, cancer, and other chronic diseases. You're lowering your glycemic load, which in turn lowers silent inflammation. Just why does a high glycemic-load diet increase silent inflammation? The increase in insulin secretion stimulates the production of AA, the building block for all pro-inflammatory eicosanoids.

Now let's redefine the four types of diets based on their daily glycemic loads.

Dietary Glycemic Load	Daily Glycemic Load (g/day)	Popular Diet Name
Very low	Less than 20	Atkins
Low	50–100	Zone
High	Greater than 200	USDA Food Pyramid, American Heart Association, and so on
Very high	Greater than 300	Typical American diet

The higher your daily glycemic load, the greater the amount of insulin your body produces. Following the USDA Food Pyramid recommendations or the American Heart Association diet will cause your body to produce two to four times the level of insulin compared to following the Zone Diet. Following the typical American diet will cause your insulin levels to rise up to six times as much as compared to the Zone Diet. Although the Atkins diet will produce two to five times less insulin than the Zone Diet, the long-term result of the Atkins diet will be increased cortisol production and the regain of any lost weight. This is why you have to keep insulin in a zone that is not too high but not too low.

THE REAL DANGERS OF VERY LOW GLYCEMIC-LOAD DIETS

You already know that high glycemic-load diets lead to excess insulin and inflammation. But if a low glycemic-load diet like the Zone is good, shouldn't a very low glycemic-load diet, like Atkins, be better?

Actually, no. These very low glycemic-load diets can also increase silent inflammation and chronic disease, although not by the mechanisms health organizations routinely warn about. The first thing that happens on a very low glycemic-load diet, like the Atkins diet, is that your body goes into an abnormal state known as ketosis. Without adequate carbohydrates in the diet, your liver doesn't have enough stored carbohydrates (called glycogen) to metabolize fats completely into water and carbon dioxide. This lack of liver glycogen alters the normal metabolism of fat and causes the liver to produce abnormal ketone bodies, which circulate in the bloodstream. The body isn't too happy about this and tends to increase urination to wash them out of the system. (It does the same thing for other dietary compounds such as caffeine and phosphorus in soft drinks.) A lot of the initial weight loss experienced on these very low-carbohydrate diets comes from shedding water, not fat. But this is not dangerous.

The real danger with very low glycemic-load diets comes from the hormonal problems they induce. The first problem is that your brain needs a certain amount of glucose in the blood to function properly. Your brain is a glucose hog. As mentioned earlier, even though the brain accounts for less than 3 percent of the mass of the human body, it guzzles more than 70 percent of the blood glucose. When blood glucose levels get too low, your brain doesn't function very well and goes into panic mode. It sends out signals (via the hormone cortisol) to start breaking down muscle mass and converting it into glucose. The process is called neo-glucogenesis. It's not a very efficient process, but it does work in the short term.

When people go on low-carbohydrate diets, such as Atkins, they will lose more weight than a person following a high-carbohydrate, low-fat diet for the first six months, and they have no short-term increased mortality from heart attacks or anything else, contrary to what critics of these diets have said. Long-term (greater than six months), however, adverse adaptive metabolic changes take place in the body. Dieters often stop losing weight, even though they are still restricting their carbohydrate intake, and then they start to gain weight. They aren't cheating, rather, they are beginning to feel the effects of excess cortisol production necessary to produce enough glucose for the brain. As I mentioned earlier, excess cortisol increases insulin resistance, which in turn converts your fat cells into fat magnets. The end result is that you regain the lost weight. This is typically what happens to those who follow the Atkins diet: they lose weight in the first six months, but then gain back the weight in the next six months. At the end of a year, they wind up with very little or no net loss of weight.

This explains why millions of people who lost weight on low-carbohydrate diets over the past thirty years gained it all back, if not more. The vast majority weren't cheaters but were simply victims of the biochemical and hormonal adaptations their body made to a very low glycemic-load diet.

If weight regain is not bad enough, here is the second hormonal danger with high-protein diets: fat-rich protein. On the Atkins diet you are encouraged to eat excessive amounts of fatty protein (steak, bacon, egg yolks, and so on). These are all great dietary sources of AA. The more AA you eat, the more silent inflammation you will generate even if you are shedding excess weight (although much is due to water loss). Increased cortisol secretion and increased silent inflammation are the real dangers of the Atkins diet.

REAL LIFE APPLICATIONS OF THE GLYCEMIC LOAD

You are probably thinking that although the concept of the glycemic load seems scientifically sound, it must be totally impossible to use in the real world. You're dead wrong. All you need to calculate the glycemic load of each meal is your hand, and your eye.

There are no such things as good or bad carbohydrates, only the differences in their glycemic load. Following the Zone Diet you can eat every carbohydrate known; you just have to know when to stop adding it your plate. But since each carbohydrate has its own glycemic load, how do you know?

Begin to think of carbohydrates as either Favorable or Unfavorable. The Favorable ones (fruits and vegetables) have low glycemic loads, whereas the Unfavorable ones (grains and starches) have high glycemic loads. This is not exactly rocket science.

The Hand-Eye Method

You only need to use your hand and eye to determine the glycemic load of your meal. Simply divide your plate into three equal sections. If you want to eat Unfavorable carbohydrates, fill one-third of the plate with them and then stop. If you are eating Favorable carbohydrates, you can fill two-thirds of plate with them and then stop. (I will shortly tell you what to put on the other third of the plate.)

You are going to have a lot of empty space on your plate if you eat Unfavorable carbohydrates, but at least you aren't going to exceed your glycemic load for that meal. You have complete freedom to what carbohydrates you want to eat, but keep in mind that by eating Favorable carbohydrates you're getting a lot more vitamins, minerals, fiber, and phytochemicals for the same glycemic load.

The Block Method

If you really want to treat food like a drug, then you need to have a slightly more structured but still simple carbohydrate accounting system. In my first book, *The Zone,* I tried to put forward the first workable (in my opinion) system for determining the glycemic load of a meal using Zone Food Blocks. The key to this system is just counting the Zone Carbohydrate Blocks to provide the upper and lower limits of an optimal glycemic load for a meal. Each Zone Carbohydrate Block contains a defined amount of carbohydrate and is separated into Favorable and Unfavorable depending on the glycemic load of that particular carbohydrate. The Favorable Zone Carbohydrate Blocks fall into the low glycemic-load carbohydrate category, whereas the Unfavorable Zone Carbohydrate Blocks fall into the inflammatory or high glycemic-load category. Listed below are some examples of Zone Carbohydrate Blocks.

Carbohydrate Source	Amount for 1 Zone Carbohydrate Block
Apple (medium)	½
Broccoli (cooked)	4 cups
Pasta (cooked)	¼ cup
Sugar cube	3

The apple and broccoli would be Favorable carbohydrates, whereas the pasta and the sugar cube would be Unfavorable carbohydrates. The key to the Zone Diet is making sure that each meal has the correct glycemic load, not too high and not too low, in order to stabilize blood glucose (and hunger) for the next four to six hours. The average woman needs only 3 Zone Carbohydrate Blocks per meal, which could be ¼ cup of pasta, 4 cups of broccoli, and ½ an apple. A better choice (lower glycemic load) would be 4 cups of broccoli and a whole apple, whereas a worse choice (higher glycemic load) would be ¾ cup of cooked pasta. If you are dealing entirely with Unfavorable Zone Carbohydrate Blocks on your plate, you are on the edge of hormonal disaster even though you are controlling carbohydrate intake. This would be like having 9 sugar cubes for your carbohydrates at that meal. Actually, the 9 sugar cubes would generate a lesser insulin response than ¾ cup of pasta! That's the power of understanding the glycemic load.

A typical male would need 4 Zone Carbohydrate Blocks per meal. This means he could eat more than the average female, but not that much more. As usual, the key is to know just when to stop adding carbohydrates to your plate.

ZONE POINTS

Over the years, I have continually tried to simplify the Zone Food Block system, and I came up with the development of Zone Points. Zone Points are simply another accounting system to keep your glycemic load under control from meal to meal. Since you are only as hormonally good as your last meal and will only be as hormonally good as your next meal, you want to have the same glycemic load at every meal. This is because the glycemic load at each meal determines the amount of insulin that will be secreted.

Zone Points are based on the glycemic load of various carbohydrates in serving sizes that will keep you satiated without being stuffed. A good rule of thumb is to make sure that your total Zone Points for any one meal are no more than 15 if you're female, and no more than 20 if you're male. A typical Zone snack would contain about 5 Zone Points. Just as with the Zone Carbohydrate Blocks, you just keep adding carbohydrates to your dish until you hit the maximum you are allowed at that meal and then stop.

Let me use the Zone Point system to illustrate why I am not a big fan of whole-grain carbohydrates, even though they are politically correct. First, most foods labeled "whole grain" really aren't. Whole-grain foods are extremely perishable. Real whole-grain products contain fats that go rancid at room temperature, and that's why they are found in the frozen section of the supermarket. When was the last time you bought a loaf of bread from the freezer section? Dried whole grains, like steel-cut oats, need to be cooked for at least 30 minutes before eating. Even though I love *real* whole grains (especially oatmeal and barley), I still consume them sparingly. Whole grains still have to be eaten with a certain degree of moderation because of their carbohydrate density, which quickly increases the glycemic load of a meal. Let me show how easy it is to overload on your glycemic load by eating whole-grain products.

Carbohydrate	Serving Size	Zone Points
Cooked pasta	1 cup	28
Potato	1 medium	28
Bagel	1 small	28
Rice	1 cup	35

Since the upper limit for a Zone meal is 15 Zone Points for a female or 20 Zone Points for a male, it is pretty easy to exceed that with even the most healthful whole-grain products. I hope you get the picture that starchy carbohydrates and grains (even whole-grain products) are probably not the best choice for the majority of your carbohydrates if insulin control is your goal.

The beauty of the Zone Points system is that you get to eat exactly the type of food you want to eat (it could even be sugar cubes) as long as you stay within your Zone Points limit for that meal. (Okay, the sugar cubes don't provide a lot of vitamins and minerals, but if that's what you want, then just know your limits.) Now let's see how a food's Zone Carbohydrate Blocks convert into Zone Points.

Carbohydrate	Amount	Zone Blocks	Zone Points
Broccoli (cooked)	4 cups	1	3
Apple	½ medium	1	5
Pasta (cooked)	¼ cup	1	7
Sugar cube	3	1	2

A typical female would need about 15 Zone Points per meal. You can see that ½ an apple (5 Zone Points), 4 cups of cooked broccoli (3 Zone Points), and ¼ cup of pasta (7 Zone Points) add up to 15. If she had a whole apple (10 Zone Points) and the 4 cups of cooked broccoli (3 Zone Points), she would have had a lower glycemic-load meal (13 Zone Points). On the other hand, consuming ¾ cup of pasta would have provided a higher glycemic-load meal (21 Zone Points) that is beyond the meal limit. Basically, the Zone Points and Zone Carbohydrate Blocks give about the same results.

As you can see from the list of foods above (a much more complete list can be found in appendices C and D), you are going to have to stock up on fruits and vegetables and reduce the amount of grains and starches you eat in order to maintain an optimal glycemic load at every meal.

The Zone Diet, however, is a little more complex than simply controlling the glycemic load at a meal. To truly maintain insulin in the Zone, you have to balance the glycemic load of a meal with the appropriate amount of low-fat protein coupled with the right type of fat. Let's look first at protein.

PROTEIN

This nutrient supplies the necessary amino acids that the body requires to repair itself, synthesize enzymes, and maintain its proper immune function. This is all good, but for the Zone Diet the importance of protein is that it also stimulates the production of glucagon, the primary hormone that maintains blood glucose levels in the brain by causing the release of stored glycogen from the liver. On the one hand, if your brain is happy (it's getting enough glucose), then you aren't hungry. On the other hand, if your brain doesn't have adequate blood glucose levels, it will throw a temper tantrum until you eat enough carbohydrates to restore its only fuel supply. By eating adequate levels of protein you don't have to eat excessive levels of carbohydrates to maintain optimal blood glucose levels, because they will be constantly released from the liver.

You don't actually need to eat much protein to ensure adequate levels of glucagon secretion. All you need is the amount that's the size and thickness of the palm of your hand. This is about 3 ounces of low-fat protein for the typical female and 4 ounces for the typical male at each meal. What is low-fat protein? Foods like fish, chicken, turkey, egg whites, very lean cuts of red meat (less than 7 percent fat), and for vegetarians soy products (tofu or soy imitation meat products). All animal protein contains some arachidonic acid (AA). The lower the fat content of the protein source, the less AA you consume and the less effort you have to expend on controlling silent inflammation. As you can see, this amount of low-fat protein is far from the protein gluttony often advocated in low-carbohydrate (i.e., high-protein) diets, like the Atkins diet.

What happens when you eat too much protein? You can get fat, since the human body has a very limited ability to store excess dietary protein as muscle; otherwise, we would all look like Arnold Schwarzenegger. All the excess protein you eat that your body doesn't immediately need gets converted into either carbohydrates or fat for storage.

FAT

Fat is the final nutrient that makes a Zone meal or snack complete. It is critical to choose the right fat if you want to keep inflammation under control. Eating the wrong kind of fat will increase your levels of AA, which will generate silent inflammation. As I already mentioned, egg yolks and fatty cuts of meat contain high levels of AA. So eating foods rich in AA is like adding kerosene to a fire. However, the most insidious inflammatory culprit in the American diet is the massive amounts of omega-6 fatty acids we consume. These fats are found in vegetable oils like soybean, corn, sunflower, and safflower. The more omega-6 fats you consume, the more likely they will get converted into AA by the body—especially if your body is already churning out high levels of insulin. This is because insulin stimulates the key enzyme that produces AA. I will discuss this in greater detail in chapter 12.

So it's really not the amount of fat, but the type of fat that becomes the culprit in the development and acceleration of silent inflammation. But how do you stop the process in its tracks? Switching from vegetable oils that are rich in omega-6 fatty acids to olive oil is a great start. Sprinkling nuts and avocado slices on your salad instead of sliced egg yolks will also help. Olive oil, nuts, and avocados are all rich in monounsaturated fats. From an inflammatory standpoint these monounsaturated fats are neutral since they cannot be synthesized into pro-inflammatory eicosanoids. The powerful effect of doing this simple reduction of omega-6 fatty acid intake was demonstrated with the Lyon Diet Heart study, which was discussed in the previous chapter.

Fat is an essential nutrient. You need a certain amount in your diet, not only to make food taste better, but also to release a hormone (cholecystokinin) from the gut that goes straight to the brain to tell it to stop eating. Fat-free diets are not only tasteless, but will fuel your hunger because you never get the "full" signal from your brain. But most important, fats can either increase or decrease the levels of inflammation. And that is the key to wellness.

On the other hand, can you eat too much fat? Of course you can. Although fat has no effect on insulin, eating excess levels of fat certainly won't make you thin. Even if you keep your insulin levels in check by following a low glycemic-load diet, eating too much fat will prevent the release of stored fat from your cells. After all, if your body has an adequate level of fatty acids floating around in the bloodstream from your last meal, why should it release any more from storage in your fat cells?

PUTTING IT ALL TOGETHER: THE ANTI-INFLAMMATION SOLUTION

The key to controlling silent inflammation lies in keeping your glycemic load high enough to avoid ketosis but low enough to avoid excess insulin secretion. You also need to eat the right amount of protein and fat. In other words, you need to keep them all in a zone. As I emphasize throughout all my Zone books, it's all about striking the right balance. What glycemic-load measurement is best for you? Since we are all genetically different, we all have slightly different glycemic loads that are optimal for our own health. But years of experience with the Zone Diet have indicated the simple methods I have described in this chapter will get you fairly close to your ideal. Most people will find that neither a low-carbohydrate nor a high-carbohydrate diet will provide the appropriate glycemic load needed to keep silent inflammation under control. In fact, the best diet for controlling silent inflammation is probably one that falls in the moderate category. This means moderate carbohydrate, moderate protein, and moderate fat. This is a pretty good description of the Zone Diet. Frankly, any diet that uses the word *high* or *low* to describe its concepts will ultimately fail to control silent inflammation because of the hormonal disturbances it creates.

SUMMARY

Following the Zone Diet for lifelong control of silent inflammation is far easier than you may think. Calculating your optimal glycemic load and balancing it with the appropriate amount of protein and fat doesn't require anything beyond your hand and your eye. The dietary rules that govern the Zone Diet are simple and are your number-one defense against silent inflammation. In the next chapter, you'll see how easy it really is to apply these rules in the real world.

Turning Your Kitchen into an Anti-Inflammatory Pharmacy

If you've been following the Zone Diet, your kitchen is probably pretty well stocked, and you can use this chapter for review. If you're concerned about the future implications of silent inflammation, you'll probably need to do a kitchen makeover. No, you don't need to call a general contractor. All you have to do is take a few foods out of your kitchen and add in a few new foods.

WHAT TO REMOVE FROM YOUR KITCHEN

Out of sight, out of mouth and mind. As you know, that's my feeling about most grains and starches. Grab any processed starch you can find (breakfast cereals, flour, crackers, pasta, bread, bagels, muffins, cookies, cake, breadsticks, granola bars, and so on) and put all these products into a trash bag. Fill another trash bag with traditional starches like rice, potatoes, and grains. But you can keep barley and steel-cut oats if you have them on hand. Now look in your pantry to see if you have products rich in sugar, such as fruit rollups, chocolate, or candy. Put these in a bag as well. Now scour your kitchen for dangerous fats: butter, margarine, Crisco, lard, and most important, vegetable oils such as soybean, corn, safflower, and sunflower. Don't even try to save them, just throw them out. Now take all these bags with unopened high glycemic-load products to the local food bank. As hard as it may be to remove these foods from your kitchen, your body will thank you later. These items are the worst offenders when it comes to raising insulin levels and increasing silent inflammation. These fall into the category of either high glycemic-load carbohydrates or pro-inflammatory fats. They are, literally, poison to your future wellness.

WHAT TO ADD TO YOUR KITCHEN

Your kitchen might be looking a little bare at this point. Not to worry. You are about to fill it up again—this time with low glycemic-load carbohydrates, such as fruits and vegetables. You'll also add the right kinds of protein and fat.

Carbohydrates

People usually buy fresh produce with the best of intentions, but time usually conspires against them. Salad greens wilt, berries become moldy, peaches become mushy, and we often end up throwing our money in the garbage. The easiest way around this is to simply buy only two or three days' worth of produce at a time. Good idea, but highly unlikely in today's world with its growing time constraints. Instead, stock up on frozen fruits and vegetables. Not only are they less expensive than fresh items, but also they are surpris-

---

ADD APPEAL TO FROZEN VEGETABLES

You can make any frozen vegetable pass for fresh if you prepare it the right way. Preheat the oven to 350°F. Spread a large piece of aluminum foil on your counter and spray it with nonstick cooking spray. Add the vegetables in the middle of the foil and drizzle on some olive oil and a few dashes of lime juice. Fold up the ends of the foil, pinching them together at the top and the sides to create a tent. Roast the vegetables for 30 minutes or until tender.

---

ingly more nutritious. This is because only the ripest fruits and veg-etables are frozen. What's more, they are frozen soon after harvest-ing, which seals in their vitamins and phytochemicals. Fresh pro-duce, on the other hand, will lose many of these nutrients when it is transported and stored.

Canned fruits and vegetables are more problematic. You have to avoid any that are floating in sweetened syrups, which are added during the canning process. (The high sugar content reduces bacte-rial growth.) Also, canned produce often contains a much lower vitamin content than frozen produce. Nonetheless, they still make a better choice for Zone carbohydrates than the high glycemic-load carbohydrates that you donated to the local food bank.

Protein

Look for low-fat sources of protein and buy them in serving-size portions. It's easy to purchase too much protein, which means you're likely to eat more than you need. Let the butcher at the supermarket become your ally. If all the meat, chicken, or fish you can find is packed in 2-pound bundles, ask the butcher to repackage it in eight ¼-pound packages. Keep one of the packages in the refrig-erator, and freeze the other seven. Or, buy in bulk to save money and repackage the meat in smaller portions yourself using freezer bags. Once you use one of the packages in the refrigerator, immedi-ately replace it with one from the freezer. This type of portion con-trol reduces the likelihood of thawing out too much protein (and eating too much), or worse, not having any protein (because you don't want to thaw a huge package). You can apply the same trick to low-fat deli meats. Just have the butcher put a piece of wax paper between every ¼ pound of deli meat.

Eggs are a great source of protein that come in convenient portion-control sizes. Let me emphasize that I'm talking about egg whites, not egg yolks, which are rich in pro-inflammatory arachi-donic acid (AA). For omelets and scrambled eggs, you may want to buy an inexpensive egg separator, or you can buy egg substitutes, such as Eggbeaters. If you eat hard-boiled eggs, make sure to eat only the white and discard the yolk.

Packaged protein like low-fat cottage cheese, low-fat cheese, and canned tuna, salmon, and sardines are also great sources of low-fat protein. They provide you readily accessible sources of low-fat protein with easy-to-control portions. For vegan meals, purchase soy protein products like tofu, tempeh, or soy imitation-meat products. You can also purchase a pure protein powder (isolated whey protein tastes the best) that can be used to make Zone smoothie shakes with mixed berries or added carbohydrates such as oatmeal on the side to give you the correct protein-to-carbohydrate balance you need to maintain long-term blood glucose control.

Having easily accessible protein sources is key to staying in the Zone because it stimulates the release of glucagon, which helps stabilize blood glucose levels. In order to maintain stable insulin levels, you need to eat before you get hungry, or within a minute or two of feeling those first hunger pangs. Opening a can of tuna or grabbing a hard-boiled egg white from your fridge mixed with some precut low glycemic-load carbohydrates and a drizzle of olive oil can make an easy-to-prepare a meal in less than two minutes. Keeping hunger at bay by controlling your blood glucose levels is the key to staving off cravings for high glycemic-load carbohydrates like bagels, cookies, and cake.

Fat

Last but not least, you have to stock your kitchen with the right kinds of fat. You've already gotten rid of the pro-inflammatory omega-6 fats, which increase levels of silent inflammation, by throwing out the vegetable oils. Removing saturated fat from your diet is just plain common sense. Now you have to increase your supply of monounsaturated fats. You should buy a bottle of extra-virgin olive oil (for dressings and seasonings) and refined olive oil (for cooking). You should also keep a stock of nuts: slivered almonds, pine nuts, and chopped cashews are all great for making pestos or topping salads. Keep at least one avocado in your fridge for slicing into salads. All of these foods are great sources of monounsaturated fats.

MAKING ZONE MEALS: THE FOUR BASIC RULES

That's it. As you can see, it's not hard to turn your kitchen into a wellness pharmacy. Once you have the right foods stocked in your freezer, refrigerator, and pantry, all you have to do is throw the right ingredients together to get yourself in the Anti-Inflammation Zone and begin reducing silent inflammation.

Following the Zone Diet just requires a little knowledge about the four basic Zone rules:

1. Plan to eat five times a day (three Zone meals and two Zone snacks).
2. Always eat breakfast within one hour after getting up.
3. Never let more than five hours go by without eating a Zone meal or snack. The best time to eat is when you aren't hungry since that means blood sugar levels are stabilized.
4. Eat a Zone snack before you go to bed to prevent nocturnal hypoglycemia.

If you follow those rules, then all you have to use is your hand and your eye to construct Zone meals and snacks as follows.

1. Divide a dinner-size plate into three equal sections. If you're having a snack, make it a dessert plate.
2. Cover one-third of your plate with some low-fat protein that is no larger or thicker than the palm of your hand. This is approximately 3 ounces of low-fat protein for the average female, and 4 ounces of low-fat protein for the average male. Protein could be in the form of chicken, turkey, fish, extra-lean cuts of beef, egg whites, or low-fat cheese products. You can also use tofu and soy imitation meat products as a protein source.

3. Cover the other two-thirds of the plate with colorful low glycemic-load carbohydrates, such as nonstarchy vegetables and fruits. *Note: If you want to use high glycemic-load carbohydrates with this approach, then fill only one-third of the plate with a volume equal to the volume of low-fat protein. If you really want to eat high glycemic-load carbohydrates, you are better off using the Zone Blocks or Zone Points system outlined in the next section.*

4. Finally, add a dash (that's a small amount) of noninflammatory monounsaturated fat. This might be a teaspoon of olive oil, a few teaspoons of slivered almonds, or a few slices of avocado.

There you have it: four basic rules for building Zone meals that are easy to follow. The only trick is to follow these rules the best you can at every meal for the rest of your life. Remember, you're only as hormonally good as your last meal. However, that means there is no guilt on the Zone Diet, since no matter how bad your last meal was, your next meal can take you right back into the Zone.

A Zone meal has the right balance of protein, carbohydrate, and fat to maintain stable insulin levels for the next four to six hours. This is how you can tell if your last meal was a Zone meal. Simply look at your watch five hours after eating. If you have no hunger and good mental acuity, it means your last meal was a Zone meal. You can always go back to that exact same meal to get the same hormonal effect.

Being in this Zone means you're using incoming calories for energy instead of storing them as fat. If you veer away from these rules, your insulin levels will no longer be in the Zone. All it takes is one meal to set you off course. On the other hand, all it takes is one meal to put you back in the Zone again. Using your diet to control insulin is like taking a drug that has to be taken at the right time and right dose. Everyone makes dietary mistakes, so don't kick yourself over them when you do. Get yourself back in the Zone as quickly as possible. Keep in mind that no matter how hormonally bad your last meal was, you only have to use your hand and your eye to get back in the Zone.

USING ZONE BLOCKS AND ZONE POINTS

Zone Blocks or Zone Points are a more precise way than the hand-eye method to determine the exact glycemic load of your meal. I first developed the Zone Carbohydrate Blocks ten years ago as a way to determine the glycemic load of a meal. Unlike protein or fat, which generate a constant metabolic response in your body based on the amount you eat, carbohydrates generate varying insulin responses based not only on the amount of carbohydrates consumed, but the glycemic index of the carbohydrate. High glycemic-load carbohydrates (grains and starches) cause a much greater insulin surge than low glycemic-load carbohydrates (nonstarchy vegetables). Fruits are intermediate, with berries being the best.

You can use either the Zone Carbohydrate Block or Zone Point methods to fill out the carbohydrate portion of your Zone meal. Either will give you greater precision than the hand-eye method. You still fill your plate with the same of amount of low-fat protein and add a dash of monounsaturated fat. The only difference is that you now add a precise amount of carbohydrates until you have reached your glycemic load allotment for that meal. This means the plate will be either overflowing (if you choose low glycemic-load carbohydrates) or very empty (if you choose high glycemic-load carbohydrates). In either case, you learn when to stop adding carbohydrates. Here are your basic Zone rules for using the Zone Blocks or Zone Points system:

- The average female should have either 3 Zone Carbohydrate Blocks or 15 Zone Points on her plate to balance out her required low-fat protein (about 3 ounces).

- The average male should have 4 Zone Carbohydrate Blocks or 20 Zone Points on his plate to balance out his required low-fat protein (about 4 ounces).

The beauty of using the Zone Blocks or Zone Points method is that you can incorporate virtually any carbohydrate into your meal as long as you adjust your portions accordingly. The higher the glycemic load of the carbohydrates, the more empty space you are going to see on your plate. Conversely, the lower the glycemic load of the carbohydrates, the more bountiful the plate is going to look.

For example, an average female with 3 ounces of low-fat protein on her plate could have 7 sugar cubes (14 Zone Points) to balance it out. Not a good meal nutritionally, but hormonally it's okay. The take-home message here is that there is no such thing as forbidden carbohydrates on the Zone Diet. If you decide to use the Food Block/Point system, follow these three rules to build each Zone meal:

1. Put a palm-size serving of low-fat protein on your plate. That should cover about one-third of your plate.
2. Add the appropriate glycemic load of carbohydrates using either the Zone Carbohydrate Block or the Zone Points method. See Appendix C for a listing of Zone Carbohydrate Blocks. See Appendix D for a listing of Zone Points.
3. Always add a dash of monounsaturated fat.

As you can see from the foods that fill your plate, the Zone Diet can be summed up in one word: moderation. Each meal is moderate in protein, carbohydrate (though with a low-glycemic load), and fat. This emphasis on moderation is what keeps your insulin levels in the Zone.

SUMMARY

If you have one eye and one hand, the Zone Diet is incredibly easy to follow for a lifetime. Yet as simple as the Zone Diet is to follow, people can always find a reason to veer away from its concept of moderation. Does this mean that all hope is lost to control silent inflammation? Not by a long shot, because you have one last powerful defense against silent inflammation. It's called high-dose fish oil.

Your Ultimate Defense Against Silent Inflammation: High-Dose Fish Oil

The single most important thing you can do to keep silent inflammation under control is this: take a daily supplement of high-dose fish oil. The Zone Diet helps to ward off silent inflammation by reducing excess insulin levels. High-dose fish oil, however, provides the ultimate boost you need to dampen down silent inflammation. It will also be your best defense against any dietary lapses you may have, such as going overboard on your glycemic load.

When I say high-dose fish oil, I mean it. You simply can't get enough fish oil from eating fatty fish like salmon, tuna, or mackerel, even if it's on a daily basis. Eating tuna salad for lunch or salmon steak for dinner will give you some benefits but not enough to truly control silent inflammation.

The Japanese do manage to maintain a state of wellness, relatively free from silent inflammation, just from consuming copious amounts of fish. Unfortunately, the massive amounts of fish, sea vegetables, and other marine creatures that the Japanese eat could never be matched by the paltry amounts of fish that Americans consume. In fact, Tufts Medical School tried to do a dietary study providing volunteers the same amount of long-chain omega-3 fatty acids (from fish and sea vegetables) as normally consumed by the Japanese. Even though the volunteers were paid and had all their meals prepared for them, the experiment lasted a total of three days.

The volunteers quit the study because they couldn't tolerate those hefty amounts of fish in their diet.

Fish oil is ultimately the healthiest fat around because it has profound anti-inflammatory properties. It might even be the healthiest medicine around, since it packs a wallop of benefits without any of the long-term side effects of anti-inflammatory drugs (such as death). In fact, the only side effect of fish oil may be that it makes you smarter. But like any drug, you have to use enough of it to gain its therapeutic benefits. The reason that high-dose fish oil is so effective in reducing silent inflammation is that it reduces arachidonic acid (AA), the building block of pro-inflammatory eicosanoids, in less than thirty days. It has the added benefit of simultaneously increasing the levels of eicosapentaenoic acid (EPA), the building block of anti-inflammatory eicosanoids. I can guarantee you that you will see a dramatic improvement in your SIP, and that you'll be back on your path to wellness.

THE FIFTEEN-SECOND RULE

Everyone wants to achieve wellness as long as they don't have to spend too much time doing it. Over the years, I have come to the conclusion that most of us are willing to pursue that wellness goal only if it takes no more than fifteen seconds out of our busy day. This is what has driven the sales of vitamins, minerals, and herbal remedies over the past decade to become a $20 billion-a-year industry. The promise is that you can take all the magic pills you need in fifteen seconds and never look back. An attractive proposal, but unfortunately no one can say with a straight face that Americans have become healthier in the last twenty years. Unfortunately, most of these magic pills from a health food store have little, if any, impact on silent inflammation. Furthermore, any potential benefits they might have are undermined by the growing rate of obesity, which has caused a rise in silent inflammation.

Fish oil, however, stands in a category all its own. Although it accounts for less than 1 percent of all supplement sales, it is the only one that is supported by robust clinical studies in diverse chronic conditions such as heart disease, cancer, immunological and inflammatory diseases, and neurological conditions such as attention deficit disorder, depression, multiple sclerosis, and Alzheimer's—if it is taken in adequate doses.

BUYER BEWARE: FISH OIL CONTAMINATION

As usual, there's always a catch. As good as high-dose fish oil is at controlling silent inflammation, it does have a drawback: contamination. Make no mistake about it, there is no fish on the face of the earth that is not contaminated. For the past two generations, we have dumped a wide range of contaminants into the ocean, including mercury, PCBs, dioxins, and flame retardants. Today more than one hundred thousand pounds of mercury are emitted from coal-burning power plants per year. That is why recent reports have indicated that virtually all freshwater fish in America have significant mercury levels. And the standard fish staple of the American diet, canned tuna fish, is in a prolonged battle in California to prevent it from being banned from supermarket sales because of its mercury levels. However, far more insidious than mercury contamination are the growing levels of PCBs and dioxins in fish. Although the production of PCBs was stopped in 1977, these chemicals remain intact in our oceans since they take decades to break down. Dioxins (the active component in Agent Orange, which was used to defoliate entire forests during the Vietnam War) will also remain in the environment for decades. These contaminants are either known carcinogens or neurotoxins. This is why American consumers are so confused about fish. On one hand, the government says to eat fish because they make us healthy, and then at the same time it tells us not to eat fish because they are contaminated.

Fish are simply at the end of the food chain in the ocean. The bigger the fish, the more toxins it contains (remember, tuna is a pretty big fish even though the size of a tuna can is small). Since these contaminants are fat-soluble, they all end up in the fish oil. This makes crude fish oil the "sewer of the sea." The vast majority of the fish oil supplements found in health food stores are only one step removed from the outflow of any major chemical processing plant.

Ironically, fish farming doesn't stop many of these problems. It actually makes them worse. The problem is that farmed fish (especially salmon) have to be fed crude fish oil in order to attain normal growth. Of course, the crude fish oil is contaminated with these toxins. This is why the levels of PCBs and dioxins in farmed fish are actually significantly greater than in wild fish.

The Japanese consume enough fish and sea vegetables to keep their levels of silent inflammation under control but at a cost. Their blood levels of toxins, such as PCBs and dioxins, are approaching the upper limits set by the World Health Organization because of the contaminated fish they're eating. Unfortunately, if you take fish oil supplements in amounts high enough to confer their anti-inflammatory health benefits, you'll also be getting a hefty dose of toxic substances. So you're left in a quandary: reduce silent inflammation and risk increased toxicity, or do nothing?

THE SOLUTION

Fortunately, you don't have to choose either. The solution to this dilemma was discovered about five years ago with the development of new manufacturing techniques that led to the development of ultra-refined EPA/DHA concentrates. Eicosapentaenoic acid (EPA) and docosahexaenoic acid (DHA) are the key omega-3 fatty acids found in fish oil. EPA has anti-inflammatory effects, and DHA provides neurological benefits. Without going into details, it takes about 100 gallons of health food–grade fish oil to make 1 gallon of an ultra-refined EPA/DHA concentrate. Think of this type of fish oil as "weapons-grade" fish oil: highly concentrated and highly purified and ready for action, and there are a handful of these products now on the market.

How can you know if a fish oil supplement is composed of these ultra-refined EPA/DHA concentrates? Well, the first thing is to never trust the advertising copy or product label. The label or product's website might promise you that the fish oil product you're purchasing is "mercury-free," "pharmaceutical-grade," or "toxin-free," but unless you have about $500,000 of testing equipment in your kitchen, you really have no way of knowing if their marketing hype is true. Your best bet is to go to an independent source with no financial interest in the product who has the sophisticated technology to analyze for these contaminants. The only organization I can recommend is the International Fish Oil Standards (IFOS) program administered by the University of Guelph in Canada. IFOS continuously tests and posts levels of toxins in fish oil samples submitted by product manufacturers. If the lot number on your fish oil is not listed on the IFOS site, then you should think twice about buying it. I strongly recommend checking out the IFOS website at www.ifosprogram.com before purchasing any fish oil product regardless of the advertising claims.

The standards set by the IFOS program for an ultra-refined EPA/DHA concentrate are rigorous:

Parameter	Upper Limit
Mercury	Less than 10 parts per billion (ppb)
Total PCBs	Less than 45 (ppb)
Total Dioxins	Less than 1 part per trillion (ppt)
Total Oxidation (TOTOX)	Less than 20 meq/L

These are incredibly rigid standards, but the minimum levels of purity in my opinion if you are going to be taking high-dose fish oil for a lifetime. As a side note, I once gave a seminar at Harvard Medical School to many of the leading researchers on the therapeutic applications of fish oil. At the end of the seminar, I asked them as true believers in the benefits of fish oil, did any one of them take fish oil personally? Not one of them did, because they were afraid of the contamination. If they are fearful of PCBs and dioxins, you should be, too. Keep in mind that these contaminants are like the ad for the roach motel—once they check into your body, they don't check out.

If you don't have Internet access, a less elegant method to determine if a fish oil might be an ultra-refined EPA/DHA concentrate is to place the product in your freezer. Pour a few teaspoonfuls of liquid into a cup or cut a few capsules open and put the liquid into the freezer for five hours. If it freezes rock-solid, then it is not an ultra-refined EPA/DHA concentrate. A true EPA/DHA concentrate would be liquid or at most a little mushy. That still doesn't mean it has very low levels of contaminants, but at least it is a good start.

Once you find a fish oil supplement composed of ultra-refined EPA/DHA concentrates, you'll probably find that it costs more than other fish oil supplements. Don't be fooled by the price of the bottle. What you are paying for is the actual amount of EPA and DHA in the bottle. If you make a quick calculation, you'll often find that the actual cost per gram of the EPA and DHA in a less refined product is often greater than the cost of the same amounts of EPA and DHA in an ultra-refined EPA/DHA concentrate (especially the liquid oil). Part of the reason is that the soft gelatin capsules cost much more than the inexpensive health-food grade fish oil in them.

So why isn't everyone selling ultra-refined EPA/DHA concentrates? The answer is that there isn't that much of it around, although supplies are continually growing. In the meantime, check the IFOS website for where to find them. It's free.

HOW MUCH FISH OIL DO YOU NEED?

You need to take the appropriate amount of fish oil to keep your SIP in the appropriate range. My research shows that the appropriate amount of EPA and DHA an individual needs ranges from 3 to 8 grams a day. This is equivalent to 1 to 3 teaspoons (or 4 to 12 capsules) of an ultra-refined EPA/DHA concentrate per day. This may seem like a lot of fish oil, but it's the amount you need to reduce your SIP to between 1.5 and 3, which is the key marker of wellness. Since the optimal dose of fish oil falls in a fairly large range, you need to find the dose that's best for you. That's why the SIP is so important.

Once you find the amount of EPA and DHA you need to keep your SIP in the Anti-Inflammation Zone, that's probably the optimal amount you need on a long-term basis. Keep in mind the amount you need does not depend on your age, weight, or sex. It depends on your unique biochemistry, your state of wellness, and your diet. The better you are at managing your insulin levels following the Zone Diet, the less EPA and DHA you'll need to control silent inflammation. Conversely, the higher your insulin levels, the more EPA and DHA you'll need to take on a daily basis to reverse silent inflammation. You can choose to follow the Zone Lifestyle Program (which includes the Zone Diet, fish oil, exercise, and meditation) or simply take fish oil alone to reduce inflammation. You do have a choice. However, if you choose to take only fish oil, you'll probably need a much higher dose than if you follow the complete program.

Based on thousands of SIP tests that I've done over the past few years, I can give the ranges of EPA and DHA that you will probably need depending on your current state of wellness. These doses give you a rough estimate of what you need to take to achieve a state of wellness. I say rough estimate because I still think you need to periodically monitor your blood to ensure that your SIP is in the appropriate range of 1.5 to 3.

Current State of Wellness	Amount of EPA and DHA Required
No existing chronic disease	2.5 grams per day
Existing obesity, heart disease, or type 2 diabetes	5 grams per day
Existing screaming pain (chronic pain)	7.5 grams per day
Existing neurological conditions	Greater than 10 grams per day

The reason why the amounts differ depending on the disease condition is that the rate of metabolic degradation of EPA and

DHA appears to be highly dependent on a particular disease condition. This means you may have to take more EPA and DHA orally to maintain a steady level in the bloodstream. If you are unable to get your SIP measured, you guesstimate the amount of EPA and DHA you need on a daily basis to reduce silent inflammation. It is preferable to get an SIP, but it is better to guesstimate the dose than forgo the fish oil.

If you are "healthy" and in the normal weight range—which means you're probably keeping your insulin levels under control—you probably need to take only 2.5 grams per day of ultra-refined EPA/DHA concentrates. This should help you achieve and maintain your SIP in the wellness range of 1.5 to 3.

As your insulin levels increase, you will generate more silent inflammation and will therefore need higher doses of EPA and DHA to achieve and maintain wellness. That's why if you're obese or have heart disease or type 2 diabetes, you also probably have elevated insulin levels, and you'll need more EPA and DHA to combat the silent inflammation induced by excess body fat.

What if your pain is no longer silent, but outright screaming pain? Those with arthritis, chronic back pain, and other inflammatory conditions that cause chronic pain need to take an even higher dose of EPA and DHA to get into the Anti-Inflammation Zone. These people also tend to have a higher SIP. Finally, if you have a neurological condition like attention deficit disorder, depression, or Alzheimer's, you will need even more EPA and DHA in order to reduce silent inflammation in the brain. That's why your grandmother may have also called fish oil "brain food."

TRICKS FOR TAKING HIGH-DOSE FISH OIL

Okay, you might believe me about the importance of high-dose fish oil, but taking that amount is a different matter. First of all, some people don't like the fish aftertaste or dislike the experience of gastric distress. Frankly, who does? These effects are primarily due to the extraneous fatty acids found in health-food-grade fish oils. Once you start using ultra-refined EPA/DHA concentrates, you'll see a dramatic reduction in these side effects, as most of the fatty acids that cause such problems have been removed in the refining process. Here are some other tricks for taking fish oil:

1. You should always take fish oil capsules with food as opposed to on an empty stomach. Intake of food causes the secretion of digestive enzymes from the pancreas that break down the fish oil for improved absorption.

2. Take fish oil capsules at night before you go to bed, along with a Zone snack.

3. Split your capsules throughout the day. If you have trouble swallowing several capsules at once, this is a good solution. Unlike vitamins and minerals, which last only a few hours in the blood, fatty acids from fish oil last several days in the blood. So you can take your dose all at once if that's easier, or you can divide it up. You'll maintain stable blood levels either way.

4. If you have to take more than four capsules a day, consider switching to a liquid fish oil. (I generally find that people will take up to four capsules per day of anything and then stop. I call this the "rule of four.") You'll also save money, since you no longer have to pay for the expensive gelatin capsules. Since ultra-refined EPA/DHA concentrates don't freeze, you should keep them in the freezer. This not only preserves them by protecting them from oxidation, but also makes the liquid taste a lot better.

   I know you are probably thinking that any type of liquid fish oil probably has a taste similar to cod liver oil, the world's most disgusting food. That's not the case with ultra-refined EPA/DHA concentrates, since most of the offending taste chemicals are removed with the toxins. But I will be honest: it is still fish oil. So keep reading down the list for additional tricks to make liquid fish oil more palatable.

5. Mix the liquid fish oil in two ounces of orange juice. The citric acid content of the orange juice dampens down the taste receptors in the mouth, so you taste very little of the fish oil. Because even this small amount of orange juice isn't very Zone-friendly, a better choice would be sucking on a piece of orange, lemon, or lime before you take the fish oil, for an even greater concentration of citric acid.

6. Have a Big Brain Shake. I developed this recipe for individuals with neurological conditions like attention deficit disorder and Alzheimer's who need very high levels of EPA and DHA in order to reduce their SIP. Frankly, I use it myself because I get a complete Zone meal and all the fish oil I need in less time than it takes to brew of cup of coffee. All you need is a good blender and the following ingredients:

1 cup 2% milk

15 to 20 grams protein powder

1 to 1½ cups thawed frozen berries

Put all the ingredients into a blender, add up to a tablespoon of liquid fish oil (which contains 7.5 grams of EPA and DHA), and blend. You can add some ice to make it more like a milkshake. The key to the Big Brain Shake is the milk globules found in the 2% milk. These are preformed emulsions into which the added EPA and DHA will immediately incorporate. These fat emulsions are an ideal delivery system to maximize the fish oil absorption with virtually no taste. The protein powder (lactose-free whey usually tastes the best) and the berries (using frozen berries is always a good choice) provide additional emulsification for any fish oil, plus make a very quick Zone meal.

CAN YOU TAKE TOO MUCH FISH OIL?

Of course you can, but not if you are monitoring your SIP periodically. If your SIP falls below 1, then take less fish oil. Usually, you would have to be taking more than the 7.5 grams of EPA and DHA to get that level. At an SIP of 0.5 or less, your risk of suffering a hemorrhagic stroke is increased. Again, to get to this potentially dangerous level, you'd have to be taking extremely high doses of fish oils. Remember, you should take the least amount of fish oil that gets you to the Anti-Inflammation Zone, and hence toward a state of wellness.

To ensure that your SIP is in the appropriate range, I recommend getting a blood test at least once a year. Also keep in mind that within two weeks after you stop taking fish oil, your SIP will climb back up to its original level. The SIP is your best clinical weapon to understand the extent of silent inflammation in your body and to determine your state of wellness. Don't be afraid to use it.

SUMMARY

If you have only fifteen seconds a day that you are willing to commit to control silent inflammation, then high-dose fish oil will be your best option. The more you follow the Zone Diet, the less high-dose fish oil you will need. The choice is yours.

Additional Supplements to Help Reduce Silent Inflammation

Embarking on the Zone Diet and taking high-dose fish oil are the two biggest steps you can take to reach the Anti-Inflammation Zone, where you begin to reverse silent inflammation. If you've started implementing this program already, then congratulations. You're well on your way toward moving back to a state of wellness. There are, though, several other support steps you need to take to fully ensure that you are controlling silent inflammation for good. Certain foods, spices, and dietary supplements—I refer to all of these as "supplements" for the purposes of this chapter—can help support the anti-inflammatory benefits of the Zone Lifestyle Program. You just need to know what to take.

I'm well aware of the huge boom taking place in the dietary supplement industry. Vitamins, minerals, herbs, and other magic potions are flying off the shelves to the tune of $20 billion a year. (Keep in mind that the total sale of prescription drugs is about $160 billion per year.) While I strongly believe that certain supplements can help you, they are not going to be your primary path to reduce silent inflammation. Consider supplements (other than high-dose fish oil) as spokes in a wheel: the more spokes, the stronger the wheel. However, the rim of that wheel is the Zone Diet plus high-dose fish oil. If the rim isn't there, then no matter how many spokes you have, you're not going to have a very good wheel.

All the anti-inflammatory supplements (foods, spices, dietary supplements) I discuss in this chapter have a direct anti-inflammatory effect by either:

- Inhibiting the formation of arachidonic acid (AA), or
- Inhibiting the enzymes that transform AA into pro-inflammatory eicosanoids.

INHIBITION OF ARACHIDONIC ACID

By inhibiting the formation of AA, you are directly choking off the production of the pro-inflammatory eicosanoids. This is the most sophisticated dietary strategy possible to reduce silent inflammation.

Fish Oil

On a scale of 1 to 10 for supplements, I give high-dose fish oil a 12. It's the number-one anti-inflammatory supplement you can take—as long as you take an ultra-refined product that has had the vast majority of the inherent toxins removed, as I discussed in the last chapter. If you only take one supplement in your life, make sure it's high-dose fish oil. The EPA found in fish oil partially inhibits the activity of the delta-5-desaturase enzyme that makes AA. This represents the primary anti-inflammatory effect of fish oil. But to achieve any significant impact on AA production, you have to provide a lot of EPA. That's why you need high-dose fish oil, which is especially rich in EPA. Your success in reducing silent inflammation will be reflected in the reduction of the AA/EPA ratio, as measured by your SIP.

My recommendations for fish oil: These are outlined in chapter 7 on page 83. Plan to take a lot of fish oil to reduce silent inflammation, but make sure that it's ultra-refined, and use the SIP to give you guidance in the exact dosage.

Sesame Oil

Although sesame oil is rich in omega-6 fatty acids, it also contains small amounts (less than 1 percent) of phytochemicals called lignans.

These lignans include sesamin, which is a direct inhibitor of the enzyme that makes AA. In this regard, sesame oil acts via the same mechanism as EPA. By inhibiting the specific enzyme used to produce AA, the building block of all pro-inflammatory eicosanoids, you reduce silent inflammation. However, unlike fish oil, sesame oil also provides a significant amount of potentially pro-inflammatory omega-6 fatty acids at the same time. So it's kind of one and one-half steps forward (providing sesamin to inhibit AA production) and one step back (providing omega-6 fatty acids to make AA). Nonetheless, the benefits of sesame oil outweigh its drawbacks if it is taken in moderate amounts.

My recommendation for sesame oil: Consume 1 to 2 teaspoonfuls a day. You can substitute sesame oil for olive oil in one of your meals.

Turmeric

Turmeric is a yellow spice that has long been used in Indian curry. Turmeric contains a phytochemical called curcumin. Like sesamin, curcumin also inhibits the enzyme that makes AA. However, curcumin doesn't have the specificity of sesamin or EPA as it also inhibits the activity of the enzyme that is necessary to make precursors of both "good" and "bad" eicosanoids. Nonetheless, like sesame oil, the benefits of turmeric as a spice outweigh any potential negative consequences.

My recommendations for turmeric: If you like curry, then you'll like the taste of turmeric and can make it a constant ally in your body. Don't be afraid to be liberal in its usage. It can be used with a wide number of dishes and recipes.

Alpha-Linolenic Acid (ALA)

Alpha-linolenic acid (ALA) is a short-chain omega-3 found in high concentrations in flaxseed oil. Like curcumin, ALA inhibits the enzyme (delta-6-desaturase) that decreases the production of the precursors of both "good" and "bad" eicosanoids. However, unlike EPA, sesamin, or curcumin, ALA has no ability to inhibit the synthesis of AA. This may be why high intakes of ALA have been linked to increases in prostate cancer. Although ALA can be theoretically synthesized into EPA, the process is very inefficient in humans.

My recommendations for ALA: Forget about taking ALA if you are taking high-dose fish oil. You will get far better anti-inflammatory effects from fish oil since the conversion of ALA into EPA is very inefficient.

Conjugated Linolenic Acid (CLA)

This is a potentially good trans-fat. It occurs naturally in dairy products and can be made synthetically. The synthetic version of CLA contains two isomers. One of the isomers acts like ALA, thereby decreasing the ultimate production of of both "good" and "bad" eicosanoids. However, one of the other isomers in the synthetic version also causes an increase in insulin resistance in humans and causes fatty livers in mice.

My recommendations for CLA: The jury is still out on this supplement, so I would avoid it for the time being.

Alcohol

You'd never think of alcohol as a dietary supplement, but it actually does a pretty good job of reducing silent inflammation if taken in moderation. In particular, the levels of C-reactive protein are lowered in individuals who drink a moderate amount of alcohol. One of the mechanisms of moderate alcohol consumption appears to be its stimulation of the conversion of omega-6 fatty acids into the building block (dihomo-gamma-linolenic acid or DGLA) necessary for the production of powerful anti-inflammatory eicosanoids. This helps explain why having one to two glasses of wine per day or the equivalent amount of other forms of alcohol appears to be cardio protective. If you consume alcohol in larger amounts, however, apparently there is an accelerated conversion of DGLA into AA, and all the benefits of moderate alcohol consumption are rapidly eradicated.

My recommendation for alcohol: Have the equivalent of two drinks a day (one glass of wine, bottle of beer, or mixed drink) if you're a male and one drink a day if you're a female. If you are going to drink alcohol, always have a protein chaser with it to prevent an overproduction of insulin. This might be an ounce of cheese for each glass of wine, or four jumbo shrimp (or chicken wings) with each bottle of beer.

ENZYMATIC INHIBITORS OF EICOSANOID SYNTHESIS

The more AA you make, the more difficult it is to control silent inflammation. In other words, an ounce of prevention (reduction of AA formation) is worth a pound of cure (inhibition of the enzymes that convert AA into pro-inflammatory eicosanoids). Nonetheless, there are a number of foods that are very useful (and tasty) to add to the Zone Diet.

Extra-Virgin Olive Oil

You've no doubt heard of the health benefits of extra-virgin olive oil. These benefits have been known for centuries. Olive oil is both rich in monounsaturated fat and low in pro-inflammatory omega-6 fatty acids. So is lard, but no one ever talks about the health benefits of lard. The true health benefits of olive oil come from a unique phytochemical called hydroxytyrosol that is found only in olive oil. Hydroxytyrosol appears to be an inhibitor of the enzymes that produce pro-inflammatory eicosanoids, just as aspirin does. This begins to explain the Crete paradox. This population consumes more than 40 percent of their calories as fat (primarily extra-virgin olive oil), but has the lowest rate of heart disease in the Mediterranean region. They are basically taking liquid aspirin.

It's good news that something as tasty as extra-virgin olive oil can have significant anti-inflammatory benefits. Unfortunately, most extra-virgin olive oils sold in America contain only trace amounts of hydroxytyrosol. Olives are a fruit, just like grapes. Different varieties of olives will have different levels of hydroxytyrosol. The higher the levels, the more desirable (and costly) the olive oil. Frankly, most of the good stuff never leaves Italy.

But don't take my word for it—try this simple taste test. Take a teaspoonful of olive oil and put it in your mouth. It should have a buttery taste, as opposed to a bland oil taste. Now swish the oil along the top of your mouth with your tongue until it hits the back of your throat. You should notice a very pepper-like taste. If you don't, then the oil contains virtually no hydroxytyrosol, which means it has virtually no health benefits. Don't despair if you find that your extra-virgin olive oil isn't so extra special. You can get the good stuff from Italy by going to www.Olio2go.com. You should expect to pay in the range of $20 to $30 a bottle, which I realize is much more than you're used to paying. But isn't the reduction of silent inflammation worth it?

My recommendation for extra-virgin olive oil: Have a total of 2–3 tea-spoons a day of true extra-virgin olive oil that's rich in hydroxytyrosol. You should have 1 teaspoonful at each meal drizzled onto low-fat protein or cooked vegetables. This is why extra-virgin olive oil (the real stuff, of course) is the primary fat recommended for the Zone Diet. If you can't get the really good stuff, then consider eating olives imported from Italy or Greece. If they are rich in hydroxytyrosol, you will notice a distinct peppery taste.

Ginger

The anti-inflammatory benefits of ginger come from a group of phytochemicals called xanthines. These xanthines are dual inhibitors of both the cyclo-oxygenase (COX) enzymes, which make pro-inflammatory prostaglandins, and also the lipo-oxygenase (LOX) enzymes, which make pro-inflammatory leukotrienes. In this regard they can be considered to be a much weaker biological equivalent of corticosteroids.

My recommendation for ginger: Use fresh ginger as a condiment as much as possible. Chop it into a stir-fry, or grate it into a salad or into a fish or chicken dish. It is possible to get capsules rich in xanthines at specialty health food stores.

Aloe Vera

Aloe vera is well known for soothing burns on the skin. The gel-like material in the aloe vera leaf works as an anti-inflammatory to calm the redness and swelling associated with the burn. The particular anti-inflammatory substance in aloe vera appears to inhibit the enzyme that makes thromboxane A_2, a particularly nasty pro-inflammatory eicosanoid. In addition, aloe vera is rich in glucomannan, which has some unique wound-healing properties. How does this translate into relieving silent inflammation? If you take it orally, it will help dampen down inflammation in the digestive tract, which in turn will help you absorb nutrients more effectively.

My recommendation for aloe vera: Take a tablespoon of organic aloe vera each day. Use it as needed to alleviate inflammation in skin burns.

ANTI-INFLAMMATORY SUPPLEMENTS VERSUS ANTIOXIDANTS

Although the health food industry is fixated on antioxidants, there is a massive difference between anti-inflammatory supplements and antioxidants. One provides powerful support in fighting silent inflammation; the other has very little medical impact.

Vitamin supplements have fallen out of favor in recent years. As more and more research findings weigh in on the lack of clinically relevant benefits from taking vitamins, the future picture looks less optimistic for them to act as magic bullets. Antioxidants such as vitamin E, vitamin C, and beta-carotene have often been touted as the keepers of eternal health. Yet under clinically controlled conditions, they don't appear to offer any significant benefits, especially regarding mortality (the only statistic that really counts). In fact, in some studies beta-carotene actually appeared to increase the likelihood of cancer. In cardiovascular studies, there were no improvements in mortality with vitamin E in the CHAOS, HOPE, and GISSI studies. On the other hand, a true anti-inflammatory supplement such as ultra-refined EPA/DHA concentrates has a dramatic impact on the reduction of death from heart disease.

Does this mean that antioxidants are a waste of time and money? Probably not, if you use them with the right diet. I believe that part of the reason antioxidant supplement studies have failed to find any benefit may be due to the fact that the subjects in the study ate a diet rich in omega-6 fatty acids. Case in point: It turns out that high levels of vitamin C can actually promote the formation of a powerful pro-inflammatory eicosanoid, which is made from omega-6 fatty acids. This means that the combination of high levels of vitamin C and omega-6 fatty acids may be downright dangerous. On the other hand, vitamin C doesn't have this effect with omega-3 fatty acids. As we learned from the Lyon Heart Diet study, when omega-6 fatty acids were aggressively removed from the diet, the results were extraordinary, with a 70 percent reduction in heart disease mortality and a complete elimination of sudden death from heart disease. From this we can conclude that controlling inflammation is a lot more important that controlling oxidation.

The truth is that the antioxidant picture is quite complex. Yes, antioxidants help neutralize free radicals. The most likely target for free radical attack is not DNA, but the polyunsaturated fatty acids in your membranes. This is important in the reduction of silent inflammation, as free radicals are the sparks that are required to make eicosanoids. If you have an excess of AA in the cell membranes, those free radicals can potentially generate massive amounts of inflammation.

Thus, the pathway between antioxidants and the reduction of silent inflammation is pretty indirect at best. You need enough antioxidants to reduce the sparks that can ignite AA into profound inflammation, but you also need enough free radicals to convert incoming food to energy and to kill invading microbes (more about this in chapter 13). Adding to this complexity is that antioxidants work together like a relay team. If one component is missing, your body isn't going to win, no matter how well the other antioxidants perform.

The most likely attack points for excess free radicals are the essential fatty acids in the membranes. The challenge is to neutralize such oxidized lipids and to remove the source of oxidation from the body. This requires three distinct types of antioxidants: fat-soluble, surface-active, and water-soluble. The members of your fat-soluble relay team are vitamin E, coenzyme Q10, and beta-carotene. As these antioxidants neutralize free radicals in the membrane, they become partially stabilized free radicals in the process. Like the game of hot potato, the goal is to keep moving the free radical into the bloodstream and eventually out into the urine.

The anchors of this antioxidant relay team, which finish the race, are the water-soluble antioxidants such as vitamin C that carry the stabilized free radicals to the liver so that they can be broken down into inert compounds and excreted from the body.

The little-understood middle members of the relay team are the surface-active antioxidants. These are not classic vitamins, but rather phytochemicals known as polyphenols. Without them, your body would have no way to shuttle free radicals from fat-soluble antioxidants to the water-soluble antioxidants. Polyphenols are crucial for this process to work, which may explain why studies haven't been able to find a benefit to taking vitamin supplements. Without adequate levels of polyphenols, you simply can't reduce excess free radical levels regardless of the amounts of other antioxidants in your body.

There are more than 4,000 known polyphenols, and the richest sources (not surprisingly) are fruits and vegetables. These polyphenols are found in high concentrations in red wine, berries, and dark-colored vegetables—and in fact it is the polyphenols that give vibrant color to fruits and vegetables. In general, the more color a fruit or vegetable has, the richer the polyphenol content. Grains and starches (especially the ones in the American diet) have relatively low levels of these polyphenols.

Just how powerful is one antioxidant-containing food compared to another? That is difficult to say, since every manufacturer of health foods makes each of its claims more outlandish than its equally lying competitor. Well, now there is a new sheriff in town, and he goes by the name of ORAC (oxygen radical absorbing capacity). ORAC is a new standardized test that was developed to compare the amount of free radical–quenching activity a particular food or antioxidant supplement really has. Fruits and vegetables with the deepest colors are often the ones with the highest ORAC levels, especially compared to vitamin E and vitamin C. But there are also a few surprising foods with high ORAC numbers. For example, the polyphenols isolated from green tea have a very high ORAC value. Likewise, herbs that have been used for centuries to preserve food, like rosemary, have even higher ORAC values. Perhaps the most surprising is that the highest ORAC value belongs to hydroxytyrosol, the polyphenol found in extra-virgin olive oil. This helps explain why extra-virgin olive oil is so healthful—not only is it an anti-inflammatory agent; it also contains the most powerful antioxidant known.

Although fish oil is truly the anti-inflammatory powerhouse out of all supplements because of its high degree of polyunsaturation, it has the potential to be oxidized in the body due to an attack by free radicals. Not only will the oxidized fatty acids in fish oil lose all of their anti-inflammatory properties, but they can actually become generators of inflammation. In fact, research has shown that those who take fish oil without taking in adequate amounts of antioxidants can develop decreased blood levels of vitamin E stores over time.

If you follow the Zone Diet with its ample amounts of fruits and vegetables, you'll have all the water-soluble and surface-active antioxidants you need from your diet. However, getting adequate levels of fat-soluble vitamins is more difficult. Therefore, I would recommend considering additional fat-soluble antioxidant supplementation to maintain your body's reserves if you are taking high-dose fish oil.

My recommendation for antioxidants: I recommend taking a supplement containing 200 IU of vitamin E and 30 mg of coenzyme Q10 every day with your fish oil. Your other option is to increase your intake of extra-virgin olive oil. According to scientists at the Norwegian Olympic Sports Clinic, this is the best antioxidative supplement they have ever tested in efforts to reduce excessive oxidation from fish oil.

If you aren't following the Zone Diet but are still taking fish oil, you should take a good multivitamin that contains water-soluble antioxidants. I also recommend a good fat-soluble antioxidant such as vitamin E, coenzyme Q10, and beta-carotene. Just to be on the safe side, always use extra-virgin olive oil with your meals. However, make sure it is the good stuff—rich in hydroxytyrosol.

SUMMARY

Never mistake supplements (other than high-dose fish oil) as your primary tools in fighting silent inflammation. Supplements can help, but they are only spokes in the wheel. The strength of the rim of that wheel is determined by your adherence to the Zone Diet and the amount of high-dose fish oil you take on a daily basis.

9

Smart Exercise to Help
Reduce Silent Inflammation

As I mentioned in the first chapter, wellness is more than just being "not sick." Fighting silent inflammation is a lifelong struggle, and you need every weapon possible at your disposal. Even though the Zone Diet and high-dose fish oil will get you 80 percent of the way to wellness, you still need to maintain a moderate level of physical activity to maximize the hormonal effects of my Zone Lifestyle Program for reducing silent inflammation.

By moderate exercise, I mean moderate. I don't want you to exercise to an extreme degree. In fact, too much exercise can be just as harmful to your body as too little. That's because it takes a toll on your body that leads to chronic silent inflammation. Yes, I know you're probably surprised by this, and maybe even a little relieved. But you need to remember that being in a state of wellness is all about balance. Balance in the foods you eat and balance in your activity levels. Push your body beyond its limits, and it will fight back by increasing inflammation and making your body more prone to illness. This is why people training for their first marathon often develop more colds, flu, and other ailments.

As an interesting aside, a friend of mine who runs a very successful anti-aging clinic in San Diego told me that nearly half of his clients are former triathletes who thought they could exercise themselves into immortality. Instead, they overexercised themselves into premature aging. Many have permanent joint problems and chronic pain due to osteoarthritis and feel (and look) much older than their years. They simply pushed their bodies beyond their limits for too many years. They are now paying the price for thinking that more was better.

While any type of exercise will cause some inflammation, the appropriate amount of exercise—coupled with the Zone Diet and high-dose fish oil—can induce an exceptionally powerful anti-inflammatory response that not only repairs the damage to your muscle tissue, but also makes the muscle stronger in the process. Thus, it will help you rejuvenate your body, not hurt it (see chapter 13 for more information).

Exercise can help ward off aging by reducing silent inflammation. It does this by alleviating insulin resistance, which in turn helps reduce visceral fat, the dangerous kind that collects on vital organs in your abdomen. It is this visceral fat that triggers the production of pro-inflammatory cytokines like interleukin-6 (IL-6), which travel to the liver to produce increased C-reactive protein (CRP) levels. Reduce this visceral fat, and you'll reduce the primary source of much of the silent inflammation in your body.

GETTING FIT VERSUS LOSING WEIGHT

Getting physically fit isn't necessarily about losing weight. It all boils down to your ability to control insulin resistance and therefore silent inflammation. If your body maintains an appropriate zone of insulin, you can still be overweight and healthy. On the other hand, if your body has to pump out greater and greater amounts of insulin due to insulin resistance in your cells, then your excess body weight is generating silent inflammation around the clock, setting you on a fast track for type 2 diabetes and heart disease.

For example, in one recent study in which overweight individuals lost weight on a calorie-restricted diet, it was only those with insulin resistance who had any decrease in their blood levels of CRP when they lost weight. This helps to explain why some overweight people have perfectly normal cholesterol levels and are at relatively little risk for heart disease. They manage to maintain their insulin levels in a healthy zone. Their weight is a cosmetic problem due to eating too many calories, but not a medical problem. Research by Stephen Blair at the Cooper Clinic in Dallas, Texas, confirms this seemingly paradoxical situation. Individuals who were physically fit but overweight were significantly less likely to develop heart disease than those who were of normal weight but less physically fit. Of course, those who were of normal weight and physically fit had even lower levels of cardiovascular risk.

How is it that some people can be healthy and overweight while others are not? It all boils down to the levels of visceral fat. Decrease this type of fat, and levels of CRP are also lowered. It is visceral fat that is mobilized by exercise. Unfortunately, exercise has a much smaller impact on subcutaneous fat, the unsightly but relatively safe fat that collects on the hips, thighs, and buttocks. In fact, I'd hazard a guess that this at least partly explains why women have a harder time losing weight via exercise than men. It's far easier to shed belly fat, which is often visceral fat, than the subcutaneous fat that is more common in females than males.

Obviously, the best course of action is to be physically fit and at a normal weight. I just don't want you to use loss of body weight as a fitness goal. First of all, you might gain a few pounds of muscle while you're reducing fat—which is a great thing, though your scale won't tell you this. This is why your body fat percentage is a far better indicator of fat loss and why I consider it to be a biomarker (although a weak one) of wellness. In Appendix E, there are simple charts that help you analyze your body fat using only a tape measure. Second, from a health standpoint, getting active will help reduce silent inflammation regardless of whether you lose any inches from your hips and thighs.

WHAT EXERCISE DOES FOR YOUR BODY

Every time you engage in physical activity, you put a certain amount of stress on your body. In aerobic activities, this means working out to a point where you begin to break a sweat. This usually happens when you get your heart rate up to 70 percent of its maximum limit for a reasonable period of time. Once this occurs, things are happening at the molecular level; in particular, you are making your cells more responsive to taking up blood glucose, thereby decreasing the amount of insulin needed to be secreted by the pancreas. If you are overweight or out of shape, then it won't take you very long to begin to increase your core temperature and break into a sweat. That's a good point to stop exercising that day. With time and consistent exercise, you will have to work out longer or with more intensity to reach the same point of exertion.

Strength training works very differently from aerobic exercise to reduce insulin levels. By building more muscle mass, your body will have an easier time extracting glucose from the bloodstream and your need for insulin will drop. Regardless of your form of exercise (aerobic versus strength), the long-term outcome is the same: reduction of excess insulin.

However, there are other hormonal changes that take place with strength training that do not occur with aerobic training. When you exercise your muscles to exhaustion, a certain level of trauma occurs. This triggers a pro-inflammatory response to treat the micro-tears in your muscles. If the pro-inflammatory response is not too severe, there will be a corresponding anti-inflammatory response to repair the muscle damage and increase muscle strength for the next bout of exercise. Part of that anti-inflammatory response is the release of growth hormone from the pituitary gland to rebuild the damaged tissue and make it stronger. This is why strength athletes are much more muscular than endurance athletes, although both have low levels of fasting insulin.

Moderate strength training should provide you with just enough micro-trauma to allow you to sufficiently recover from your workouts to repair and rebuild your muscles before your next strength workout. As you age, the time for this repair process increases. This is why young athletes can do intense two-a-day workouts, whereas older athletes should do moderate strength training every other day. The amount of recovery time ultimately depends on your innate anti-inflammatory responses, which can be enhanced by being in the Anti-Inflammation Zone. However, no matter how good your dietary program, excessive exercise increases inflammation to such an extent that it overwhelms the body's ability to produce sufficient levels of anti-inflammatory eicosanoids needed for recovery. The end result is you're still sore and weak from your last workout on the day of your next workout.

The most important thing is to listen to your body. If it's still sore from your last workout when you're about to begin your next one, you've probably pushed it too hard and your body is still churning out inflammatory mediators. Rest some more, and cut back a bit on your next workout.

HOW TO BURN FAT FASTER

To burn fat, you have to lower insulin levels, since insulin inhibits the release of stored fat from the adipose tissue. This is true as you exercise, but it is also true as you watch TV. Exercise just speeds up the fat-burning process. All exercise burns the same number of calories, but not necessarily the same amount of fat. Let's look at running. If you increase your running pace from, say, 5.5 miles per hour to 6.5 miles per hour, you will burn both more fat and more calories if you cover the same distance. However, if you then increase your pace from 6.5 miles per hour to 7.5 miles per hour, you'll actually burn less fat in proportion to the total calories burned. That's because your muscles need adequate amounts of oxygen to metabolize fat to chemical energy (adenosine triphosphate or ATP) needed for muscle contractions. As you go beyond a certain exercise intensity, this growing lack of oxygen transfer to the muscle cells makes them more dependent on burning stored glucose for ATP production. You are still burning calories, but more of these are coming from a low-octane fuel (glucose) and less is coming from a high-octane fuel (fat). The combination of the Zone

Diet plus high-dose fish oil increases your oxygen transfer capacity so that you can keep using high-octane fat for ATP production at increasingly higher exercise intensities.

BURNING CALORIES VERSUS PRODUCING ATP

One of the more difficult concepts to get across to athletes, coaches, dietitians, and physicians is the differences between burning calories and producing ATP from calories. ATP is the chemical that is required not only for muscle contraction, but also for virtually all of our metabolism. ATP is made on an as-needed basis from either glucose or fat. Your production of ATP is far greater from a calorie of fat than from a calorie of glucose. In the Anti-Inflammation Zone, you are primarily burning fat for ATP production as opposed to glucose. This means you are also making all the ATP you need, even though fewer calories are being expended. This is why diabetics, world-class athletes, or just plain normal people require far fewer calories on the Zone Diet than calculated from the usual metabolic equations. It is because they are producing more ATP from less calories.

Furthermore, doing high-intensity aerobic exercise in an effort to burn fat faster can set you up for muscle injury due to the excess impact on your joints. Every time you lift both feet off the ground (as you do when you run), each foot transmits three times your weight through your ankles, legs, knees, and hips as it hits the surface. This is why I recommend brisk walking over running to minimize potential damage to your joints and minimize increased inflammation.

Strength training, on the other hand, uses primarily glucose for ATP production. Therefore, you will always burn less fat during a strength-training workout than an aerobic workout. However, this is more than compensated by increased muscle mass that can extract excess glucose from the blood throughout the day. This effectively lowers the need for extra insulin secretion and thus allows more effective burning of fat throughout the day.

Realize that 80 percent of your insulin-lowering ability will come from your diet, and only 20 percent from exercise. The amount of fat burning from exercise drops even further if you are following a high glycemic-load diet. This is because excess insulin produced by a high glycemic-load diet blocks the release of stored fat for its potential use as energy. This explains why many people (especially women) who spend an extraordinary number of hours in the gym have very little to show for their efforts. However, following the Zone Diet maximizes the fat-burning benefits of exercise.

THE UNAPPRECIATED BENEFITS OF EXERCISE

Of course, 99 percent of people do exercise in order lose weight faster. Actually, their goal is lose to excess body fat faster. Well, here is some sad news. Losing body fat is a slow, long process. Frankly, to lose more than one pound of fat a week is a difficult task. Fortunately, there are plenty of other reasons why you want to be incorporating exercise into your daily life regardless of the fat loss benefits.

Let's start with strength training first. The primary benefit is maintaining muscle mass while you age, and in the process maintaining your immune function as you age. Between ages twenty and forty, you will lose about 40 percent of your muscle mass, and then about 1 percent every year thereafter. The good news is that your body maintains the ability to synthesize new muscle as you age. You have the same ability to build new muscle up through your seventies and eighties as you did in your twenties and thirties. Although we maintain the ability to synthesize new muscle mass as we age, we have to combat the increase in the rate of degradation of muscle that occurs with aging. The most likely reason behind this muscle loss is an increased level of cortisol, which rapidly tears down existing muscle mass and converts it into glucose. This also happens if you follow a very low glycemic-load diet, like the Atkins diet.

Thus, you are going to naturally lose muscle mass if you take no steps to maintain it. You have to continually do strength training to keep a constant stimulus to induce the cascade of events that leads to the synthesis of new muscle mass. If a lifetime of strength training doesn't seem to be your cup of tea, then consider that without enough muscle, you'll get sicker more often. The reason? Your body stores all its amino acid reserves in your muscle cells including the amino acid glutamine—a critical component for certain immune cells called macrophages and neutrophils described in more detail in chapter 13. During times of acute stress, such as an infection, your body secretes excess cortisol in order to break down muscle cells to supply adequate levels of glutamine to your immune system.

If you don't have adequate amounts of muscle, then you're not going to have adequate levels of glutamine in a crisis, and your immune system is going to suffer. This is one reason that so many elderly people die from infections shortly after bone fractures. When they have a major injury such as a bone fracture, their body breaks down what little muscle it has to release enough glutamine to help repair the bone. This leaves practically no glutamine reserves to fend off infections. Thus, these patients are far more susceptible to pneumonia, staph, and other infections that run rampant in the nursing homes and hospitals where they are often recovering. Strength training at any age becomes a great defense to ensure the adequate levels glutamine reserves you need for maximum immunity and for reducing silent inflammation. The result is maintenance of wellness for as long as possible.

Just as the unexpected benefit of strength training is maintaining proper immune function, the unexpected benefit of aerobic exercise is that it builds your brain. Aerobic exercise can improve your overall brain function by activating a hormone called brain-derived neurotrophic factor (BDNF) to repair and potentially trigger the development of new nerve cells in the brain. Just as muscle cells need amino acids from protein-rich foods to repair themselves and grow, nerve cells in the brain require a very specialized type of long-chain omega-3 fatty acid as a fuel source. This fatty acid, docosahexaenoic acid (DHA), is found in rich amounts in fish oil. The DHA in fish oil works hand in hand with BDNF to keep your neurons and brainpower primed over time.

For years it was thought that the brain couldn't regenerate nerve cells. Now we know that under the right conditions, it can be done. The stimulus for that nerve growth is BDNF. Aerobic exercise stimulates the release of BDNF. BDNF is a like a master mason, but in order to build the structure, he needs some bricks. The bricks for the building of new nerves come from having adequate levels of DHA in the diet. So if you want to remain sharp as a tack as you age, do daily aerobic exercise and take your fish oil.

THE ANTI-INFLAMMATION ZONE EXERCISE PLAN

By now, you should be convinced that there is more to exercise than simply fat loss, and that you have to exercise on a lifetime basis. You have to treat exercise like a drug to be taken at the right dose and at the right time. Here is your Anti-Inflammation Zone exercise prescription:

- Exercise aerobically six days a week.
- Do strength training three days a week.
- On the three days you don't do strength training, do stretching.

Although stretching won't help you lose fat, build muscle, or decrease silent inflammation, it will prevent the nagging injuries that can keep you from exercising. As you age, your tendons and ligaments become shorter, thus limiting your range of motion, especially as you strength train. Consider stretching to be a cheap insurance policy against exercise-induced inflammation.

Now you probably want to know how to do it with the least amount of time and effort. If you feel you don't have the time to exercise, let me tell you—it's going to be a lot easier than you think. That's because your exercise partner in this plan will be your favorite TV program.

STEP ONE: GET YOUR EQUIPMENT READY

The most important piece of equipment for your Anti-Inflammation Zone exercise program is a TV, which you are going to use for timing. Other essential pieces of equipment are a towel (for use during stretching) and some full unopened soup cans or empty milk jugs (for strength training). So far, your expenses are pretty limited.

Although eventually you may want to purchase a set of light weights, you should consider starting out using one-pound cans of fruits or vegetables and empty plastic milk jugs that can be partially filled with water. I recommend starting with very light amounts of weight if you are just beginning the strength-training program that I am about to describe. You can always increase the weight if the exercises get too easy. It is better to start with too little weight than too much, since overexertion will increase inflammation.

If you do invest in a set of dumbbells, then I recommend getting three pairs of different weights. If you're a female beginning with weights, you might want to start with pairs of 1-pound, 2-pound, and 5-pound dumbbells. If you're a male, you might want to start with 5-pound, 7.5-pound, and 10-pound dumbbells. Before you buy any dumbbells, you should go to a fitness store to see how much you can easily lift. Pick up a dumbbell and do a bicep curl slowly. (See page 114 for more details on this exercise.) Repetitions should be slow. For each one, do a slow count to six on the way up, hold for two seconds, and then do a slow release for a count of six while squeezing or flexing the muscle. If you can do fewer than eight repetitions of curls, then that would be a good intermediate weight. You may be surprised at how little weight you can lift doing these slow repetitions. Once you find your intermediate weight, get another set of dumbbells that's about two pounds lighter and a third set that's two pounds heavier than the intermediate weight. You should be able to get a set of three pairs of dumbbells for $30 to $60. Also, you will be doing most of these weight-bearing exercises in front of your TV, so you should consider purchasing dumbbells that have a plastic or rubberized neoprene coating that won't ruin the floor of your family room. These are also easier to roll off to the side or under the couch for storage.

STEP TWO: TURN ON YOUR TV

That's right. These exercises are supposed to be done while you're watching your favorite program. Rather than making extra time to exercise, why not squeeze in a workout when you're doing something you enjoy? What's more, the commercials built into these shows are perfect timers for switching from aerobics to strength training and back again. A typical 30-minute sitcom is divided into segments of two 11-minute segments of programming and three 3-minute segments of commercials. You can use these segments as timers to tell you when to switch from aerobic to weight training. At the end of the show, you'll have done about 20 minutes of aerobic training and about 10 minutes of strength training or 10 minutes of stretching.

Once your dumbbells (or towel) are in front of you, you're ready to begin at the start of your TV program. During the two 11-minute segments of your aerobic training, you'll be marching in place. I want to give you a no-brainer activity that you can do without distracting yourself too much from your TV show. You can increase the intensity of your marching by either increasing the speed or lifting your knees higher as you progress in your workout. Alternatively, you can use a step platform to step up on and then step down from during your marching.

STEP AEROBICS

You've no doubt seen a step aerobic class if you've ever been to a gym. It may have looked complicated and scary if you never took a class yourself. People leaping across the steps, crossing over, and hopping up and down, to and fro. It's enough to make you twist your ankle just watching them. The truth is, you don't need to do a complicated dance routine on the step to get a good workout. Simply step up on your right foot, placing the foot flat on the step and then bring your left foot up, placing it flat down next to your right foot. To step down, bring your right foot flat down first, followed by your left foot. Once you get comfortable with this motion, shift feet, bringing your left foot up first followed by your right foot. Start out with just the basic step before adding risers to lift the height of the step.

You can purchase a step and risers (which range in cost from $35 to $100, depending on the product) from any sports equipment store or an online sports catalog, such as Sports Unlimited (www.sport sunlimitedinc.com).

During commercial breaks, you'll be doing your strength-training exercises (or towel stretching on alternate days). The goal of strength training is to exercise a particular muscle group to exhaustion, but not to a level of overexertion that would leave the muscles sore the next day. The technique I recommend is to use a slow rise (concentric phase) with weights to contract the muscle and a slow lowering (eccentric phase) of the weights to relax and elongate the muscle. I want you to take 6 seconds to raise the weight for the contraction phase, 2 seconds to hold it at the top, and 6 seconds to lower the weight for the relaxation phase. One complete lifting and lowering of the weights counts as a repetition. Since each repetition should take about 15 seconds, it will take about 2 minutes to complete eight repetitions of one exercise. You should do two exercises during each commercial break and finish the second exercise to completion even if the show comes back on. You can then resume the aerobic activity of marching in place or stepping up and down on a box. Aim for two to three upper-body and two to three lower-body exercises in each strength-training session.

The form of slow repetitions used in the strength-training exercises not only makes you focus on the muscle group of interest and use correct form, but also forces you to lift a lot less weight than you normally would on faster repetitions. All of this will help prevent injury. I like to think of it as Tai Chi with light weights.

Here's how to do a correct repetition. First, you need to focus on breathing. Correct breathing is vital when you lift weights, since it ensures that adequate oxygen is getting to your muscles as they exert themselves. Before you begin each repetition, inhale deeply. Now exhale as you slowly lift the weight for a count of six. Hold the weights for 2 seconds, breathing normally. (Don't hold your breath!) Exhale just before you begin to lower the weight. Lower the weights slowly on a count of six, inhaling deeply. Hold the weight at the beginning position, breathing normally, for 2 seconds. Inhale deeply again, and repeat the exercise again until you have completed eight repetitions. Here's a helpful hint: you know you are reaching fatigue when you find yourself taking short, shallow breaths to complete the lifting phase of your final repetition. If you can get through the eight repetitions without using short breaths, you need to increase your weight.

Leah Garcia, a longtime Zone advocate who is also a certified personal trainer, TV sports commentator, and former professional mountain bike champion, has put together a simple but effective strength-training program with stretching exercises that can be done in any hotel room for business and leisure travelers. I have adapted the concepts of her program for the Anti-Inflammation Zone exercise program.

On the days you do a strength-training workout, pick up to three exercises from the upper-body routines and up to three from the lower-body group. Choose different exercises each time. The variety will keep you from getting bored and will allow you to exercise the widest range of muscle groups. Each of the exercises listed should be done with proper form to not only avoid injury, but also to better the results.

Upper-Body Routines	Lower-Body and Back Routines
Shoulder press	Narrow squat
Two-arm overhead triceps press	Wide squat
Biceps curl	Reverse lunge
Triceps dip	Hamstring press
Lateral front shoulder raise	Crunch

Here's a description of each exercise, accompanied by a photo of Leah demonstrating it.

UPPER-BODY ROUTINES

SHOULDER PRESS

The shoulder press develops and increases strength in the front and side heads of the deltoids, as well as in the triceps. This is a great exercise for people who lift objects above their heads and want an increased range of motion.

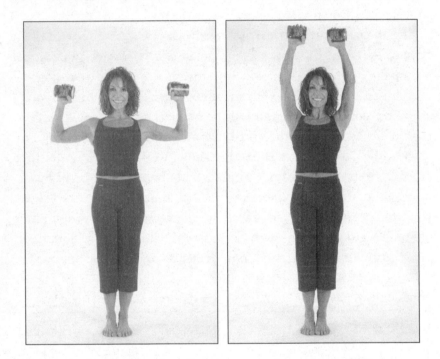

Stand upright with your shoulders squared and your legs and feet together. Hold a weight (soup can or partially filled plastic milk jug) in each hand, with your palms facing the ceiling. Your hands are only slightly above your shoulder height. Your elbows are bent (creating a field goal position with your arms). Exhale as you press the soup cans (or dumbbells) toward the ceiling, extending your arms so that your elbows straighten, but don't lock. Concentrate on keeping your shoulder blades pushed toward your back. Hold the weights for 2 seconds, and then inhale as you lower the weights to the starting position.

TWO-ARM OVERHEAD TRICEPS PRESS

The overhead triceps press strengthens the muscles that work in opposition to the biceps and improve connective tissue strength. Triceps essentially allow you to straighten the arm and twist the wrist upward. Developing the entire triceps muscle will reduce the much lamented "arm wattle" and allow you to press objects with force.

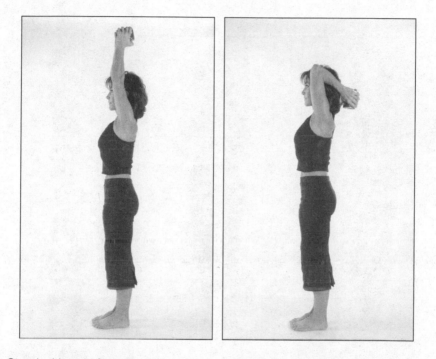

Stand with your feet together. Hold the soup can (or dumbbell) between both hands high above your head. Keep your shoulders dropped down and your neck and head extended. Exhale as you bend your arms from the elbows, lowering the weight behind your head and tucking it toward your body. Hold this position for 2 seconds, and then inhale as you raise the weight to the starting position, focusing on working the back of your arms.

BICEPS CURL

The curl exercise increases strength in the biceps brachii, the muscle that helps lift and curl the arm and twist the wrist downward. Working the biceps will balance the upper arm and ultimately help with grip strength.

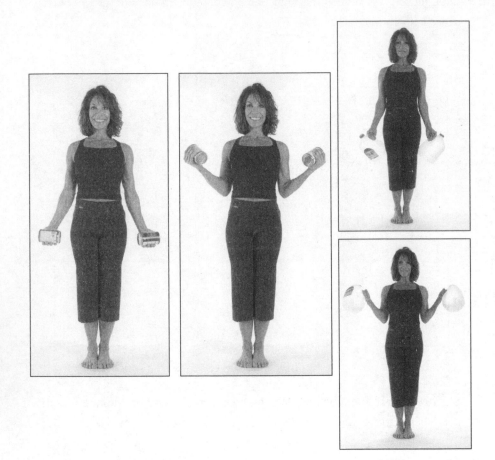

Stand upright, with your shoulders squared and legs and feet together. Hold a weight in each hand with palms facing outward. Curl both arms upward, exhaling as you lift the weights toward your shoulders. Flex the biceps at the top of the movement, keeping your shoulders stable and body neutral. Inhale as you slowly lower the weights back to the starting position. (Avoid swinging the weights downward too swiftly.)

TRICEPS DIP

This exercise is both a triceps movement and a chest exercise. The movement will develop the thickness of the triceps, especially around the elbow. When executed with proper form and a slow buildup, the dip will define, tone, and improve strength in the upper arms and the chest.

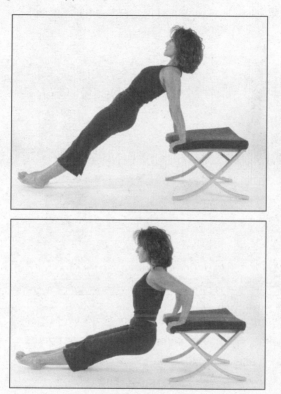

Stand with your back against the seat of a sturdy chair. Hold the edge of the seat with the palms of your hands facing down. Extend your feet forward while grabbing the chair so that your legs are angled straight out in front of you. Keep your shoulders aligned directly above your elbows and wrists. Your arms should be extended, but not locked at the elbows, and your chest should be lifted toward the ceiling with your shoulders tucked in. Inhale as you slowly lower your hips by bending from the elbows, keeping the hips as close to the chair as possible. Continue until your upper arms are parallel with the floor, but do not sit all the way down on the floor. Hold this position for 2 seconds, and then exhale slowly as you press up by straightening your arms back to the starting position.

LATERAL FRONT SHOULDER RAISE

The purpose of this exercise is to develop the deltoid muscles, decreasing the probability of shoulder aches and pains and helping you maintain a full range of motion.

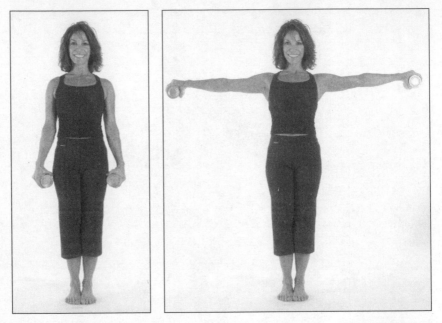

Stand upright, with your shoulders squared and your legs and feet together. Hold soup cans (or dumbbells) in your hands as they rest at your sides with your palms facing in toward the body. Keeping your arms straight, lift the weights up and out to your sides until the weights reach the level of your shoulders. Make sure your palms face downward during the movement. Hold for 2 seconds, and rotate the weights to the front of your chest, keeping the arms straight and extended, then inhale slowly as you lower the weights to your starting position. For an advanced exercise, return to the side position and hold before lowering the weights.

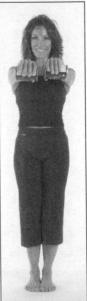

LOWER-BODY ROUTINES

NARROW SQUAT

This exercise builds strength in the legs, especially the thighs, hamstrings, glu-teus, and lower back. There are few movements in life that do not involve leg effort—from sports to walking comfortably up and down stairs. The lower body is the foundation to balance and general activity. Using all the muscles involved in a squat will make you stronger and faster.

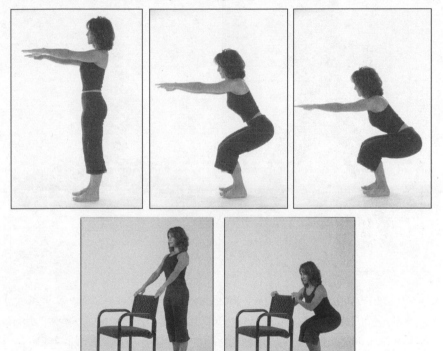

Stand with your feet slightly less than shoulder-width apart. Straighten and extend your arms in front of your body while keeping your shoulders pushed back. Inhale as you bend your knees and lower your hips until your thighs are parallel with the floor. Don't lock your knees. You can do a modified squat, going halfway down, if you're a beginner. Exhale as you push from the heels to rise back to your starting position. A variation of this exercise is to hold on to the back of a chair for support.

WIDE SQUAT

The wide squat increases strength and development in the quadriceps and, with the toes turned out, you will develop and tone the inside of the thighs. This is an appropriate exercise for anyone who wants to add variety to the traditional narrow squat and mimic a lifelike position of squatting to pick up objects off of the floor.

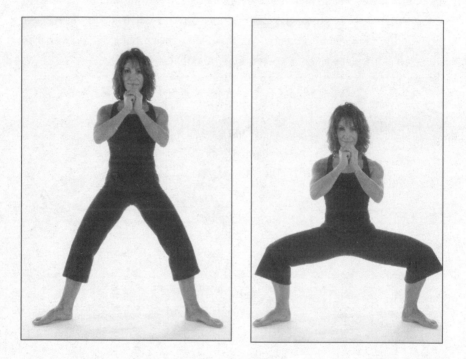

Stand with your feet wider than shoulder-width apart and with your toes angled slightly out. Bring your hands under your chin or place them on your hips. Inhale as you bend your knees and lower your hips until they parallel the thighs as closely as possible. Keep your back straight, chin up, and shoulders and pelvis square during the movement. Exhale slowly as you press up from the heels to the starting position.

To increase the difficulty of this exercise, hold a partially filled water jug or dumbbell in both hands at waist level near your belly button during the movement. Or to modify, hold on to the back of a chair for support.

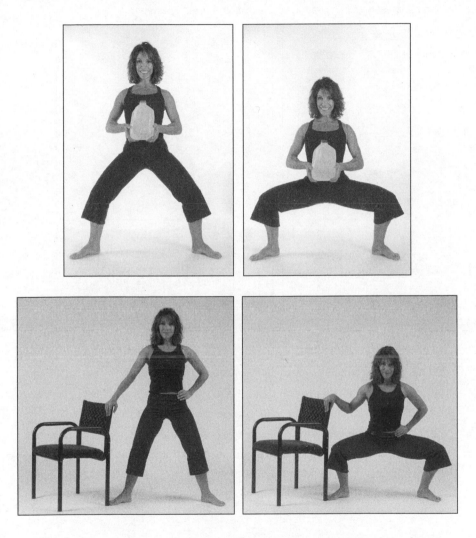

REVERSE LUNGE

The lunge exercise develops the front of the thighs and gluteus, and helps overall balance and agility. The reverse lunge is critical to getting up and down from a kneeling position and to maintaining healthy knees.

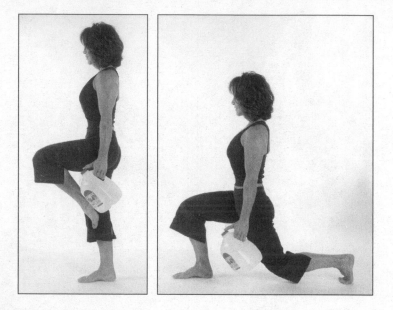

Stand straight and tall, with your feet close together. Hold a partially filled water jug or dumbbell in each hand. Keep your shoulders squared and your back straight. Inhale as you take a large step backward with your left leg, bending the knee toward a kneeling position. Do not touch your knee to the floor. The right knee should be bent and positioned above the ball of your foot. Exhale as you push off with the right leg, rising back up to the starting position. Do a set of four repetitions with each leg.

To modify this exercise, position hands on hips instead of holding weights, or hold onto the back of a chair for support.

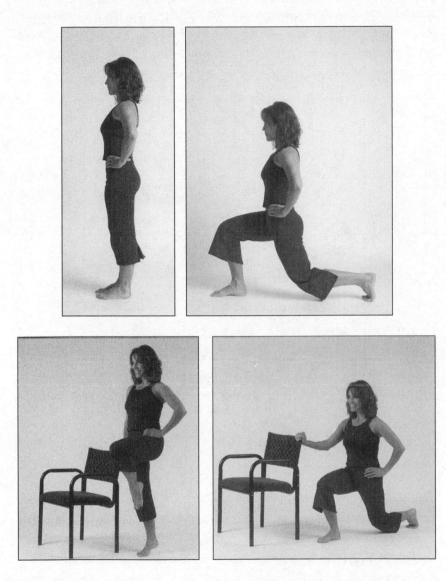

HAMSTRING PRESS

Strong hamstrings protect the alignment of the legs, making sure that there is no muscular imbalance between the front and the back side. The more developed the hamstring, the more your legs are going to meet in the middle and touch each other, allowing for a strong foundation to the upper torso. The hamstrings are also critical muscles for acceleration, stepping up, and jumping activities.

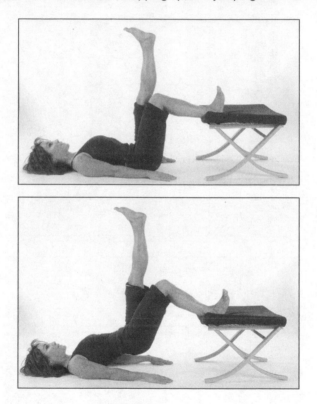

Lie flat on the ground near a stool or ottoman, with hands by your side. Place both feet on the stool with feet flexed and toes pointing up toward the ceiling. Keeping your right leg still, raise your left leg straight into the air for a count of six so that it forms a right angle with your body (but don't lock your left knee). Flex your left foot, lift your buttocks off the floor, and hold the position for 2 seconds. Lower your buttocks back down to the floor, then bring your left foot down onto the stool slowly for a count of six. Repeat three more times on the left leg, concentrating on the straight up-and-down movement of your leg. Now switch legs and do four repetitions on your right leg.

CRUNCH

The basic crunch is one in a series of many exercises to strengthen the abdominals. The function of the abdominals is to flex and rotate the spinal column, to draw the sternum toward the pelvis, and to lift the ribs and draw them together. With proper strength, flexibility, and tone, they will help maximize performance in most sports and life activities, including improvement in your posture, overall alignment, and intestinal health.

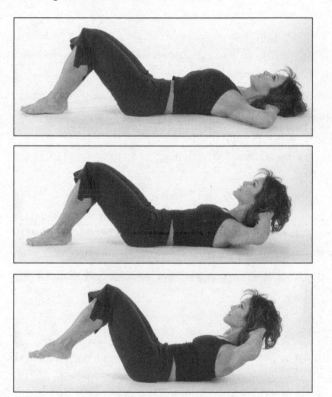

Lie face-up on the floor, placing your hands and fingertips beside your head with your elbows facing outward. Your knees should be bent and your feet should be flat on the floor and hip-distance apart. Exhale and push your lower back into the floor as you slowly roll your shoulders up for a count of six; keep your knees and hips motionless. Maintain this position for 2 seconds while holding in your abdominals. Keep your head and neck relaxed. Inhale as you lower your shoulders back to the starting position. To create a more challenging crunch, lift your feet slightly off the floor.

STRETCHING

Even using light poundage, the slowness of the above strength-training exercises will exhaust your muscles. You need to give them time to repair and rebuild new tissue. This is why on alternate days, I want you to do stretching exercises. You'll extend and elongate the tendons and ligaments that are needed to maximize any increase in strength. Just as with the strength-training exercises, the stretches will be incorporated into your aerobic activity during commercial breaks. You can wear the same comfortable clothes and sneakers. The only extra thing you'll need is a hand towel to help you extend your range of motions in each stretch.

Unlike strength training, in which you aim for slow movements in order to exhaust a particular muscle group, stretching requires you to reach a maximum position and then hold that position relatively motionless for 30 seconds. Here are some basic rules for stretching:

- Lengthen the body throughout each movement.
- Imagine someone is gently stretching you from an opposite direction (this is how the towel helps).
- Although you shouldn't bounce, you can reach a bit further and deepen the stretch as you hold for 30 seconds, as long as you maintain good form.
- Never force, pull, or bounce during a stretch.

Here are a number of effective stretches to try during the commercial breaks. Take a minute for each stretch (30 seconds to get into position and 30 seconds to maintain the stretch) and you should be able to get through most—if not all—of these stretches during the three 3-minute commercial breaks.

STRETCHES

- Standing side stretch
- Standing twist stretch
- Chest and shoulder stretch

- Triceps stretch
- Seated hamstring stretch
- Back stretch
- Quad stretch
- Glute stretch
- Lateral floor side stretch

STANDING SIDE STRETCH

Stand tall with your feet together. Reach your arms straight up toward the ceiling, holding the towel taut in both hands. Keep your shoulder blades down while stretching up and out with the towel. Squeeze in your abdominals and reach out and over your right side as if you are bending around a big ball. Hold the position for a count of 30 seconds, all the while reaching for more length through the torso. Repeat on the other side.

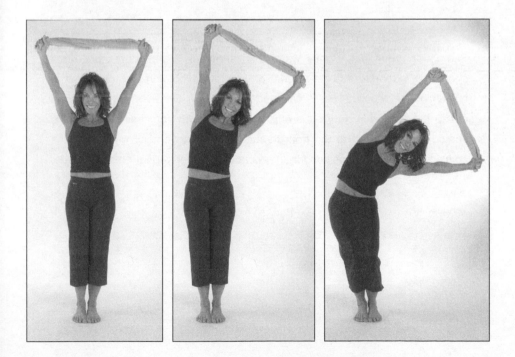

STANDING TWIST STRETCH

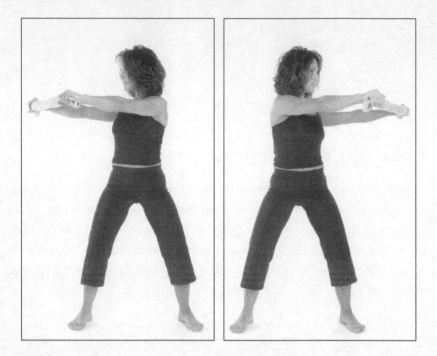

Stand with your feet slightly wider than shoulder width apart. Your arms should be extended straight in front of your body, holding the towel taut in both hands. Keep your pelvis centered to the front. Slowly swing your arms out to the right side and focus on the movement of your spine. The pelvis should stay centered to the front throughout the movement, enhancing the spinal twist. Hold the position for 30 seconds, and then repeat on the left side.

CHEST AND SHOULDER STRETCH

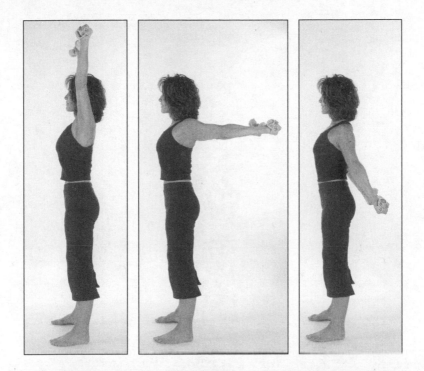

Stand tall, with your feet shoulder width apart. Reach your arms straight up over your head, holding the towel taut in both hands. Inhale as you lift your arms slightly behind your head, keeping your shoulders low and your neck long. Use the towel's length to extend the stretch. Exhale as you reach your individual range of motion. Eventually, as you increase flexibility, you'll be able to rotate your arms up, over, and behind your body until you come in contact with your backside. Hold each segment of the movement for 15 seconds before moving to the next level. Continue for at least 30 seconds of total stretch time.

TRICEPS STRETCH

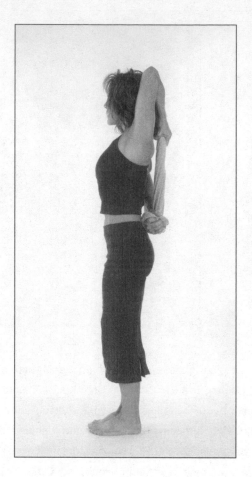

Stand tall with your feet together and towel in one hand. Hold the towel with one hand behind your neck, with that elbow pointing toward the ceiling. Grab the towel behind your waist with the opposite hand, creating an oppositional pull. Hold the shoulder stable while gently pulling down on the towel with one hand and lifting with the elbow (toward the ceiling) from the other.

SEATED HAMSTRING STRETCH

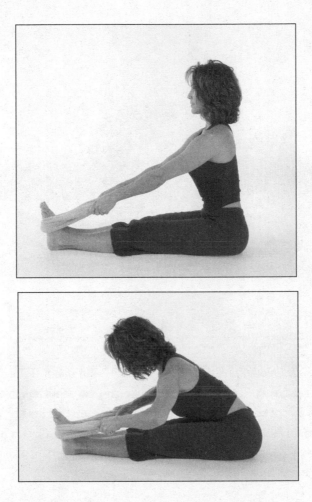

Sit upright on the floor with back straight. Holding the towel at both ends, tuck it under your feet and press your feet together. Avoid locking your knees by bending them slightly. Keep your back as straight as possible so that the exercise does not turn into a back stretch. Maintain your focus on the back of the legs. Use the towel to pull your feet toward your body, stretching the hamstrings and buttocks. Breathe through the stretch and hold this position for 30 seconds.

BACK STRETCH

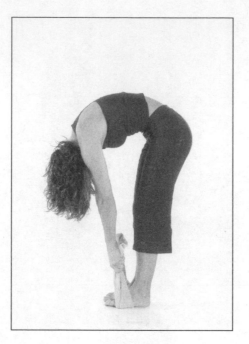

Stand relaxed, holding one end of the towel in each hand. Gently bend forward from the spine, rounding the back, dropping the shoulders, and keeping your knees unlocked. Place the towel under your feet. Still holding onto both ends of the towel in a bent-over position, bring your head upward and look forward. Arch your back toward the ceiling. Breathe through the exercise. Hold for 30 seconds.

QUAD STRETCH

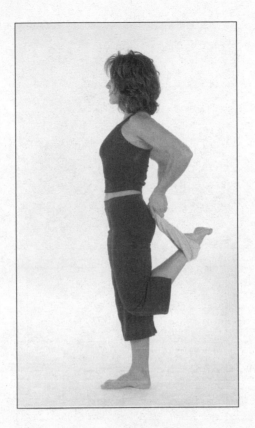

Stand flat footed. Bend one foot up toward your buttocks, keeping your hips as square as possible (avoid hiking one hip up). Place the towel under the foot and hold with both hands behind the back. Inhale and lift slightly on the towel. Exhale and simultaneously push your knee straight down toward the floor, focusing on the area above the knee and through the upper leg. Note that this is a balance exercise as well. You might need to hold onto a sturdy chair at first. Hold the position for 30 seconds, then repeat with the other leg.

GLUTE STRETCH

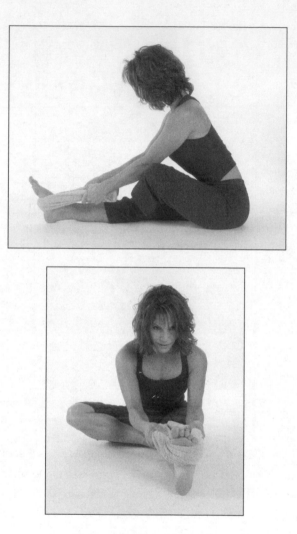

Sit on the floor and extend your right leg straight out in front of you. Cross your left foot over your extended right knee (or ankle or thigh, depending on your flexibility). Hold the back and spine as straight as possible, reaching your head straight up from your neck. Rope the towel around your extended right foot and gently pull your chest (back and spine lengthened) toward your toes, keeping the hips square on the floor. You will feel the stretch to the deep muscles within the gluteus. Hold the position for 30 seconds. Repeat on the opposite leg.

LATERAL FLOOR SIDE STRETCH

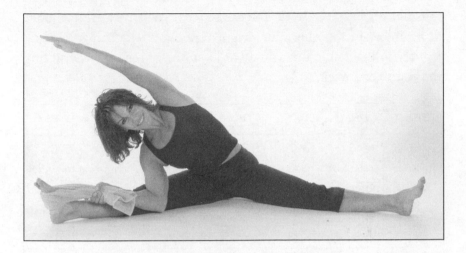

Sit with your hips squarely on the floor, legs spread wide apart and back straight. Focus on the floor as it makes contact with your buttocks, legs, inner thighs, back of the knees, calves, and heels. Wrap the towel around your right foot and hold it in your right hand. Now bend to the right side. Pull on the towel with your right hand and reach your left arm over your head, while still maintaining a square pelvis. Exhale and continue to reach over the top of the head with the upper arm, creating length and flexibility throughout both sides of the body. Imagine that you are bending up and over an invisible ball. Hold the position for 30 seconds, then repeat on the other side.

A SAMPLE WEEKLY WORKOUT PLAN

Here's what a typical Anti-Inflammation Zone exercise routine should look like on any given week. You can see that you have a great amount of flexibility in choosing your weight-training or stretching exercises. Just try to make sure that you do at least one of each exercise during the course of a week.

DAY 1	DAY 2	DAY 3	DAY 4	DAY 5	DAY 6	DAY 7
3 minutes weight training	3 minutes stretching	3 minutes weight training	Rest Day	3 minutes stretching	3 minutes weight training	3 minutes stretching
11 minutes walking in place	11 minutes step aerobics	11 minutes walking in place		11 minutes walking in place	11 minutes step aerobics	11 minutes walking in place
3 minutes weight training	3 minutes stretching	3 minutes weight training		3 minutes stretching	3 minutes weight training	3 minutes stretching
11 minutes walking in place	11 minutes step aerobics	11 minutes walking in place		11 minutes step aerobics	11 minutes walking in place	11 minutes step aerobics
3 minutes weight training	3 minutes stretching	3 minutes weight training		3 minutes stretching	3 minutes weight training	3 minutes stretching

SUMMARY

There you have it, your complete Anti-Inflammation Zone exercise prescription. Thirty minutes a day, six days a week. The biggest challenge, in my opinion, is finding six different TV programs that you like to watch in a given week. If that is too difficult, there is always the Weather Channel or CNN. As good as exercise is, I want you to remember the 80/20 rule: 80 percent of your success in combating silent inflammation will come from your diet and the other 20 percent will come from exercise. Just as following the Zone Diet and taking high-dose fish oil is a lifetime anti-inflammatory diet program, so is exercise. On the flip side, a high glycemic-load diet will wipe out many of the hormonal benefits of even the best possible exercise program.

10

Decreasing the Collateral Damage of Silent Inflammation: Cortisol Reduction Strategies

One of the most insidious consequences of silent inflammation is the chronic increase in cortisol levels that it causes. There is no way you can be in a state of wellness if your cortisol levels are too high. Silent inflammation is a direct result of excess production of pro-inflammatory eicosanoids. In an effort to shut down these eicosanoids, your body's primary hormonal defense mechanism is to secrete more cortisol. Unfortunately, cortisol is too powerful for its own good. It not only shuts down "bad" pro-inflammatory eicosanoids but also the "good" anti-inflammatory ones as well. That might be okay if the damage stopped there, but it's only the beginning of the collateral hormonal damage caused by excess cortisol.

Cortisol is produced by your body in response to long-term stress. When you are under any type of stress, whether physical or emotional, your body pumps out cortisol in an attempt to shut off the production of pro-inflammatory eicosanoids. Stress is defined as disruption to your body's normal equilibrium. It might be due to an acute injury, chronic disease, excess exercise, change in temperature or humidity, lack of sleep, or chronic anxiety. Whatever the cause, at the molecular level the end result is an increase in silent inflammation.

We often think of cortisol as a stress hormone, but in reality it is an anti-stress hormone whose job is to deal with the inflammatory responses that chronic stress is generating in your body. It is meant to be a short-term response to stress, and it works quite well in this capacity. The hormonal mechanism that evolved for cortisol was never intended to handle long-term stress coming from silent inflammation. Cortisol was meant to shut down the immune system to recover from a short-term, though potentially deadly, infectious disease or a fear of being eaten by a wild animal.

But what happens if you have high levels of silent inflammation on a long-term basis? In an attempt to shut down this silent inflammation, your body pumps out more and more cortisol, keeping its levels chronically elevated. Chronically high cortisol can lead to a host of health ills, from insulin resistance, to nerve cell death, to a depressed immune system. As a result, you gain weight, lose your intellectual potential, and become predisposed to illness.

While it's true that we have far fewer threats to our lives these days, we tend to have more lifelong problems, such as stressful jobs, chronic health conditions, and mood disorders. The result is a hormonal mess for many of us.

Cortisol output is normally governed by our circadian rhythms. Levels are at their lowest between midnight and 2 A.M. and slowly begin to rise to awaken us out of sleep. They peak between 6 A.M. and 8 A.M. and then gradually decrease throughout the day, dropping off to their lowest point during sleep. That is, of course, if you have no extra stress to muck things up.

Far too often, though, you have a stressful blip that disturbs this cycle. Usually, cortisol production shifts back in gear after you get past that blip. But if you have certain bad habits in your lifestyle on a permanent basis, you might have chronically high cortisol levels. These bad habits include:

- Prolonged or intense exercise
- Stuffing yourself with large meals
- Skipping meals
- Excess intake of stimulants, such as caffeine

- Being overweight
- Low blood sugar from a very low-carbohydrate diet

THE DANGERS OF EXCESS CORTISOL

Increased cortisol sends a signal to your body that it needs to prepare for a possible flight from danger. This triggers an immediate breakdown of muscle to make more blood glucose (neo-glucogenesis). To prevent nonessential organs in the body from using this precious blood glucose, a transient insulin resistance develops with a corresponding rise in insulin levels in the bloodstream.

Constant stress means constant secretion of cortisol. As your body adapts to chronic stress, you become hyperinsulinemic, thereby creating more visceral fat. This fuels a new round of cortisol secretion, and the end result is you get fatter (especially in the abdominal region) and wind up with chronic silent inflammation.

As your body keeps producing excess cortisol, it cuts back on its production of other hormones, such as testosterone. Without adequate levels of testosterone, it is impossible to maintain, let alone build, muscle. Making matters worse, a deficiency in testosterone dampens libido (in both men and women), so that sex becomes far less enticing. Excess cortisol also destroys your short-term memory, which makes sense in times of acute stress (like combat, severe accidents, or physical abuse) because it allows you to repress very tragic events. Under long-term stress, however, this short-term memory loss is far more problematic and can lead to a decreased ability to recall a wide number of memories, including pleasant ones.

Like insulin, cortisol levels tend to increase naturally in our bodies as we age. But this increase occurs in a unique way. As I have mentioned, the normal circadian rhythm of cortisol is for it to peak in the morning, with a sharp drop-off in the afternoon. As we get older, the increase in overall cortisol is much more gradual, because the hormone remains elevated in the evening instead of dropping sharply. As a result of this elevation, it may be more difficult to get to sleep at night, which can lead to late-night cravings, especially for carbohydrates.

Lack of sleep itself can have a devastating effect on cortisol. Studies show that if you decrease your sleep from 8 hours to 6½ hours per night, within a week you'll experience a significant increase in cortisol levels and a corresponding increase in insulin levels. In addition to all the psychological stressors we have today, most of us are chronically sleep deprived. The average American clocks in only 7 hours of sleep a night, down from the 9 hours we were getting a century ago.

LONG-TERM INCREASED CORTISOL = ADRENAL BURNOUT

Producing too much cortisol for months or years can eventually lead to burnout of your adrenal glands, the glands that sit on top of your kidneys and pump out both adrenaline and cortisol. If after being chronically overtaxed your adrenal glands eventually fail to produce enough cortisol, then you're in real trouble, because you no longer have your primary hormonal tool to reduce silent inflammation. This is similar to what happens to the pancreas when it continually overproduces insulin in response to continuing insulin resistance in cells. Eventually, the pancreas fails to function properly and can no longer produce enough insulin to bring down elevated blood glucose levels. The result is type 2 (adult-onset) diabetes. This only accelerates the generation of silent inflammation throughout the body and rapidly increases the likelihood of heart attacks, blindness, kidney failure, and amputation. With adrenal burnout, you have no internal mechanism to stop the overproduction of pro-inflammatory eicosanoids, and aging begins to accelerate.

CORTISOL-REDUCTION STRATEGIES

I am sure you've now received the message loud and clear that excess cortisol is bad. Now, what should you do about it? Since excess cortisol is caused by the excess production of "bad" pro-inflammatory eicosanoids, the best way to lower your levels is to reduce the same eicosanoids. This means the reduction of silent inflammation.

If you're following the Zone Diet (which stabilizes blood glucose levels) and taking high-dose fish oil (which reduces AA levels), you're taking your first steps to reducing excess cortisol. By maintaining stable blood sugar and insulin levels, your body will secrete less cortisol when you're stressed. The EPA in the fish oil reduces the production of AA, which chokes off the production of pro-inflammatory eicosanoids. Without these "bad" eicosanoids, your body has less need to secrete excess cortisol. High-dose fish oil also increases the production of serotonin, the "feel-good" hormone in your brain, which allows you to adapt to stress more effectively. The stress is still there, but now your ability to handle the collateral damage that comes from it is significantly increased.

Unlike our Paleolithic ancestors, we have a pretty good idea when emotional and physical stresses are coming. This gives you the opportunity to plan in advance. This is especially true with respect to your diet. If you know you're going to be under stress, you have to double your efforts to stick to the Zone Diet. This will prevent you from having the increased carbohydrate cravings that come with stress, because you'll be keeping your insulin levels stable.

How many times in the past have you given in to cravings for high glycemic-load carbohydrates such as candy bars, potato chips, and pizza during stressful situations? This type of emotional eating will quickly replenish a rapidly dropping blood glucose level caused by increased cortisol. However, this form of self-medication puts you on a vicious cycle of rapid increases in blood sugar and insulin, followed by a rapid decrease, followed by craving for more carbohydrates. The result is that your body will continue to pump out even more cortisol to try to maintain adequate blood sugar levels (by tearing down more muscle to convert into glucose) for the brain.

Trying to rigidly maintain the Zone Diet in times of great stress is not the easiest job. Therefore, the best hormonal strategy to rapidly address a particularly stressful period is to double your usual intake of fish oil. The results will be almost immediate. Once the stress passes, you can simply go back to your standard dose of fish oil.

High-dose fish oil and the Zone Diet remain your primary tools for combating the collateral damage induced by excess cortisol. But there also remains one other tool that has been time tested. It's called relaxation.

RELAXATION STRATEGIES

Probably the best relaxation technique is being independently wealthy and living on a ranch in Wyoming. Unfortunately, this is not a very practical approach for most of us. What we all can do is to decrease cortisol levels though relaxation techniques. The goal is to get your mind to focus on absolutely nothing, but you actually have to learn a set of skills to do this. If practiced correctly, various relaxation techniques can generate a beneficial physiologic response in the body and result in lowered cortisol levels.

We may think of meditation as something for only the very mystical or highly religious. In reality, we all practice some form of meditation when we induce a state of relaxation. Any activity or focused breathing technique that lets you clear your mind of troubling thoughts (in fact, all thoughts) will automatically begin reducing cortisol levels. Some people can meditate effectively when they go fly-fishing. I used to wonder what the benefits were of simply flicking a fishing line into a running stream over and over again. Then I realized that it is a great way to lull the mind into a state of relaxation. Others may find comfort in staring at intricate patterns on a fallen leaf, a technique called mindful awareness. Some of us, however, may benefit from a more formal meditation technique that involves focusing on breathing and muscle relaxation techniques. Developing any of these skills will enable you to relax your body any time you're feeling stressed and reduce excess cortisol.

Herbert Benson, a researcher at Harvard Medical School, coined the term *relaxation response* to define the physiological changes that occur in your body when you meditate effectively. (This is the opposite of the "stress response," which induces excess production of cortisol.) Benson outlined ways to elicit the relaxation response, which helps to lower your blood pressure, heart rate, and breathing rate. If you can elicit this relaxation response once a day, you'll be better able to decrease your cortisol levels and keep levels from rising too high when you're under stress.

I'll be the first to admit that setting aside twenty minutes a day to think about nothing can be pretty hard work. I think it's much easier to incorporate thirty minutes of daily exercise in front of the TV, or to make three daily Zone meals. And of course, the easiest thing is to set aside fifteen seconds a day to take a high enough dose of fish oil. Nonetheless, if you can do a form of relaxation on a regular basis, you will reduce cortisol levels and feel happier and more refreshed. There are three simple techniques for getting the beneficial physiological responses that counteract cortisol secretion. Choose whichever one you prefer.

1. **Meditation Made Easy:** Sit comfortably and pick a focus word or short phrase that's meaningful to you. If this sounds too mystical, then just repeat the number one over and over. This might not be too inventive, but it works. Close your eyes and relax your muscles. Now breathe slowly and naturally, repeating your focus word or phrase to yourself as you exhale. Try to breathe from your diaphragm (deep breathing) as opposed to using only your lungs. Throughout, assume a passive attitude. Don't worry if you are performing the technique correctly, and let any negative thoughts or worries pass through your mind without thinking about them. If an extraneous thought comes into your mind, let it pass, and then go back to thinking of nothing while continually repeating the word or phrase. Continue for twenty minutes. You may open your eyes to check the time, but don't use an alarm. It will disrupt your relaxation.

2. **Progressive Muscle Relaxation:** Sit in a comfortable chair with back and head support, or lie on a cushioned mat on the floor. (Don't lie in bed since you may fall asleep.) Tense each of your muscles one at a time; inhale and slowly exhale as you release the tension from your muscles. Begin with your face by wrinkling your forehead and shutting your eyes as tight as you can. Exhale and release. Then tense your neck and shoulders by drawing your shoulders up into a shrug. Exhale and release. Work your way down to your arms, hands, and fingers. Contract your stomach. Exhale and release. Arch your back and release. Tense your hips and buttocks. Exhale and release. Point and flex your toes. Exhale and release.

Now tense all your muscles at once. Take a deep breath, hold it, and exhale slowly as you relax the muscles, letting go of the tension. Feel your body at rest and enjoy this state of relaxation for several minutes. When you're first learning this technique, you may want to make a tape recording with the instructions to remind yourself which muscles to tense and relax. You can play the recording while you're doing the technique to make sure you don't skip any muscle groups.

3. **Traditional Meditation:** Sit comfortably in an upright position with your head, neck, and back erect but not tensed. Choose a single object of focus like your breathing or your favorite word or portion of a prayer. Concentrate on the qualities of that object—the sounds and sensations it elicits—and try to avoid any other thoughts that enter into your awareness. If they do, let them pass out of your consciousness.

You can sit cross-legged on the floor or in a stiff-backed chair. You can do this indoors or outside in a natural setting, such as a garden. Focus mentally on the air flowing in and out of your body as you breathe. Appreciate the beauty of nature as you transcend your own problems, but do it with your eyes closed to prevent a continuing flow of visual data to the brain.

All of this may sound a little too touchy-feely. After all, we live in a high-tech world and generally want some physical proof that our efforts are actually paying off. You can now actually measure your success eliciting the relaxation response using a new piece of software called HeartMath (www.heartmath.com). The software program measures your heart rate during meditation and then, through a complex analysis of your heart frequency patterns, it provides a computer screen readout of your success. You can consider this software to be your high-tech meditation coach, and with that computer support you begin to take meditation out of the mystical and into the medical world.

SUMMARY

Although meditation probably won't have as much of an effect on reducing cortisol as the Zone Diet or high-dose fish oil, it may provide the significant last boost you need. This boost may be necessary to truly get your cortisol levels back to a manageable level. Only then will you be able to enter the Anti-Inflammation Zone and move rapidly back toward a state of wellness.

11

Seven Days in the Anti-Inflammation Zone

Let me emphasize once again that the Anti-Inflammation Zone is not a diet. It is a metabolic state of hormonal control that you induce by following the Zone Lifestyle Program. This includes the Zone Diet, supplemental fish oil, an anti-inflammation exercise plan, and relaxation strategies through meditation. Following all these components will give you total control over your hormones and enable you to reverse silent inflammation. Since this struggle against inflammation is a lifelong one, staying in the Anti-Inflammation Zone needs to be a lifelong goal.

If you follow my Zone Lifestyle Program, it will take about thirty days before you can see significant changes in your clinical biomarkers of wellness, such as the SIP. You should, though, begin to feel the differences within the first week. Here are some of the benefits you'll see after a week in the Anti-Inflammation Zone:

1. You will think more clearly throughout the day as you stabilize your blood glucose levels.
2. You will notice a surge in physical energy, as you are able to access stored body fat for energy by decreasing insulin levels.
3. Your clothes will fit better even though you haven't lost a lot of weight. That is, you'll have lost primarily fat, and the first fat your body likes to shed is concentrated in your abdominal area.

4. You will handle stress more effectively by lowering excess levels of cortisol.

All of these changes indicate that you are moving toward the Anti-Inflammation Zone, your pathway back to wellness. As with any drug, you get benefits only as long as you keep taking that drug. The Zone Lifestyle Program truly functions as a drug to get you to the Anti-Inflammation Zone. As long as you use it, the benefits will be readily apparent. The day you stop, you will begin to see a steady increase in silent inflammation that takes you further from wellness.

The Zone Lifestyle Program is pretty much the same for men and women. The only difference is the amount of food you need to consume. Because of greater muscle mass, men have to eat more total calories than women (life is never fair), but both men and women need to pay close attention to their maximum glycemic loads at each meal and snack.

You will also see that many of the meals include extra-virgin olive oil, sesame oil, turmeric, and even some alcohol to further enhance the meal's anti-inflammatory properties. By following this seven-day template, you'll also have a step-by-step guide for following the Zone Lifestyle Program every day for the rest of your life. But first, give it a week. You have to eat, so you might as well eat smart. You'll also find that squeezing in a fitness routine in front of your favorite TV program and setting aside twenty minutes to meditate (i.e., think of nothing) are not that challenging.

ZONE LIFESTYLE PROGRAM FOR WOMEN

DAY 1

BREAKFAST

Oriental Vegetable Omelet

1 teaspoon olive oil

¼ cup scallions, thinly sliced diagonally

1 cup sliced drained canned mushrooms

½ cup sliced red and green bell peppers

½ cup drained canned chickpeas

3 cups bean sprouts

½ teaspoon minced garlic

3 tablespoons cider vinegar

½ teaspoon grated fresh gingerroot*

1 tablespoon soy sauce

⅛ tablespoon Worcestershire sauce

¾ cup egg substitute

In large nonstick sauté pan heat ½ teaspoon of the oil. Stir-fry the scallions for 1 minute over medium-high heat. Add the mushrooms and cook another 2 minutes, then add the peppers, chickpeas, sprouts, garlic, vinegar, ginger, soy sauce, and Worcestershire sauce and cook 3 to 5 minutes, or until bean sprouts are tender.

In a second large nonstick sauté pan heat the remaining ½ teaspoon oil over medium-high heat. Pour in the egg substitute. As it cooks, push the cooked portions toward the center of pan with a spatula. When the eggs are set, remove the omelet to a warmed serving plate and place the filling from the first pan into one side of the omelet. Fold over the other side and serve.

*Note: When a recipe calls for fresh gingerroot (available in most grocery stores or Asian markets), it is not advisable to substitute ground ginger. The flavors are very different.

LUNCH

Garden Salad Topped with Sautéed Scallops and Bacon

1 teaspoon olive oil

1 ounce Canadian bacon, diced

3 ounces bay scallops

3 teaspoons cider vinegar

½ teaspoon grated fresh gingerroot

½ teaspoon chopped fresh mint

¼ cup chicken stock

2 cups shredded lettuce

⅓ cup mandarin orange slices

½ cup diced red onion

¼ cup kidney beans, rinsed

¼ cup chickpeas, rinsed

Heat ⅓ teaspoon of the olive oil in a medium nonstick sauté pan over medium-high heat. Sauté the bacon, scallops, 1 teaspoon of the vinegar, and ¼ teaspoon of the ginger for 4 minutes, or until the bacon and scallops are cooked through.

To make the dressing, in a small bowl whisk together the remaining ⅔ teaspoon oil, ¼ teaspoon ginger, 2 teaspoons vinegar, mint, and chicken stock. Combine the remaining ingredients in a large salad bowl. Add the bacon and scallops. Pour on the dressing and toss to coat.

LATE AFTERNOON SNACK

2 hard-boiled eggs

¼ cup hummus (contains fat)

Paprika

Slice the eggs in half, discard the yolks, and fill each egg white with half the hummus. Top with paprika to taste.

DINNER

Indian Shrimp with Apples and Yogurt

1 teaspoon olive oil

3 ounces small shrimp, shelled, deveined, and cooked

2 teaspoons cider vinegar

⅛ teaspoon minced fresh gingerroot

½ teaspoon minced garlic

1 tablespoon minced cilantro

Dash hot pepper sauce

¼ teaspoon turmeric

⅛ teaspoon ground coriander

⅛ teaspoon ground cumin

½ cup plain low-fat yogurt

¾ cup minced onion

½ Granny Smith apple, diced

5 cups romaine lettuce

Heat the oil in a medium nonstick sauté pan over medium heat. Add the shrimp, vinegar, herbs, and spices. Cook 1 to 2 minutes, or until the shrimp are opaque. In a second nonstick sauté pan heat yogurt, onion, and apple over low heat until heated through. Do not boil. Add the shrimp mixture and stir to mix. Form a bed of romaine on a serving plate and top with shrimp mixture. Have apple for dessert.

LATE NIGHT SNACK

¼ cup low-fat cottage cheese

⅓ cup light fruit cocktail or ½ cup pineapple or ½ cup blueberries or ½ chopped apple or ⅓ cup applesauce or 1 block Zone-favorable fruit

1 macadamia nut or 3 almonds

FISH OIL SUPPLEMENTATION

Take 2.5 grams of EPA and DHA. If you are using ultra-refined EPA/DHA concentrate, this would be either four 1-gram capsules or 1 teaspoon of liquid.

EXERCISE PROGRAM

Do Day 1 of the Sample Weekly Workout Plan found on page 134.

MEDITATION PROGRAM

Do 20 minutes of Meditation Made Easy, as described on page 143.

DAY 2

BREAKFAST

Breakfast Fruit Salad

¾ cup low-fat cottage cheese

½ cup fresh or reduced-sugar cubed canned pineapple

⅔ cup mandarin orange slices, canned in water, drained

3 macadamia nuts, crushed

Place the cottage cheese in a bowl. Fold in the pineapple, oranges, and nuts.

LUNCH

Savory Lentils with Goat Cheese

¾ cup dried lentils, rinsed and drained

¼ teaspoon salt

¼ teaspoon freshly ground black pepper

2¼ tablespoons chopped roasted red peppers

1 clove garlic, minced

1½ tablespoons chopped fresh cilantro

1½ tablespoons chopped red onion

2 tablespoons chopped chives

⅛ teaspoon paprika

¾ teaspoon cumin

1 teaspoon extra-virgin olive oil

Juice of 1 lime

3 ounces goat cheese, at room temperature

2 radicchio leaves for garnish

In a medium saucepan place the lentils, salt, and black pepper in 1½ cups water.
Cover and bring to a boil over medium heat and simmer for 20 minutes, or until

the lentils are tender but still have texture. Remove from the heat and drain. In a medium bowl mix the lentils, roasted peppers, garlic, cilantro, onion, and chives. In a small bowl combine the paprika, cumin, olive oil, and lime juice. Toss together with the lentil mixture. Before serving, fold in goat cheese. Arrange radicchio leaves on a plate. Spoon the lentil salad onto the radicchio and serve.

LATE AFTERNOON SNACK

Raspberry Protein Smoothie

7 grams protein powder

1 cup frozen raspberries, defrosted

1 teaspoon slivered almonds

Blend the ingredients in a blender until smooth.

DINNER

Ginger Chicken

1 teaspoon olive oil

3 ounces boneless, skinless chicken breast, cut lengthwise into thin strips

2 cups broccoli florets

1½ cups snow peas

¾ cup chopped yellow onion

1 teaspoon grated fresh gingerroot

½ cup grapes

In a wok or large nonstick pan heat the oil over medium-high heat. Add the chicken and sauté, turning frequently, until lightly browned, about 5 minutes. Add the broccoli, snow peas, onion, ginger, and ¼ cup water. Continue cooking, stirring often, until the chicken is done, the sauce is reduced to a glaze, and the vegetables are tender, about 20 minutes. If the pan becomes too dry during the cooking, add water 1 tablespoon at a time. Serve the grapes for dessert.

LATE NIGHT SNACK

Tuna with Hummus

1 ounce canned tuna fish packed in water

¼ cup hummus

Drain the tuna fish. Mix with the hummus.

FISH OIL SUPPLEMENTATION

Take 2.5 grams of EPA and DHA. If you are using ultra-refined EPA/DHA concentrate, this would be either four 1-gram capsules or 1 teaspoon of liquid.

EXERCISE PROGRAM

Do Day 2 of the Sample Weekly Workout Plan found on page 134.

MEDITATION PROGRAM

Do 20 minutes of Progressive Muscle Relaxation, as described on page 144.

DAY 3

BREAKFAST

Curried Asparagus Omelet

---

1 teaspoon olive oil

½ teaspoon minced garlic

½ to 1 teaspoon curry powder

⅛ teaspoon Worcestershire sauce

⅛ teaspoon turmeric

Salt and pepper, to taste

1½ cups seeded, chopped tomato

2 cups chopped mushrooms

½ cup asparagus, cut into 1-inch pieces, steamed

1½ cups chopped onion

¾ cup egg substitute

1 teaspoon chopped fresh parsley

In a medium nonstick sauté pan heat ½ teaspoon of the olive oil over medium heat. Add the garlic and sauté until lightly browned, about 2 minutes. Stir in the curry powder, Worcestershire sauce, turmeric, salt, and pepper. Cook 1 minute to heat through. Add the tomato, mushrooms, asparagus, and onion. Cook until softened, about 5 minutes. Cover and remove from the heat.

In a second nonstick sauté pan heat the remaining ½ teaspoon oil. Pour the egg substitute into second sauté pan and cook until set. Place the omelet on a serving plate, spoon the asparagus mixture onto half of the omelet, and fold other half over. Sprinkle with parsley and serve immediately.

LUNCH

Grilled Turkey Salad with Mandarin Oranges

---

1 teaspoon olive oil

3 ounces turkey breast chunks

1 cup finely sliced celery

¾ cup finely sliced red onion

¼ cup Zoned French Dressing (see recipe on page 158)

½ peach, diced

⅓ cup mandarin orange slices, canned in water, drained

⅛ teaspoon turmeric

1 tablespoon chopped fresh mint

1½ cups chopped romaine lettuce

Heat ⅓ teaspoon of the olive oil in a small sauté pan over medium heat. Add the turkey and stir-fry until cooked through, about 8 minutes. In a salad bowl combine the remaining ⅔ teaspoon oil, turkey, celery, onion, dressing, peach, oranges, turmeric, and mint. Toss lightly to coat. On a lunch plate place the lettuce, top with turkey salad, and serve.

Zoned French Dressing*

8 teaspoons cornstarch

¾ cup finely minced onion

¼ cup tomato puree

¼ cup canned kidney beans, rinsed and minced

1¾ cups water

¼ cup cider vinegar

2 tablespoons balsamic vinegar

⅛ teaspoon Worcestershire sauce

1 teaspoon dried tarragon

1 teaspoon dried oregano

1 teaspoon dried parsley flakes

3 teaspoons minced garlic

1 teaspoon dried basil

½ teaspoon chili powder

2 teaspoons paprika

1 teaspoon dried dill

In a small bowl mix the cornstarch with a little cold water to dissolve it. Combine all ingredients in a small saucepan, turn the heat to medium-low, and bring the mixture to a simmer, constantly stirring until the dressing thickens, about 5 minutes. Cool the dressing for 10 to 15 minutes, then blend it in a food processor or blender until smooth. Transfer the dressing to a storage container, cool, cover, and refrigerate.†

*Note: Each ½ cup of Zoned French Dressing contains 1 Carbohydrate Zone Block. There are no Protein or Fat Blocks in this dressing recipe. This recipe is used as a component in other Zone recipes. Each time you make a Zone-favorable meal, use this dressing as a replacement for 1 Carbohydrate Zone Block.

†Note: This dressing may be refrigerated for up to 5 days, or if you prefer, the dressing may be frozen and defrosted for later use. Although the dressing is freeze-thaw stable, after it has been frozen and defrosted it may need to be stirred to reincorporate the small amount of moisture that forms on the dressing during the freezing and thawing process.

LATE AFTERNOON SNACK

Tomato and Low-Fat Mozzarella Salad

⅛ teaspoon extra-virgin olive oil

Balsamic vinegar, to taste

1 clove garlic, minced

2 tomatoes, diced or sliced

1 ounce skim mozzarella cheese, diced or sliced

1 teaspoon chopped fresh basil leaves

Place tomatoes on a plate. In a small bowl whisk together the olive oil, vinegar, and garlic. Pour the dressing over the tomatoes. Top with the mozzarella and basil.

DINNER

Quick and Delicious Salmon Patties

3 ounces canned pink salmon

2 egg whites

1 ounce slow-cooking oatmeal, dry

¼ onion, diced

Garlic salt, to taste

Pepper, to taste

1 teaspoon olive oil

½ apple

Using a fork, flake the salmon in a medium bowl. Add the egg whites, oatmeal, onion, garlic salt, and pepper and mix well with clean hands. Shape the mixture into a patty. Heat the olive oil in a medium sauté pan over medium heat, add the salmon patty, and cook for 3 to 5 minutes on each side, or until golden brown. Serve immediately. Have the apple for dessert.

LATE EVENING SNACK

Low-Fat Yogurt and Nuts

½ cup plain low-fat yogurt

1 teaspoon slivered almonds or 1 macadamia nut

FISH OIL SUPPLEMENT

Take 2.5 grams of EPA and DHA. If you are using ultra-refined EPA/DHA concentrate, this would be either four 1-gram capsules or 1 teaspoon of liquid.

EXERCISE PROGRAM

Do Day 3 of the Sample Weekly Exercise Plan found on page 134.

MEDITATION PROGRAM

Do 20 minutes of Traditional Meditation, as described on page 144.

DAY 4

BREAKFAST

Seven-Minute Breakfast

1 ounce lean Canadian bacon

Olive oil spray

1 whole egg

2 egg whites

1 slice French Meadow bread, lightly toasted

1 teaspoon olive oil

1 pear

In a dry nonstick skillet over medium heat prepare the Canadian bacon according to instructions. Remove it to a plate. Lightly spray the pan with olive oil spray and fry or scramble the egg and egg whites. Add them to the plate. Drizzle the toast with the olive oil and serve it on the side with the pear.

LUNCH

Chicken Waldorf Salad

3 ounces chicken breast

Vegetable broth and/or water for cooking

Curry powder, to taste

Cumin, to taste

Turmeric, to taste

½ cup grapes

½ cup chopped Granny Smith apple

1 cup chopped celery

1 cup sliced red pepper

1 tablespoon light mayonnaise

2 tablespoons yogurt

Nutmeg, to taste

Cinnamon, to taste

Black pepper, to taste

In a small saucepan place the chicken. Pour in enough vegetable broth to cover the chicken and add curry powder, cumin, and turmeric. Bring the liquid to a simmer over medium heat and poach the chicken until it's cooked through, about 10–15 minutes. Cool the chicken and cut it into small chunks.

In a big bowl combine the chicken, grapes, apple, celery, and red pepper. Stir in the mayonnaise, yogurt, nutmeg, cinnamon, and black pepper and serve.

LATE AFTERNOON SNACK

Cottage Cheese and Salsa

¼ cup low-fat cottage cheese

½ cup mild or spicy salsa

1 tablespoon guacamole

Mix the ingredients together.

DINNER

Sautéed Green Beans with Tofu

1 teaspoon olive oil

½ teaspoon Worcestershire sauce

⅛ teaspoon celery salt

6 ounces extra-firm tofu, cut into 1-inch pieces

2 cups green beans, cut into 2-inch pieces

1½ cups chopped onion

½ teaspoon minced garlic

2 teaspoons cider vinegar

⅛ teaspoon nutmeg

⅛ teaspoon cinnamon

⅛ teaspoon lemon herb seasoning

⅛ teaspoon ground double-superfine mustard

½ teaspoon soy sauce

Salt and pepper, to taste

Heat ⅔ teaspoon of the oil in a medium nonstick sauté pan over medium heat. Add the Worcestershire sauce, celery salt, and tofu and stir-fry until the tofu is browned and crusted on all sides, about 5 minutes.

In a second nonstick sauté pan over medium heat heat the remaining ⅓ teaspoon oil and add the green beans, onion, garlic, vinegar, nutmeg, cinnamon, lemon herb seasoning, mustard, soy sauce, salt, and pepper. Sauté about 5 minutes until the beans are crisp-tender. Place the beans on a serving plate and top with the tofu.

LATE NIGHT SNACK

> 4-ounce glass wine
> 1 ounce cheese

FISH OIL SUPPLEMENT

Take 2.5 grams of EPA and DHA. If you are using ultra-refined EPA/DHA concentrate, this would be either four 1-gram capsules or 1 teaspoon of liquid.

EXERCISE PROGRAM

Take a rest day.

MEDITATION PROGRAM

Do 20 minutes of Meditation Made Easy, as described on page 143.

DAY 5

BREAKFAST

Spicy Shrimp and Mushroom Omelet

1 teaspoon olive oil

1 cup sliced asparagus spears

⅛ teaspoon minced garlic

¼ teaspoon dried parsley

⅛ teaspoon dry mustard

⅛ teaspoon dried basil

⅛ teaspoon cayenne pepper

⅛ teaspoon turmeric

Salt and pepper, to taste

¾ cup chopped onion

2 cups chopped mushrooms

1½ ounces shrimp, chopped

½ cup egg substitute

1 kiwifruit, peeled and sliced

In a medium nonstick sauté pan heat the oil over medium-high heat. Add the asparagus, herbs, and spices and sauté for 1 minute, then add the onion and mushrooms. Cook for 3 to 5 minutes, or until the vegetables are tender. Remove the vegetables and keep them warm.

Place the shrimp in the sauté pan and sauté for 1 minute, or until opaque. Pour in the egg substitute and stir to distribute the shrimp throughout the egg. Cook until the omelet is almost set, about 2–3 minutes. Remove the omelet to a serving plate. Spoon the mushroom mixture onto the omelet and fold it over. Garnish the plate with the kiwi slices and serve.

LUNCH

Taco Burger

---

3 ounces lean (90% fat-free) ground beef

½ cup mild or spicy salsa

1 teaspoon olive oil

¼ cup cooked black beans, rinsed

⅛ cup chopped onion

½ teaspoon minced garlic

½ teaspoon Worcestershire sauce

⅛ teaspoon celery salt

1 tablespoon lemon- or lime-flavored spring water

2 cups shredded lettuce

1 taco shell, broken into pieces

1 ounce low-fat Monterey Jack cheese, shredded

In a small bowl, combine the ground beef and ¼ cup of the salsa. Form into a patty. Heat ⅔ teaspoon of the oil in a medium nonstick sauté pan over medium heat and fry until it's cooked through, turning it once.

In a second nonstick sauté pan heat the remaining ⅓ teaspoon oil. Add the beans, onion, garlic, remaining ¼ cup salsa, Worcestershire sauce, celery salt, and spring water and cook until heated through. Place the lettuce on a plate, add the patty, sprinkle with the taco pieces, and top with the bean mixture and the cheese.

LATE AFTERNOON SNACK

Waldorf Salad

1 cup sliced celery

¼ apple, diced

1 teaspoon light mayonnaise

1 pecan half, crushed

1 ounce part-skim or "soft" cheese

In a small bowl combine the celery, apple, and mayonnaise. Sprinkle the pecan pieces on top and serve the cheese on the side.

DINNER

Salmon with Fruity Asian Salsa

1 teaspoon olive oil

4½ ounces salmon steak

2 teaspoons soy sauce

1 teaspoon minced fresh gingerroot

½ teaspoon chopped fresh dill

Dash hot pepper sauce

½ cup mild or spicy salsa

½ cup canned pineapple cubes

½ Granny Smith apple, cored and diced

Preheat oven to 350°F. Brush a small baking dish with the oil and place the salmon steak in the baking dish. Sprinkle with the soy sauce, ginger, dill, and hot pepper sauce. Cover with aluminum foil and bake 30 to 35 minutes, or until the salmon is cooked through. In a small bowl, combine the salsa and fruit. Place the fish on one side of a serving plate and the salsa beside it.

LATE NIGHT SNACK

Low-Fat Yogurt and Nuts

½ cup plain low-fat yogurt

1 teaspoon slivered almonds or 1 macadamia nut

FISH OIL SUPPLEMENT

Take 2.5 grams of EPA and DHA. If you are using ultra-refined EPA/DHA concentrate, this would be either four 1-gram capsules or 1 teaspoon of liquid.

EXERCISE PROGRAM

Do Day 5 of the Weekly Exercise Program found on page 134.

MEDITATION PROGRAM

Do 20 minutes of Progressive Muscle Relaxation, as described on page 144.

DAY 6

BREAKFAST

Breakfast in a Bowl

1 cup plain, nonfat yogurt

¼ cup nonfat cottage cheese

1 tablespoon slow-cooking oatmeal, dry

1 tablespoon slivered almonds

4 teaspoons vanilla extract

Allspice, to taste

Blend all the ingredients together in a medium bowl and refrigerate overnight to soften the oats.

LUNCH

Grilled Chicken Salad

1 cup green leaf or romaine lettuce, washed, dried, and torn into
    large pieces

1 cup broccoli florets

1 green bell pepper, cored, seeded, and cut into thin strips

¼ cup kidney beans

1 medium tomato, sliced

1 teaspoon extra-virgin olive oil

2 teaspoons vinegar (or more to taste)

1 tablespoon lemon juice

1 teaspoon Worcestershire sauce

½ teaspoon freshly ground pepper, or to taste

3 ounces grilled skinless chicken breast, cut into bite-sized chunks

½ medium pear

In a medium bowl toss together the lettuce, broccoli, green pepper, kidney beans, and tomato. In a small bowl whisk together the olive oil, vinegar, lemon juice, Worcestershire sauce, and ground pepper. Toss the dressing with the vegetables until well combined and top with the chicken chunks. Serve the pear for dessert.

LATE AFTERNOON SNACK

Spinach Salad

Spinach (side-salad size)
2 hard-boiled egg whites, sliced
⅓ cup mandarin orange slices, canned in water, drained
⅛ teaspoon olive oil
Balsamic vinegar, to taste

Place the spinach on a plate. Top with the egg whites and oranges. Whisk together the olive oil and vinegar and pour over the salad.

DINNER

Hot and Sour Stir-Fry Pork and Cabbage

1 teaspoon olive oil

3 ounces lean pork loin, cut into large dice

½ cup chicken stock

1 teaspoon cornstarch

1 tablespoon soy sauce

1 tablespoon cider vinegar

½ cup chopped scallions

⅛ teaspoon black pepper

2 tablespoons diced jalapeño peppers

2 teaspoons minced garlic

2 teaspoons minced fresh gingerroot

¾ cup cauliflower florets

1 cup sliced onion

2 cups shredded cabbage

½ pear, cored and sliced

In a medium glass bowl combine the oil, pork, stock, cornstarch, soy sauce, vinegar, scallions, peppers, garlic, and ginger. Cover and marinate in the refrigerator for 30 minutes.

Place the pork mixture in a medium nonstick sauté pan, turn the heat to medium, and sauté until the pork is browned on both sides, about 15 minutes. Add the cauliflower, onion, and cabbage and saute until the vegetables are tender, about 15 minutes. Place the pork and vegetables on a large dinner plate, garnished with the pear slices, and serve immediately.

LATE NIGHT SNACK

Tomato and Low-Fat Cottage Cheese

¼ cup low-fat cottage cheese

2 tomatoes, sliced

6 peanuts

FISH OIL SUPPLEMENT

Take 2.5 grams of EPA and DHA. If you are using ultra-refined EPA/DHA concentrate, this would be either four 1-gram capsules or 1 teaspoon of liquid.

EXERCISE PROGRAM

Do Day 6 of the Weekly Exercise Plan found on page 134.

MEDITATION PROGRAM

Do 20 minutes of Traditional Meditation, as described on page 144.

DAY 7

BREAKFAST

Florentine Filled Omelet Crepes

¾ cup egg substitute

⅛ teaspoon celery salt

⅛ teaspoon nutmeg

⅛ teaspoon cinnamon

1 teaspoon olive oil

4 cups sliced mushrooms

¾ cup chopped onion

Salt and pepper, to taste

4 tablespoons balsamic vinegar

5 cups fresh spinach*

1 kiwifruit, peeled and sliced

In a small bowl combine the egg substitute, celery salt, nutmeg, and cinnamon. In a large nonstick sauté pan heat ⅔ teaspoon of the oil over medium-high heat. Pour the egg mixture into the sauté pan. When the eggs are browned on one side, flip them with a spatula and brown the other side.

Heat the remaining ⅓ teaspoon oil in a second nonstick sauté pan over medium-high heat. Add the mushrooms, onion, salt, and pepper and cook for 3 to 5 minutes, or until softened. Add the balsamic vinegar and spinach and cook until the spinach is just wilted. Place the omelet onto a serving plate, spoon the vegetable mixture onto the omelet, and fold the omelet over. Garnish with the kiwi slices and serve.

*Note: Fresh spinach often has sand on it, so be sure to wash it carefully before cooking.

LUNCH

Thai Turkey Soup

4½ ounces lean ground turkey

1½ cups bean sprouts

½ cup sliced scallions

1 teaspoon olive oil

3 teaspoons minced garlic

½ teaspoon grated fresh gingerroot

2 tablespoons soy sauce

3 cups chicken stock

1 tablespoon finely diced hot chili pepper

2 cups spinach leaves

¼ cup cooked fine egg noodles

½ cup light fruit cocktail

Combine the turkey, sprouts, scallions, oil, garlic, ginger, soy sauce, stock, and chili pepper in a medium saucepan. Bring to a boil over medium heat, reduce the heat, and simmer for 15 minutes. Add the spinach and noodles and simmer for 1 minute. Spoon the soup into a serving bowl. Serve the fruit cocktail in a side dish.

LATE AFTERNOON SNACK

Veggies and Dip

---

2 ounces firm tofu

⅛ teaspoon olive oil

Dry onion soup mix, to taste

1 cup celery, sliced for dipping

1 green pepper, sliced for dipping

In a small bowl blend the tofu, olive oil, and soup mix. Serve with the veggies.

DINNER

Spicy Tofu with Scallions and Radishes

1 teaspoon olive oil

1 teaspoon minced fresh gingerroot

6 ounces extra-firm tofu, cut into 1-inch cubes

1 tablespoon lemon juice

4 teaspoons soy sauce

1½ teaspoons white wine

1 teaspoon minced garlic

Salt and pepper, to taste

¾ cup finely diced jalapeño and red bell pepper (mix to the desired heat)

5 cups torn fresh spinach

1 cup thinly sliced radishes

1½ cups seeded, diced tomatoes

1 cup chopped scallions

1½ cups canned or fresh mushroom slices

Heat the oil and ½ teaspoon of the ginger in a medium sauté pan over medium-high heat. Add the tofu and stir-fry until it is browned on all sides, about 6 minutes. In a small bowl, whisk together the lemon juice, 1 tablespoon water, soy sauce, wine, garlic, salt, pepper, and remaining ½ teaspoon ginger. Combine the peppers, spinach, radishes, tomatoes, scallions, and mushrooms in a medium bowl. Pour in the soy sauce mixture and toss to coat. Add the tofu and spoon onto a serving dish.

LATE NIGHT SNACK

Berries and Low-Fat Cheese

½ cup blueberries or 1 cup strawberries

1 ounce low-fat mozzarella cheese

6 peanuts

FISH OIL SUPPLEMENT

Take 2.5 grams of EPA and DHA. If you are using ultra-refined EPA/DHA concentrate, this would be either four 1-gram capsules or 1 teaspoon of liquid.

EXERCISE PROGRAM

Do Day 7 of the Weekly Exercise Program found on page 134.

MEDITATION PROGRAM

Do 20 minutes of Meditation Made Easy, as described on page 143.

ZONE LIFESTYLE PROGRAM FOR MEN

DAY 1

BREAKFAST

Oriental Vegetable Omelet

1 ⅓ teaspoons olive oil

¼ cup scallions, thinly sliced diagonally

1 cup sliced drained canned mushrooms

½ cup sliced red and green bell peppers

½ cup drained canned chickpeas

3 cups bean sprouts

½ teaspoon minced garlic

3 tablespoons cider vinegar

⅛ teaspoon grated fresh gingerroot*

1 tablespoon soy sauce

⅛ tablespoon Worcestershire sauce

1 cup egg substitute

In large nonstick sauté pan heat ⅔ teaspoon of the oil. Stir-fry the scallions for 1 minute over medium-high heat. Add the mushrooms and cook another 2 minutes, then add the peppers, chickpeas, sprouts, garlic, vinegar, ginger, soy sauce, and Worcestershire sauce and cook 3 to 5 minutes, or until bean sprouts are tender.

In a second large nonstick sauté pan heat the remaining ⅔ teaspoon oil over medium-high heat. Pour in the egg substitute. As it cooks, push the cooked portions toward the center of pan with a spatula. When the eggs are set, remove the omelet to a warmed serving plate and place the filling from the first pan into one side of the omelet. Fold over the other side and serve.

*Note: When a recipe calls for fresh gingerroot (available in most grocery stores or Asian markets), it is not advisable to substitute ground ginger. The flavors are very different.

LUNCH

Garden Salad Topped with Sautéed Scallops and Bacon

1⅓ teaspoons olive oil

1 ounce Canadian bacon, diced

4½ ounces bay scallops

3 tablespoons cider vinegar

½ teaspoon grated fresh gingerroot

½ teaspoon chopped fresh mint

¼ cup chicken stock

2 cups shredded lettuce

⅔ cup mandarin orange slices

½ cup diced red onion

¼ cup kidney beans, rinsed

¼ cup chickpeas, rinsed

Heat ⅓ teaspoon of the olive oil in a medium nonstick sauté pan over medium-high heat. Sauté the bacon, scallops, 1 teaspoon of the vinegar, and ¼ teaspoon of the ginger for 4 minutes, or until the bacon and scallops are cooked through.

To make the dressing, in a small bowl whisk together the remaining 1 teaspoon oil, ¼ teaspoon ginger, 2 teaspoons vinegar, mint, and chicken stock. Combine the remaining ingredients in a large salad bowl. Add the bacon and scallops. Pour on the dressing and toss to coat.

LATE AFTERNOON SNACK

2 hard-boiled eggs

¼ cup hummus (contains fat)

Paprika

Slice the eggs in half, discard the yolks, and fill each egg white with half the hummus. Top with paprika to taste.

DINNER

Indian Shrimp with Apples and Yogurt

1⅓ teaspoons olive oil

4½ ounces small shrimp, shelled, deveined, and cooked

2 teaspoons cider vinegar

⅛ teaspoon minced fresh gingerroot

½ teaspoon minced garlic

1 tablespoon minced cilantro

Dash hot pepper sauce

¼ teaspoon turmeric

⅛ teaspoon ground coriander

⅛ teaspoon ground cumin

½ cup plain low-fat yogurt

¾ cup minced onion

1 Granny Smith apple, diced

5 cups romaine lettuce

Heat the oil in a medium nonstick sauté pan over medium heat. Add the shrimp, vinegar, herbs, and spices. Cook 1 to 2 minutes, or until the shrimp are opaque. In a second nonstick sauté pan heat yogurt, onion, and apple over low heat until heated through. Do not boil. Add the shrimp mixture and stir to mix. Form a bed of romaine on a serving plate and top with shrimp mixture.

LATE NIGHT SNACK

¼ cup low-fat cottage cheese

⅓ cup light fruit cocktail or ½ cup pineapple or ½ cup blueberries or ½
   chopped apple or ⅓ cup applesauce or 1 block Zone-favorable
   fruit

1 macadamia nut or 3 almonds

FISH OIL SUPPLEMENT

Take 2.5 grams of EPA and DHA. If you are using ultra-refined EPA/DHA concentrate, this would be either four 1-gram capsules or 1 teaspoon of liquid.

EXERCISE PROGRAM

Do Day 1 of the Sample Weekly Workout Plan found on page 134.

MEDITATION PROGRAM

Do 20 minutes of Meditation Made Easy, as described on page 143.

DAY 2

BREAKFAST

Breakfast Fruit Salad

1 cup low-fat cottage cheese

½ cup fresh or reduced-sugar cubed canned pineapple

1 cup mandarin orange slices, canned in water, drained

4 macadamia nuts, crushed

Place the cottage cheese in a bowl. Fold in the pineapple, oranges, and nuts.

LUNCH

Savory Lentils with Goat Cheese

1 cup dried lentils, rinsed and drained

¼ teaspoon salt

¼ teaspoon freshly ground black pepper

2 ¼ tablespoon chopped roasted red peppers

1 clove garlic, minced

1½ tablespoons chopped fresh cilantro

1½ tablespoons chopped red onion

2 tablespoons chopped chives

⅛ teaspoon paprika

¾ teaspoons cumin

1⅛ teaspoons extra-virgin olive oil

Juice of 1 lime

4 ounces goat cheese, at room temperature

2 radicchio leaves for garnish

In a medium saucepan place the lentils, salt, and black pepper in 1½ cups water.
Cover and bring to a boil over medium heat and simmer for 20 minutes, or until the

lentils are tender but still have texture. Remove from the heat and drain. In a medium bowl mix the lentils, roasted peppers, garlic, cilantro, onion, and chives. In a small bowl combine the paprika, cumin, olive oil, and lime juice. Toss together with the lentil mixture. Before serving, fold in goat cheese. Arrange radicchio leaves on a plate. Spoon the lentil salad onto the radicchio and serve.

LATE AFTERNOON SNACK

Raspberry Protein Smoothie

7 grams protein powder

1 cup frozen raspberries, defrosted

1 teaspoon slivered almonds

Blend the ingredients in a blender until smooth.

DINNER

Ginger Chicken

1⅛ teaspoons olive oil

4 ounces boneless, skinless chicken breast, cut lengthwise into thin strips

2 cups broccoli florets

1½ cups snow peas

¾ cup chopped yellow onion

1 teaspoon grated fresh gingerroot

1 cup grapes

In a wok or large nonstick pan heat the oil over medium-high heat. Add the chicken and sauté, turning frequently, until lightly browned, about 5 minutes. Add the broccoli, snow peas, onion, ginger, and ¼ cup water. Continue cooking, stirring often, until the chicken is done, the sauce is reduced to a glaze, and the vegetables are tender, about 20 minutes. If the pan becomes too dry during the cooking, add water 1 tablespoon at a time. Serve the grapes for dessert.

LATE NIGHT SNACK

Tuna with Hummus

1 ounce canned tuna fish packed in water
¼ cup hummus

Drain the tuna fish. Mix with the hummus.

FISH OIL SUPPLEMENTATION

Take 2.5 grams of EPA and DHA. If you are using ultra-refined EPA/DHA concentrate, this would be either four 1-gram capsules or 1 teaspoon of liquid.

EXERCISE PROGRAM

Do Day 2 of the Sample Weekly Workout Plan found on page 134.

MEDITATION PROGRAM

Do 20 minutes of Progressive Muscle Relaxation, as described on page 144.

DAY 3

BREAKFAST

Curried Asparagus Omelet

1⅓ teaspoons olive oil

½ teaspoon minced garlic

½ to 1 teaspoon curry powder

⅛ teaspoon Worcestershire sauce

⅛ teaspoon turmeric

Salt and pepper, to taste

1½ cups seeded, chopped tomato

4 cups chopped mushrooms

1 cup asparagus, cut into 1-inch pieces, steamed

1½ cups chopped onion

1 cup egg substitute

1 teaspoon chopped fresh parsley

In a medium nonstick sauté pan heat ⅔ teaspoon of the olive oil over medium heat. Add the garlic and sauté until lightly browned, about 2 minutes. Stir in the curry powder, Worcestershire sauce, turmeric, salt, and pepper. Cook 1 minute to heat through. Add the tomato, mushrooms, asparagus, and onion. Cook until softened, about 5 minutes. Cover and remove from the heat.

In a second nonstick sauté pan heat the remaining ⅔ teaspoon oil. Pour the egg substitute into second sauté pan and cook until set. Place the omelet on a serving plate, spoon the asparagus mixture onto half of the omelet, and fold other half over. Sprinkle with parsley and serve immediately.

LUNCH

Grilled Turkey Salad with Mandarin Oranges

1⅓ teaspoons olive oil

4 ounces turkey breast chunks

1 cup finely sliced celery

⅓ cup finely sliced red onion

½ cup Zoned French Dressing (see recipe on page 186)

1 peach, diced

⅓ cup mandarin oranges slices, canned in water, drained

⅛ teaspoon turmeric

1 tablespoon chopped fresh mint

1½ cups chopped romaine lettuce

Heat ⅓ teaspoon of the olive oil in a small sauté pan over medium heat. Add the turkey and stir-fry until cooked through, about 8 minutes. In a salad bowl combine the remaining 1 teaspoon oil, turkey, celery, onion, dressing, peach, oranges, turmeric, and mint. Toss lightly to coat. On a lunch plate place the lettuce, top with turkey salad, and serve.

Zoned French Dressing*

8 teaspoons cornstarch

¾ cup finely minced onion

¼ cup tomato puree

¼ cup canned kidney beans, rinsed and minced

1 ¾ cups water

¼ cup cider vinegar

2 tablespoons balsamic vinegar

⅛ teaspoon Worcestershire sauce

1 teaspoon dried tarragon

1 teaspoon dried oregano

1 teaspoon dried parsley flakes

3 teaspoons minced garlic

1 teaspoon dried basil

½ teaspoon chili powder

2 teaspoons paprika

1 teaspoon dried dill

In a small bowl mix the cornstarch with a little cold water to dissolve it. Combine all ingredients in a small saucepan, turn the heat to medium-low, and bring the mixture to a simmer, constantly stirring until the dressing thickens, about 5 minutes. Cool the dressing for 10 to 15 minutes, then blend it in a food processor or blender until smooth. Transfer the dressing to a storage container, cool, cover, and refrigerate.[†]

*Note: Each ½ cup of Zoned French Dressing contains 1 Carbohydrate Zone Block. There are no Protein or Fat Blocks in this dressing recipe. This recipe is used as a component in other Zone recipes. Each time you make a Zone-favorable meal, use this dressing as a replacement for 1 Carbohydrate Zone Block.

†Note: This dressing may be refrigerated for up to 5 days, or if you prefer, the dressing may be frozen and defrosted for later use. Although the dressing is freeze-thaw stable, after it has been frozen and defrosted it may need to be stirred to reincorporate the small amount of moisture that forms on the dressing during the freezing and thawing process.

LATE AFTERNOON SNACK

Tomato and Low-Fat Mozzarella Salad

⅓ teaspoon extra-virgin olive oil

Balsamic vinegar, to taste

1 clove garlic, minced

2 tomatoes, diced or sliced

1 ounce skim mozzarella cheese, diced or sliced

1 teaspoon chopped fresh basil leaves

Place tomato on a plate. In a small bowl whisk together the olive oil, vinegar, and garlic. Pour the dressing over the tomatoes. Top with the mozzarella and basil.

DINNER

Quick and Delicious Salmon Patties

4½ ounces canned pink salmon

2 egg whites

1 ounce slow-cooking oatmeal, dry

¼ onion, diced

Garlic salt, to taste

Pepper, to taste

1⅓ teaspoons olive oil

1 apple

Using a fork, flake the salmon in a medium bowl. Add the egg whites, oatmeal, onion, garlic salt, and pepper and mix well with clean hands. Shape the mixture into a patty. Heat the olive oil in a medium sauté pan over medium heat, add the salmon patty, and cook for 3 to 5 minutes on each side, or until golden brown. Serve immediately. Have the apple for dessert.

LATE EVENING SNACK

Low-Fat Yogurt and Nuts

½ cup plain low-fat yogurt
1 teaspoon silvered almonds or 1 macadamia nut

FISH OIL SUPPLEMENTATION

Take 2.5 grams of EPA and DHA. If you are using ultra-refined EPA/DHA concentrate, this would be either four 1-gram capsules or 1 teaspoon of liquid.

EXERCISE PROGRAM

Do Day 3 of the Sample Weekly Exercise Plan found on page 134.

MEDITATION PROGRAM

Do 20 minutes of Traditional Meditation, as described on page 144.

DAY 4

BREAKFAST

Seven-Minute Breakfast

1 ounce lean Canadian bacon

Olive oil spray

1 whole egg

4 egg whites

1 slice French Meadow bread, lightly toasted

1⅓ teaspoons olive oil

1 pear

½ cup of grapes

In a dry nonstick skillet over medium heat prepare the Canadian bacon according to package instructions. Remove it to a plate. Lightly spray the pan with olive oil spray and fry or scramble the egg and egg whites. Add them to the plate. Drizzle the toast with the olive oil and serve it on the side with the fruit.

LUNCH

Chicken Waldorf Salad

4 ounces chicken breast

Vegetable broth and/or water for cooking

Curry powder, to taste

Cumin, to taste

Turmeric, to taste

½ cup grapes

1 cup chopped Granny Smith apple

1 cup chopped celery

1 cup sliced red pepper

4 teaspoons light mayonnaise

2 tablespoons yogurt

Nutmeg, to taste

Black pepper, to taste

Cinnamon, to taste

In a small saucepan place the chicken. Pour in enough vegetable broth to cover the chicken and add curry powder, cumin, and turmeric. Bring the liquid to a simmer over medium heat and poach the chicken until it's cooked through, about 10–15 minutes. Cool the chicken and cut it into small chunks.

In a big bowl combine the chicken, grapes, apple, celery, and red pepper. Stir in the mayonnaise, yogurt, nutmeg, black pepper, and cinnamon and serve.

LATE AFTERNOON SNACK

Cottage Cheese and Salsa

¼ cup low-fat cottage cheese

½ cup mild or spicy salsa

1 tablespoon guacamole

Mix the ingredients together.

DINNER

Sautéed Green Beans with Tofu

1⅓ teaspoons olive oil

½ teaspoon Worcestershire sauce

⅛ teaspoon celery salt

8 ounces extra-firm tofu, cut into 1-inch pieces

2 cups green beans, cut into 2-inch pieces

1½ cups chopped onion

½ teaspoon minced garlic

2 teaspoons cider vinegar

⅛ teaspoon nutmeg

⅛ teaspoon cinnamon

⅛ teaspoon lemon herb seasoning

⅛ teaspoon ground double-superfine mustard

½ teaspoon soy sauce

Salt and pepper, to taste

½ apple

Heat ⅔ teaspoon of the oil in a medium nonstick sauté pan over medium heat. Add the Worcestershire sauce, celery salt, and tofu and stir-fry until the tofu is browned and crusted on all sides, about 5 minutes.

In a second nonstick sauté pan over medium heat heat the remaining ⅔ teaspoon oil and add the green beans, onion, garlic, vinegar, nutmeg, cinnamon, lemon herb seasoning, mustard, soy sauce, salt, and pepper. Sauté about 5 minutes until the beans are crisp-tender. Place the beans on a serving plate and top with the tofu.

LATE NIGHT SNACK

4-ounce glass wine

1 ounce cheese

FISH OIL SUPPLEMENT

Take 2.5 grams of EPA and DHA. If you are using ultra-refined EPA/DHA concentrate, this would be either four 1-gram capsules or 1 teaspoon of liquid.

EXERCISE PROGRAM

Take a rest day.

MEDITATION PROGRAM

Do 20 minutes of Meditation Made Easy, as described on page 143.

DAY 5

BREAKFAST

Spicy Shrimp and Mushroom Omelet

1⅓ teaspoons olive oil

1 cup sliced asparagus spears

⅛ teaspoon minced garlic

¼ teaspoon dried parsley

⅛ teaspoon dry mustard

⅛ teaspoon dried basil

⅛ teaspoon cayenne pepper

⅛ teaspoon turmeric

Salt and pepper, to taste

¾ cup chopped onion

2 cups chopped mushrooms

1½ ounces shrimp, chopped

¾ cup egg substitute

2 kiwifruits, peeled and sliced

In a medium nonstick sauté pan heat the oil over medium-high heat. Add the asparagus, herbs, and spices and sauté for 1 minute, then add the onion and mushrooms. Cook for 3 to 5 minutes, or until the vegetables are tender. Remove the vegetables and keep them warm.

Place the shrimp in the sauté pan and sauté for 1 minute, or until opaque. Pour in the egg substitute and stir to distribute the shrimp throughout the egg. Cook until the omelet is almost set, about 2–3 minutes. Remove the omelet to serving plate. Spoon the mushroom mixture onto the omelet and fold it over. Garnish the plate with the kiwi slices and serve.

LUNCH

Taco Burger

4½ ounces lean (90% fat-free) ground beef

½ cup mild or spicy salsa

1⅓ teaspoons olive oil

½ cup cooked black beans, rinsed

⅓ cup chopped onion

½ teaspoon minced garlic

½ teaspoon Worcestershire sauce

⅛ teaspoon celery salt

1 tablespoon lemon- or lime-flavored spring water

2 cups shredded lettuce

1 taco shell, broken into pieces

1 ounce low-fat, Monterey Jack cheese, shredded

In a small bowl, combine the ground beef and ¼ cup of the salsa. Form into a patty. Heat ⅔ teaspoon of the oil in a medium nonstick sauté pan over medium heat and fry the patty until it's cooked through, turning it once, about 8 minutes in all.

In a second nonstick sauté pan heat the remaining ⅔ teaspoon oil. Add the beans, onion, garlic, remaining ¼ cup salsa, Worcestershire sauce, celery salt, and springwater and cook until heated through. Place the lettuce on a plate, add the patty, sprinkle with the taco pieces, and top with the bean mixture and the cheese.

LATE AFTERNOON SNACK

Waldorf Sald

1 cup sliced celery

¼ apple, diced

1 teaspoon light mayonnaise

1 pecan half, crushed

1 ounce part-skim or "soft" cheese

In a small bowl combine the celery, apple, and mayonnaise. Sprinkle the pecan pieces on top and serve the cheese on the side.

DINNER

Salmon with Asian Fruity Salsa

1⅓ teaspoons olive oil

6 ounces salmon steak

2 teaspoons soy sauce

1 teaspoon minced fresh gingerroot

½ teaspoon chopped fresh dill

Dash hot pepper sauce

½ cup mild or spicy salsa

½ cup canned pineapple cubes

1 Granny Smith apple, cored and diced

Preheat oven to 350°F. Brush a small baking dish with the oil and place the salmon steak in the baking dish. Sprinkle with the soy sauce, ginger, dill, and hot pepper sauce. Cover with aluminum foil and bake 30 to 35 minutes, or until the salmon is cooked through. In a small bowl, combine the salsa and fruit. Place the fish on one side of a serving plate and the salsa beside it.

LATE NIGHT SNACK

Low-Fat Yogurt and Nuts

½ cup plain low-fat yogurt

1 teaspoon slivered almonds or 1 macadamia nut

FISH OIL SUPPLEMENT

Take 2.5 grams of EPA and DHA. If you are using ultra-refined EPA/DHA concentrate, this would be either four 1-gram capsules or 1 teaspoon of liquid.

EXERCISE PROGRAM

Do Day 5 of the Weekly Exercise Program found on page 134.

MEDITATION PROGRAM

Do 20 minutes of Progressive Muscle Relaxation, as described on page 144.

DAY 6

BREAKFAST

Breakfast in a Bowl

1 cup plain, nonfat yogurt

½ cup nonfat cottage cheese

2 tablespoons slow-cooking oatmeal, dry

4 teaspoons slivered almonds

4 teaspoons vanilla extract

Allspice, to taste

Blend all the ingredients together in a medium bowl and refrigerate overnight to soften the oats.

LUNCH

Grilled Chicken Salad

1 cup green leaf or romaine lettuce, washed, dried, and torn into
   large pieces

1 cup broccoli florets

1 green bell pepper, cored, seeded, and cut into thin strips

¼ cup canned kidney beans, rinsed and drained

1 medium tomato, sliced

1 tablespoon extra-virgin olive oil

2 teaspoons vinegar (or more to taste)

1 tablespoon lemon juice

1 teaspoon Worcestershire sauce

½ teaspoon freshly ground pepper, or to taste

4 ounces grilled skinless chicken breast, cut into bite-sized chunks

1 medium pear

In a medium bowl toss together the lettuce, broccoli, green pepper, kidney beans, and tomato. In a small bowl whisk together the olive oil, vinegar, lemon juice, Worcestershire sauce, and ground pepper. Toss the dressing with the vegetables until well combined, and top with the chicken chunks. Serve the pear for dessert.

LATE AFTERNOON SNACK

Spinach Salad

Spinach (side-salad size)
2 hard-boiled egg whites, sliced
⅓ cup mandarin orange slices, canned in water, drained
⅛ teaspoon olive oil
Balsamic vinegar, to taste

Place the spinach on a plate. Top with the egg whites and oranges. Whisk together the olive oil and vinegar and pour over the salad.

DINNER

Hot and Sour Stir-Fry Pork and Cabbage

1½ teaspoons olive oil

4 ounces lean pork loin, cut into large dice

½ cup chicken stock

1 teaspoon cornstarch

1 tablespoon soy sauce

1 tablespoon cider vinegar

½ cup chopped scallions

⅛ teaspoon black pepper

2 tablespoons diced jalapeño peppers

2 teaspoons minced garlic

2 teaspoons minced fresh gingerroot

¾ cup cauliflower florets

¾ cup sliced onion

2 cups shredded cabbage

1 pear, cored and sliced

In a medium glass bowl combine the oil, pork, stock, cornstarch, soy sauce, vinegar, scallions, peppers, garlic, and ginger. Cover and marinate in the refrigerator for 30 minutes. Place the pork mixture in a medium nonstick sauté pan, turn the heat to medium, and sauté until the pork is browned on both sides, about 15 minutes. Add the cauliflower, onion, and cabbage and sauté until the vegetables are tender, about 15 minutes. Place the pork and vegetables on a large dinner plate, garnished with the pear slices, and serve immediately.

LATE NIGHT SNACK

Tomato and Low-Fat Cottage Cheese

¼ cup low-fat cottage cheese

2 tomatoes, sliced

6 peanuts

FISH OIL SUPPLEMENT

Take 2.5 grams of EPA and DHA. If you are using ultra-refined EPA/DHA concentrate, this would be either four 1-gram capsules or 1 teaspoon of liquid.

EXERCISE PROGRAM

Do Day 6 of the Weekly Exercise Plan found on page 134.

MEDITATION PROGRAM

Do 20 minutes of Traditional Meditation, as described on page 144.

DAY 7

BREAKFAST

Florentine Filled Omelet Crepes

1 cup egg substitute

⅛ teaspoon celery salt

⅛ teaspoon nutmeg

⅛ teaspoon cinnamon

1⅓ teaspoons olive oil

4 cups sliced mushrooms

¾ cup chopped onion

Salt and pepper, to taste

4 tablespoons balsamic vinegar

5 cups fresh spinach*

2 kiwifruits, peeled and sliced

In a small bowl combine the egg substitute, celery salt, nutmeg, and cinnamon. In a large nonstick sauté pan heat ⅔ teaspoon of the oil over medium-high heat. Pour the egg mixture into the sauté pan. When the eggs are browned on one side, flip them with a spatula and brown the other side.

Heat the remaining ⅔ teaspoon oil in a second nonstick sauté pan over medium-high heat. Add the mushrooms, onion, salt, and pepper and cook for 3 to 5 minutes, or until softened. Add the balsamic vinegar and spinach and cook until the spinach is just wilted. Place the omelet onto a serving plate, spoon the vegetable mixture onto the omelet, and fold the omelet, over. Garnish with the kiwi slices and serve.

*Note: Fresh spinach often has sand on it, so be sure to wash it carefully before cooking.

LUNCH

Thai Turkey Soup

---

6 ounces lean ground turkey

1½ cups bean sprouts

½ cup sliced scallions

1⅛ teaspoons olive oil

3 teaspoons minced garlic

½ teaspoon grated fresh gingerroot

2 tablespoons soy sauce

3 cups chicken stock

1 tablespoon finely diced hot chili pepper

2 cups spinach leaves

¼ cup cooked fine egg noodles

1 cup light fruit cocktail

Combine the turkey, sprouts, scallions, oil, garlic, ginger, soy sauce, stock, and chili pepper in a medium saucepan. Bring to a boil over medium heat, reduce the heat, and simmer for 15 minutes. Add the spinach and noodles and simmer for 1 minute. Spoon the soup into a serving bowl. Serve the fruit cocktail in a side dish.

LATE AFTERNOON SNACK

Veggies and Dip

---

2 ounces firm tofu

⅛ teaspoon olive oil

Dry onion soup mix, to taste

1 cup celery, sliced for dipping

1 green pepper, sliced for dipping

In a small bowl blend the tofu, olive oil, and soup mix. Serve with the veggies.

DINNER

Spicy Tofu with Scallions and Radishes

1⅓ teaspoons olive oil

1 teaspoon minced fresh gingerroot

8 ounces extra-firm tofu, cut into 1-inch cubes

1 tablespoon lemon juice

4 teaspoons soy sauce

1½ teaspoons white wine

1 teaspoon minced garlic

Salt and pepper, to taste

¾ cup finely diced jalapeño and red bell pepper (mix to the desired
   heat)

5 cups torn fresh spinach

1 cup thinly sliced radishes

1½ cups seeded, diced tomatoes

1 cup chopped scallions

1½ cups canned or fresh mushroom slices

Heat the oil and ½ teaspoon of the ginger in a medium sauté pan over medium-high heat. Add the tofu and stir-fry until it is browned on all sides, about 6 minutes. In a small bowl whisk together the lemon juice, 1 tablespoon water, soy sauce, wine, garlic, salt, pepper, and remaining ½ teaspoon ginger. Combine the peppers, spinach, radishes, tomatoes, scallions, and mushrooms in a medium bowl. Pour in the soy sauce mixture and toss to coat. Add the tofu and spoon onto a serving dish.

LATE NIGHT SNACK

Berries and Low-Fat Cheese

½ cup blueberries or 1 cup strawberries

1 ounce low-fat mozzarella cheese

6 peanuts

FISH OIL SUPPLEMENT

Take 2.5 grams of EPA and DHA. If you are using ultra-refined EPA/DHA concentrate, this would be either four 1-gram capsules or 1 teaspoon of liquid.

EXERCISE PROGRAM

Do Day 7 of the Weekly Exercise Program found on page 134.

MEDITATION PROGRAM

Do 20 minutes of Meditation Made Easy, as described on page 143.

SUMMARY

After one week of following the Zone Lifestyle Program, I guarantee you that you will start enjoying the benefits described in the beginning of this chapter. If you like those changes, then just imagine a lifetime of those benefits. That's what you can expect once you squarely position yourself in the center of the Anti-Inflammation Zone.

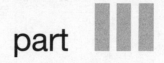

The Science Behind Silent Inflammation

Eicosanoids: The Good, the Bad, and the Neutral

Strange, mysterious, and almost mystical, eicosanoids are the key to wellness because they control the levels of silent inflammation in your body. Yet as important as eicosanoids are, most physicians know nothing about them. If your doctor is unaware of them, then you're likely to be, too—unless you've read one of my previous books about the Zone. My Zone technology has always been about eicosanoids and how the diet affects them. Control these hormones, and you control your future.

Eicosanoids were the first hormones produced by living organisms, dating back to about 550 million years ago. However, our story doesn't begin until 1929 when researchers stumbled upon the discovery that if fat was totally removed from the diet, the test animals soon died. Adding back certain fats (then called vitamin F) was found to enable fat-deprived animals to live. Eventually, as technologies advanced, researchers realized that these essential fats were composed of two classes of fatty acids: omega-6 and omega-3. Unfortunately, the body cannot synthesize them, so they have to be supplied by the diet.

Having these essential fatty acids in the diet is only the first of many steps toward making eicosanoids, as they have to be metabolized into longer-chain molecules that serve as the actual building blocks of eicosanoids. In fact, the word *eicosanoids* is derived from the Greek word for twenty (*eicosa*), since all of these hormones are synthesized from essential fatty acids that are twenty carbon atoms in length.

Ulf von Euler discovered the first eicosanoid in 1936. It was isolated from the human prostate gland (an exceptionally rich source of eicosanoids). Because it was thought at that time that all hormones had to originate from a discrete gland, it made perfect sense to name this new hormone a *prosta*glandin. With time it became clear that every living cell in the body could make eicosanoids, and that there was no discrete organ or gland that was the center of eicosanoid synthesis. In essence, you have 60 trillion eicosanoid "glands."

The breakthrough in eicosanoid research occurred in 1971, when John Vane finally discovered how aspirin (the wonder drug of the twentieth century) actually worked: It changed the levels of eicosanoids. The 1982 Nobel Prize in Physiology or Medicine was awarded to Vane and his colleagues Bengt Samuelsson and Sune Bergelson for their discoveries of the critical role that eicosanoids play in human disease.

If eicosanoids are so important, why are they virtually unknown to the medical community? First of all, these hormones have a very short life span. In just a few seconds, they are created and sent off to carry out a mission, and then they self-destruct. This makes them extremely difficult to study. Second, they are cell-to-cell messengers that don't circulate in the bloodstream, making them a challenge to sample. Finally, they work at vanishingly low concentrations, making them almost impossible to detect. Despite these barriers, more than 87,000 articles on eicosanoids have been published. So, at least the basic research community is interested in eicosanoids, even if your doctor never learned about them in medical school.

Eicosanoids encompass a wide array of hormones, many unknown by most medical researchers. The different classes of eicosanoids are shown below:

- Prostaglandins
- Thromboxanes
- Leukotrienes

- Lipoxins
- Aspirin-triggered epi-lipoxins
- Hydroxylated fatty acids
- Isoprostanoids
- Epoxyeicosatrienoic acids
- Endocannabinoids

There are hundreds of eicosanoids, and more are being discovered on a yearly basis. But for all of their actions, the most important to us is their role in inflammation.

EICOSANOIDS AND INFLAMMATION

As I discuss throughout this book, eicosanoids are the central players in the inflammatory response. They turn it on and can turn it off. Just to make it simple, I call those eicosanoids that turn on the inflammatory response "bad" and the ones that turn off the inflammatory response "good." Obviously, you need some balance of "good" and "bad" eicosanoids to survive. It's only when the ratio of these two opposing groups gets out of kilter that you develop silent inflammation and eventually end up with chronic disease.

Herein lies the power of the Silent Inflammation Profile (SIP). It can tell you with frightening precision the relative balance of the building blocks of "good" and "bad" eicosanoids in your body. As I mentioned in chapter 4, if your SIP is too high (greater than 3), then you have silent inflammation. The higher your SIP, the greater your overproduction of "bad" eicosanoids, and the further you are from a state of wellness.

There are two ways you can modify the balance of eicosanoids in your body to control silent inflammation. One way is to take anti-inflammatory drugs (such as aspirin, Motrin, COX-2 inhibitors, and corticosteroids) for the rest of your life. Considering that almost as many Americans die from taking the correct dosage of anti-inflammatory drugs as die from AIDS, this is probably not a good long-term strategy. The other way to control silent inflammation is with your diet—in particular, the Zone Diet coupled with high-dose fish oil. The only side effects of the second choice are beneficial: It will make you smarter and thinner as well as healthier.

SYNTHESIS OF ESSENTIAL FATTY ACIDS

To understand the importance of the Zone Diet in controlling these eicosanoids and reestablishing an appropriate eicosanoid balance, you have to understand how the actual building blocks of eicosanoids are made. To begin with, all eicosanoids ultimately are produced from essential fatty acids that the body cannot make, and therefore must be consumed as part of the diet. These essential fatty acids are classified as either omega-3 or omega-6, depending upon the position of the double bonds within them. This is important, because the positioning of these double bonds dictates the fatty acid's three-dimensional structure in space and ultimately determines the way your body responds physiologically to the eicosanoids derived from that fatty acid. However, typical essential fatty acids are only 18 carbons in length and must be further elongated to 20-carbon fatty acids by the body before eicosanoids can be made. It is just not the number of carbon atoms that count, but also their configuration. How your diet can manipulate the formation of dietary essential fatty acids into the actual 20-carbon atom precursors of eicosanoids is a somewhat complex story. Nonetheless, it is the foundation for understanding the Zone Diet.

OMEGA-6 FATTY ACIDS

Omega-6 fatty acids are the key players in this eicosanoid drama. They have the potential for great good or great harm. In many ways, they are like Dr. Jekyll and Mr. Hyde. On the other hand, the eicosanoids that come from the omega-3 fatty acids don't do much of anything. They are basically neutral. So why do I constantly tout the importance of EPA? Because it plays the key role in determining whether the omega-6 fatty acids end up being the building blocks for "good" or "bad" eicosanoids.

The vast majority of omega-6 fatty acids in your diet come from linoleic acid, which contains two double bonds. Common sources are vegetable oils such as corn oil, soybean oil, safflower oil, and sunflower oil. These are the oils that are now ubiquitous in the American diet.

The first step in this biochemical journey from seemingly inno-cent vegetable oils to "bad" eicosanoids starts with inserting another double bond in linoleic acid in just the right position to begin bending inward and forming gamma-linolenic acid (GLA) from linoleic acid, as shown below:

Linoleic Acid

↓

Gamma-Linolenic Acid (GLA)

Up to this point nothing nefarious has happened. Actually, you want your body to produce GLA. It's a key fatty acid that can make powerful anti-inflammatory ("good") cicosanoids. But it also has the potential to produce equally powerful pro-inflammatory ("bad") eicosanoids.

Once you get linoleic acid transformed into GLA, the ball starts to move with growing momentum toward eicosanoids, both "good" and "bad," as GLA can be rapidly converted into dihomo-gamma-linolenic acid (DGLA), as shown below:

Gamma-Linolenic Acid (GLA)

↓

Dihomo-Gamma-Linolenic Acid (DGLA)

That is potentially great news, since DGLA is the building block for most of the "good" eicosanoids that have powerful anti-inflammatory effects. If omega-6 fatty acid metabolism stopped here, life would be good. Unfortunately, there is no free lunch when it comes to eicosanoids. This is because DGLA is also the substrate for another enzyme known as delta-5-desaturase (D5D) that produces the arachidonic acid (AA) that is the building block for all of the pro-inflammatory eicosanoids, as shown below:

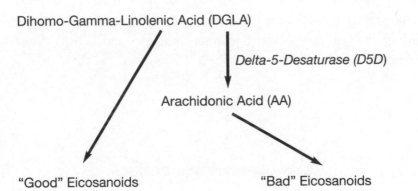

Dihomo-Gamma-Linolenic Acid (DGLA)

Delta-5-Desaturase (D5D)

Arachidonic Acid (AA)

"Good" Eicosanoids   "Bad" Eicosanoids

The problem lies in the dietary intake of excessive amounts of vegetable oils that are rich in omega-6 fatty acids. By sheer brute force, the high levels of linoleic acid in these vegetable oils will ultimately increase the production of AA and therefore increase silent inflammation, which in turn accelerates aging and causes chronic disease.

Understanding the critical importance of the D5D enzyme and silent inflammation marked the actual beginnings of the Zone Diet more than twenty years ago, just after the Nobel Prize in Physiology or Medicine had been awarded for understanding eicosanoids. I reasoned that if I could control the activity of this one enzyme, I could alter the balance of "good" and "bad" eicosanoids on a lifetime basis.

All that I had to find was an appropriate natural inhibitor of the D5D activity. And I had just the right nutrient. It was the long-chain omega-3 fatty acid EPA. I figured if you give a person enough GLA (to increase DGLA levels) with the right amount of EPA (to inhibit the production of AA from DGLA), it would automatically ensure that you would quickly be making more "good" anti-inflammatory eicosanoids and fewer "bad" pro-inflammatory eicosanoids. In fact, I was so confident twenty years ago, I was already beginning to outline my acceptance speech for the Nobel Prize. Unfortunately, life is never that simple.

In those early days in the 1980s, I thought that simply controlling the dietary intake of EPA and GLA would be all that I needed to control eicosanoids. I could always get EPA from fish oil (although it wasn't very high quality then), and all I had to do was to find enough GLA. There was the problem. There wasn't very much of it, and no one was growing the richest source of it—borage. Not to be turned off by that fact, my brother Doug and I cornered the entire world's borage market (it wasn't too hard) and then went to the plains of upper Canada to grow it. (Of all the places in the world, borage grows very well in this climate.) Now that there were available sources of both EPA and GLA, all I had to do was pick the right ratio of EPA to GLA and I would be off to fame and fortune. So I started out with a 4:1 ratio and made some soft gelatin capsules containing both fish oil (the source of EPA) and borage oil (the source of GLA). I then found some friends who were willing to be guinea pigs. I gave them my standard phrase, "Trust me." Much to the surprise of my friends (and to my great relief), many of the physiological benefits I predicted occurred within weeks, if not days.

After several months, however, I noticed that strange things seemed to be happening. Virtually everyone who took the combinations of EPA and GLA initially felt much better. After all, they were now making more "good" and fewer "bad" eicosanoids, since I was changing the DGLA/AA balance in each of their 60 trillion cells. With time, some individuals mentioned that they saw a drop-off in the early benefits they first experienced. Nonetheless, they still felt better than before they started. However, there was another group who saw their initial benefits erode completely, and they actually began to feel worse than when they started. Some of my friends were no longer quite so friendly, until I figured out what was happening. I called it the "spillover" effect.

Spillover Effect

Initially, as the ratio of DGLA to AA improves, the person begins making more "good" eicosanoids and fewer "bad" ones. Everything just keeps getting better and better. But there will be some point in time, depending on your genetics, that the DGLA to AA ratio begins to degrade as more of the DGLA gets converted into AA. It turns out that the dosage of EPA I was using was providing only partial inhibition of the D5D activity, so that with time more and more AA would be made. (Until the recent advent of ultra-refined EPA/DHA concentrates, it was simply impossible to get enough EPA into the person without a significant overload of contaminants such as mercury, PCBs, and dioxins.) The initial increase in DGLA levels by supplying GLA was overwhelming the amount of EPA being supplied to inhibit the D5D enzyme. The end result was a growing accumulation of AA. Interestingly, this spillover effect seemed to occur more often in females than in males. So much for my idea that "one size fits all" on the ideal ratio of EPA to GLA.

So I decided that if one size does not fit all, I had better start making a wide array of different EPA and GLA combinations and fine-tune them for each individual. But how could I do this? Fortunately, eicosanoids do leave a biochemical audit trail that gives an insight into their actual balance in different organs in the body. That's what led me to develop the Silent Inflammation Report I discussed in chapter 2. I used this questionnaire to provide me with an assessment of each individual in order to fine-tune his or her ratios of activated essential fatty acids. (Now the SIP blood test makes it even more precise, because it is based on blood chemistry, not observation.)

By 1988, I thought I had finally gotten this concept down to a science, so to speak. It was a much more complex science than I had originally thought, but one still governed by some basic biochemical rules. However, what finally gave me the insight into the complexity of the eicosanoid modulation was my work with elite athletes.

THE HISTORY OF THE ZONE DIET

I began working with elite athletes (primarily the Stanford swimming teams) to see if my multiple combinations of EPA and GLA would enhance their performance. I could continually switch the athletes from one combination to another to prevent the spillover effect. It required weekly communication with each individual swimmer, but I had great results with them during the summer of 1989. But once they went back to eating dormitory food in the fall, the benefits evaporated almost overnight. The coaches were calling me asking why their swimmers who had done so well in the summer were now cramping up and being constantly fatigued. I racked my brain trying to understand what had gone wrong or what had changed to explain this sudden shift in their performance. Then it struck me. Perhaps the high glycemic-load dorm food might be increasing their insulin levels, and this might be a connection.

A trip to the bowels of the MIT library confirmed my suspicion. There I found old research on rats that demonstrated that a high level of insulin (stimulated by eating carbohydrates) activates the D5D enzyme. Therefore, all the performance benefits I had carefully crafted for each athlete by manipulating their ratios of EPA and GLA were being undermined by the surge of insulin caused by their elevated carbohydrate intake. This excess in insulin secretion stimulated the D5D enzyme to increase the production of AA at the expense of DGLA. For these athletes, the result was that a highly favorable DGLA to AA ratio created during the summer quickly became a very undesirable ratio once they returned to dormitory food. I quickly came to the realization that I would never be able to control eicosanoid levels completely without controlling insulin first. It was back to the drawing board.

So now I had to take into account how the metabolism of

DGLA essential fatty acids was modified by the effect of insulin on the D5D, as shown below:

Dihomo-Gamma-Linolenic Acid (DGLA)

Delta-5-Desaturase (D5D)
Activated by Insulin
Inhibited by EPA

Arachidonic Acid (AA)

Since insulin is an activator of the D5D enzyme, it explained the growing number of studies that were linking excess insulin with heart disease. D5D was increasing silent inflammation by increasing AA production. It wasn't that insulin was a cause of heart disease, but rather it caused an increase in silent inflammation, especially in the presence of excess dietary omega-6 fatty acids.

Unfortunately, I knew the only way to control insulin requires controlling the protein-to-carbohydrate ratio at every meal. This means you have to treat food as if it were a drug to be taken at the right dosage and the right time. Of course, my next challenge was to figure out what the optimal protein-to-carbohydrate ratio should be. (I obviously had not done a great job of predicting the ideal EPA to GLA ratio.) I had to start from scratch and get creative. I felt that a good beginning was to attempt to estimate the protein-to-carbohydrate ratio consumed by neo-Paleolithic man some 10,000 to 40,000 years ago, since our genes haven't changed that much since then.

Again, I got lucky with the medical literature. Boyd Eaton of Emory University had already considered this question well before me and set out to answer it. Using anthropological data and comparing a large number of existing hunter-gatherer tribes, he estimated the average protein-to-carbohydrate ratio in neo-Paleolithic diets to be about 3 grams of protein for every 4 grams of carbohydrate, or a protein-to-carbohydrate ratio of 0.75.

I figured this was a good starting point. I began developing a diet that would keep the protein-to-carbohydrate ratio in a range between 0.5 and 1.0 at *every* meal with the bulk of the carbohydrates being low glycemic-load ones, such as vegetables and fruit (the only carbohydrates that existed 10,000 years ago). By doing so, I reasoned that the balance of insulin and glucagon would be maintained from meal to meal. I called this dietary approach the Zone Diet. In essence, the Zone Diet was developed to enhance the ability of EPA to reduce AA formation. This is why the Zone Diet has always been first and foremost an anti-inflammatory diet, not simply a weight-loss program.

To fully control silent inflammation, you need both the supplementation of high-dose fish oil rich in EPA and a balance of protein to carbohydrate at every meal. What about GLA to make necessary levels of DGLA? It turns out that the more successful you are in controlling the activity of the D5D enzyme, the less likely that DGLA would spill over into AA. Thus the low levels of linoleic acid in the Zone Diet would be sufficient to maintain DGLA levels to produce adequate levels of anti-inflammatory eicosanoids. Furthermore, the more you control insulin by the diet, the less fish oil you need to control silent inflammation. On the flip side, the less you control insulin by diet, the more fish oil you need to control silent inflammation.

If EPA is so important for controlling silent inflammation by inhibiting the D5D activity, why even worry about DHA, since it contains twenty-two carbon atoms and can't be made into a classical eicosanoid? First, it turns out that DHA is critical for brain function. Second, DHA acts as a reservoir that can be retro-converted into EPA. Third, DHA can alter genetic expression by binding to certain transcription elements on the DNA that can help increase the sensitivity of cells to insulin. Finally, although DHA cannot be synthesized into a classical eicosanoid, it can be made into a newly discovered class of powerful anti-inflammatory eicosanoids known as resolvins. Bottom line: if you are going to take EPA, make sure you are also taking DHA to cover all of your hormonal bets. I believe the best ratio of EPA to DHA, based on the published data, is about 2:1.

VEGETARIANS AND EPA

Although there are no vegetarian sources of EPA, there are certain algae that make DHA. This vegetarian source of DHA can also be retro-converted into EPA. The process is not that efficient, but at least it provides a mechanism by which vegetarian sources can provide adequate levels of EPA as well as DHA. This retro-conversion of DHA into EPA is far more efficient than trying to synthesize EPA and DHA from other vegetable sources, such as flaxseed oil.

Even though the eicosanoids derived from EPA are neutral, EPA plays a critical role in getting you to the Anti-Inflammation Zone by inhibiting the activity of the D5D enzyme, thereby restricting the flow of omega-6 fatty acids into AA. As long as you are consuming very moderate amounts of omega-6 fatty acids with equal amounts of EPA, then the omega-6 fatty acids in your diet tend to accumulate at the level of DGLA that increases the production of powerful "good" anti-inflammatory eicosanoids. But EPA is still a relatively weak inhibitor of the D5D activity, so you don't want to overwhelm it by consuming high levels of vegetable oil such as soy, corn, or safflower that are rich in omega-6 fatty acids. In fact, it makes good sense to get some extra nutritional help from other natural D5D inhibitors, such as the lignans from sesame oil, or spices such as turmeric.

The total amount of omega-3 and omega-6 fatty acids you need on a daily basis to control silent inflammation is still relatively low. This means you have to add some additional fat to your diet to help slow the rate of entry of carbohydrates to control insulin secretion. This fat should be primarily monounsaturated fat. Monounsaturated fats can't be made into eicosanoids ("good" or "bad"). By having no effect on eicosanoids, monounsaturated fats can provide the necessary amount of fat for controlling the entry rate of carbohydrates into the bloodstream. They do this without disturbing the hormonal balances that you are trying to maintain to achieve ultimate wellness.

DO THE DRUG COMPANIES KNOW THIS?

Don't kid yourself. Although your physician may know nothing about eicosanoids and very little about inflammation (other than it's bad), the drug companies do. They have already spent billions of dollars trying to develop eicosanoid-modifying (i.e., anti-inflammatory) drugs. Eicosanoids as drugs, however, have a very limited role in the world of pharmaceuticals. They are not only too difficult to work with (they have to be injected), but also are simply too powerful to be used as a drug because they are not meant to circulate in the bloodstream.

The reason you never hear the drug companies talking about diet (and especially high-dose fish oil) in treating inflammation is that they make the assumption that it is impossible to reduce AA levels in the cells. They have chosen to fight the battle against inflammation by decreasing the activity of the enzymes that make pro-inflammatory eicosanoids derived from AA. This is a little like closing the barn door after the horses have gotten out, and it's known in pharmacology as *going downstream*. My approach is the opposite: simply *go upstream* and reduce the amount of AA (and also increase the levels of DGLA) in every cell in the body. This not only restricts the amount of pro-inflammatory eicosanoids that can be synthesized, but also increases the number of anti-inflammatory eicosanoids that can be made from DGLA.

To understand the fundamental differences in how these two approaches control inflammation, you have to know a little about how eicosanoids are actually made.

HOW EICOSANOIDS ARE SYNTHESIZED

Eicosanoids are cell-to-cell regulators. Rather than responding to some master hormone, each cell responds to changes in its immediate environment by releasing eicosanoids. The first step in generating a cellular response is the actual release of an essential fatty acid from the phospholipids in the cell membrane. The enzyme responsible for the release of the essential fatty acid is called phospholipase A_2. Depending on whether the fatty acid is released, you will either make "good" eicosanoids (from DGLA), "bad" eicosanoids (from AA), or neutral eicosanoids (from EPA).

Since there is no feedback loop to stop the production of eicosanoids, the only way to inhibit their release from the membrane is by producing cortisol from the adrenal gland, which causes the synthesis of a protein (lipocortin) that inhibits the action of phospholipase A_2. By inhibiting this enzyme, which releases essential fatty acids from the cell membranes, you choke off the supply of the substrate required for all eicosanoid synthesis. Obviously, if you are overproducing cortisol (or taking corticosteroid drugs), you'll bring all eicosanoid synthesis to a crashing halt, which can cause the shutdown of your immune system. In fact, if you give a single injection of corticosteroids to healthy individuals, within twenty-four hours their white blood cells (lymphocytes) will be very similar to those in AIDS patients. No wonder when patients hear that they will be taking steroids, they know they are in bad shape.

Once any long-chain essential fatty acid containing 20-carbon atoms (AA, DGLA, or EPA) is released from the cell membrane, the horse is now definitely out of the barn, because the enzymes that make eicosanoids are primed to act on these free fatty acids. There are two primary pathways from which it can be made into an eicosanoid. The first is via the cyclo-oxygenase (COX) pathway, which makes prostaglandins and thromboxanes. The second is through the lipo-oxygenase (LOX) pathway that makes leukotrienes, hydroxylated fatty acids, and lipoxins.

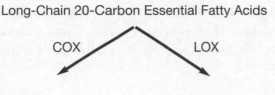

Long-Chain 20-Carbon Essential Fatty Acids

COX   LOX

Prostaglandins   Leukotrienes

Thromboxanes   Hydroxylated fatty acids

Lipoxins

The development of drugs to inhibit one of these two pathways has been the focus of pharmaceutical companies because once the essential fatty acid has been released, some type of eicosanoid is going to be made. If you make the assumption that you can't reduce AA, then you have to put all your hopes on inhibiting the various enzymes that make pro-inflammatory eicosanoids. As you will see later, this is a very dangerous game to play. Certain drugs can inhibit only the COX pathway for eicosanoid formation, whereas others can inhibit only the LOX enzymes. The best-known COX pathway inhibitor is aspirin. Other drugs known as nonsteroidal anti-inflammatory drugs (NSAIDs) also inhibit the COX enzyme. The common names for these NSAIDs are Motrin, Advil, Aleve, and others. The new classes of prostaglandin inhibitors are called COX-2 inhibitors, and they inhibit only a small subclass of the COX enzymes. All of these drugs have side effects, because they are in effect dumb bombs that leave a lot of collateral damage. This is because often the COX enzymes that they inhibit are the same ones required to make "good" eicosanoids. As an example, the COX-2 inhibitors don't seem to cause the stomach damage as do typical COX inhibitors, but they also don't appear to have any benefits in reducing heart attacks. (In fact one COX-2 Inhibitor, Vioxx, was recently pulled off the market because it appears to increase heart attacks.)

However, the ugly secret of all COX inhibitors is that if the free AA can't be made into a prostaglandin, it will then be quickly acted upon by the LOX enzymes to make a different type of eicosanoid, which may even be worse. In many ways once AA is released from the membrane, it is like a live hand grenade just waiting to go off.

LOX Enzymes

Unlike inhibitors of the COX enzymes, there are very few inhibitors of the LOX enzymes. Since leukotrienes (particular LTB_4) represent the primary mediators of inflammation, any free AA often ends up becoming a pro-inflammatory eicosanoid, no matter how many COX inhibitors you might be taking.

WHY GOING UPSTREAM IS GOOD MEDICINE

Drug companies are committed to developing new patentable drugs—ones that affect the downstream COX and LOX enzymes that control eicosanoid production from AA. Unfortunately, there are a bewildering number of pro-inflammatory eicosanoids that can be derived from AA.

Going upstream is the opposite: simply change the balance of the precursors of eicosanoids in the membrane by decreasing AA and increasing DGLA. You can easily do this by the combination of high-dose fish oil and the Zone Diet. By going upstream, if the fatty acid is released, it is more likely that DGLA will be released than AA. This is basically a biological lottery. The end result is more "good" eicosanoids and fewer "bad" ones. This is simply a much more sophisticated strategy to manipulate eicosanoids and therefore inflammation. I don't think I am smarter than the thousands of scientists in drug companies; I just have a very different point of view of how to reach the goal of reduction of inflammation, and especially the reduction of silent inflammation. But it is truly amazing that at every international eicosanoid conference that I attend, virtually none of the researchers has ever considered the possibility that you can actually change the levels of eicosanoid precursors in the cell membrane. Of course, since the drug companies are the primary sponsors of these conferences, their lack of awareness should not be too surprising.

MAKING EVEN MORE "GOOD" EICOSANOIDS

Being in the Anti-Inflammation Zone means you have set yourself up to make more "good" eicosanoids by decreasing the amounts of AA, thus choking off the production of "bad" eicosanoids. At the same time, you are also increasing the levels of DGLA, thus increasing the production of "good" eicosanoids.

That's good, but can you do even better? Of course you can. Here are two approaches to further enhance the production of anti-inflammatory eicosanoids.

The first is to add extra inhibitors of the D5D enzyme to your diet as an added insurance policy to further reduce any potential DGLA spillover into AA. Sesame oil contains such inhibitors, but in very low concentrations, so you would have to eat a lot of it. Unfortunately, sesame oil is also rich in omega-6 fatty acids that can be converted into AA. The answer lies in isolating out the D5D inhibitors from sesame oil while leaving all the omega-6 fatty acids behind. It is a difficult job, but it can be done.

The second approach is truly unique, as it uses aspirin to induce a new series of "good" eicosanoids known as aspirin-triggered epi-lipoxins. Aspirin binds irreversibly to the COX enzymes, preventing any formation of prostaglandins or thromboxanes. For years it was thought this was its only mode of action. Then Charlie Serhan of Harvard Medical School discovered that aspirin actually induces the formation of a whole new series of eicosanoids (aspirin-triggered lipoxins) that have profound anti-inflammatory properties. And the most powerful of these anti-inflammatory eicosanoids come from DHA and to a lesser extent EPA. How much aspirin do you need? Probably not more than a baby aspirin a day if you are taking high-dose fish oil.

SUMMARY

If you want to control silent inflammation on lifetime basis, you have to control the balance of "good" and "bad" eicosanoids. Anti-inflammatory drugs are simply dumb bombs that can cause tremendous amounts of collateral damage, often causing more long-term damage than short-term good. On the other hand, the combination of high-dose fish oil and the Zone Diet can rapidly change the balance of the precursors of eicosanoids in every one of your 60 trillion cells so that you can produce more "good" and fewer "bad" eicosanoids. You are what you eat when it comes to eicosanoids.

Why Inflammation Hurts, How Inflammation Heals

As I mentioned at the beginning of this book, doctors often have a tough time explaining inflammation to their patients. The primary reason is that it is highly complex. Inflammation actually consists of two parts: the pro-inflammatory "attack" phase and the anti-inflammatory "rejuvenation" phase. In the first phase, your body wages an immunological battle, which generates pain, swelling, and redness. This attack phase is relatively well understood by medical researchers. The second phase, in which your body has to rejuvenate all the damage incurred during the immunological battle, is not as well understood. Yet, this second phase is the most fascinating part of inflammation because it holds the key to maintaining wellness.

The true key to wellness is to dampen down the pro-inflammatory phase in order to eliminate silent inflammation and simultaneously boost the anti-inflammatory rejuvenation phase to continuously renew the body. You can induce both of these actions by getting into the Anti-Inflammation Zone. Sounds too good to be true? Let's see how the science of inflammation backs up that concept.

IMMUNOLOGICAL LINK TO INFLAMMATION

Every army needs soldiers, and your immunological army is no different. The soldiers that are critical to the "attack" phase fall into five distinct battle groups; (1) chemical mediators, (2) complement systems, (3) eicosanoids, (4) cytokines, and (5) immunological attack cells. Like any good army, these soldiers are housed in their own barracks until called to action. Once they get the signal, they immediately launch into combat in an exceptionally coordinated way.

The first *chemical mediator* sent into battle is histamine. Histamine, which causes you to sneeze during allergy season, is a quick-acting alarm system to alert your other troops that an attack on the body has been launched. Its primary function is to dilate nearby blood vessels to trigger other immune soldiers into action and enable them to reach the site of injury quickly. It also stimulates immediate defensive measures, such as contracting the airways in the lungs and increasing the secretion of mucus from your nose.

A lot of things can activate histamine release other than ragweed. Here is a short list:

- Bacterial toxins
- Heat
- UV radiation
- Trauma
- Proteolytic enzymes released from invading or damaged cells
- Allergens

Regardless of the trigger, histamine is released and then is quickly inactivated by the body. Other initial inflammatory mediators, such as serotonin and bradykinin, work alongside histamine and activate what is known as the *complement system.* This system is extremely complex and made up of twenty proteins that, when activated by the chemical mediators, act to amplify the signals to the rest of your immunological army to be ready for action. The proteins of the complement system get to the injured site through the vasodilating action of histamine on the vascular lining of the site of the attack.

THE ROLE OF "BAD" EICOSANOIDS

Once these complement system proteins get to the site, the key players, *eicosanoids,* now enter the battlefield. They have the real job of opening the blood vessels to let the battleships (immunological cells) onto the battlefield. Pro-inflammatory "bad" eicosanoids (prostaglandins) are released into battle to increase vascular permeability, cause fever (heat is a great way to kill invaders), and trigger noticeable pain. Other pro-inflammatory eicosanoids (leukotrienes) further increase the permeability of the blood vessels (giving rise to swelling) and also put down chemical signals, like flares, to the immunological cells to reveal the enemy's location. Like histamines, leukotrienes also cause bronchial constriction and mucus secretion, but they are a thousand times more powerful. Thus, each step of the inflammation cascade ups the ante.

The increase in the vascular permeability induced by pro-inflammatory eicosanoids explains why inflammation induces swelling. It also explains the redness and heat associated with inflammation, which are both due to increased blood flow. So now you know what causes three (swelling, redness, and heat) of the four classical signs of inflammation. But what about pain? Where does that come from?

Not surprisingly, pain is also triggered by eicosanoids. (That's how anti-inflammatory drugs relieve pain—by reducing the production of "bad" eicosanoids.) Pain is a necessary warning signal to you that you need to protect the injured part of the body by immobilizing or resting it. But how does the information get from the site of trouble to the brain?

First, the swelling of the tissue itself is enough to touch off surrounding nerve endings. This is especially true in spaces that have a very limited ability to expand, such as the area under a fingernail or in the teeth gums. (Now you know why torture techniques such as driving bamboo slivers under fingernails or drilling teeth without anesthetics work so well.) Just to make sure your brain gets the message, the same pro-inflammatory eicosanoids that promote swelling also increase the sensitivity of the nerve fibers. The medical term for this increased sensitivity to pain is *hyperalgesia*. But all you really care about is that it hurts.

Note: I'm talking here about inflammation that causes screaming pain, not silent inflammation. The inflammatory process, however, is pretty similar in both classic inflammation and silent inflammation. The real difference is simply intensity. In silent inflammation, the output of pro-inflammatory eicosanoids is below the threshold of pain perception. The end result is that you don't get the warning signal and therefore don't respond as you would if you had screaming pain. Thus, the pro-inflammatory attack phase relentlessly continues with silent inflammation.

THE ROLE OF IMMUNE CELLS

Once pro-inflammatory eicosanoids hit the battlefield to open the vascular wall, the heavy hitters come into action: the *immune cells*. These white blood cells (macrophages and neutrophils) are activated for battle when they receive a signal from pro-inflammatory *cytokines,* whose release is stimulated by the pro-inflammatory eicosanoids. The pro-inflammatory cytokines also help you conserve energy for the upcoming battle by depressing your appetite (it takes energy to digest food) and increasing your need for sleep. They also cause the release of other inflammatory proteins that can help in the final battle, including our old friend C-reactive protein. This is how C-reactive protein is associated with inflammation, but at a stage that is much further down the line from the initial stimulus caused by the production of pro-inflammatory eicosanoids.

After they are activated by the cytokines, immune cells have to squeeze through the blood vessels onto the battlefield. (This is made easier by the actions of pro-inflammatory eicosanoids, such as leukotrienes.) Once at the target site, the white blood cells begin their attack by first attaching to the offending target, then engulfing it, killing it, and digesting the remains of the vanquished enemy. No remains are left behind. (Immunological war can be hell.)

Your white blood cells also employ free radicals to kill target cells, but, unfortunately, this form of destruction is nonspecific. It kills nearby healthy cells as well as the offending targets. Antioxidants, which fight free radicals, can help prevent damage to these healthy cells. Too many antioxidants, however, can reduce the ability of the white cells to destroy the alien invaders. This is why taking high levels of antioxidant supplements can lead to a suppressed immune system. You want enough antioxidants to control free radicals but not enough to wipe them all out—a tricky proposition. This is why I'm not a strong advocate for megadoses of antioxidant supplements. Anti-inflammatory nutrients (such as fish oil, sesame oil, and extra-virgin olive oil) are far more beneficial because they modulate the initial inflammatory response without compromising the ability of your white cells to launch an all-out free radical attack when required.

You should now be able to see how pro-inflammatory eicosanoids orchestrate your initial inflammation response. Constant inflammation due to microbial invaders is a surefire way to accelerate the aging process. This is why great advances in longevity in the last century have come not from pharmaceuticals, but from improved public health practices (like clean water) that decrease the constant microbial assault on our bodies.

Unfortunately, this improvement in public health has little effect on silent inflammation. This low-level inflammation is caused by an inflammatory response that was never completely turned off. It just occurs at a slower pace and lower intensity that is below the threshold of pain but still causes you to develop chronic diseases at an earlier age. We might live longer than people did in the past, but our quality of life is not as great as it could be. But what if that same inflammatory process can be harnessed to improve the way the body repairs itself? Could this turn back the clock on aging?

HOW INFLAMMATION HEALS

Here's where the second "rejuvenation" phase of the inflammatory process comes in. This phase of the inflammation process can be considered to be true anti-inflammation. Whereas pro-inflammation degrades the invaders and surrounding tissue, anti-inflammation heals and repairs the tissue. The balancing of these two parts of the inflammation response is the key to maintaining wellness.

At alternative medicine conferences, speakers often discuss unleashing the innate healing processes in the body. What they are really trying to describe is the second phase of the inflammatory process, the healing or rejuvenation phase. This process actually consists of four distinct stages: recall, resolution, regeneration, and repair. As you might expect, it is much easier to win a war than to repair and even enhance the battlefield after victory. If you can, then you are truly a remarkable general. The Zone Lifestyle Program is the battle plan for reaching the Anti-Inflammation Zone, and you are the commander of that healing process.

Recall

The recall phase starts with calling off the attack dogs, pro-inflammatory eicosanoids, which it launched to fight the battle. It does this by releasing cortisol, the hormonal fireman that douses the flames of "bad" eicosanoids. The trouble is, cortisol also shuts down the "good" anti-inflammatory eicosanoids, and so it also inhibits healing.

The release of cortisol is caused by the interaction of the pro-inflammatory cytokines with the brain that starts the cascade of hormonal responses that ends with increased production of cortisol from the adrenal glands. Unfortunately, unlike the precise location of inflammation, this newly secreted cortisol goes everywhere. Therefore the parts of the body that aren't affected by inflammation are now bathed in cortisol, which shuts down their normal eicosanoid production whether they like it or not.

Although cortisol is considered a stress hormone, it should really be viewed as an anti-stress hormone because it shuts down inflammation. The trouble is that when you have constant silent inflammation, cortisol is constantly being secreted. The result is that you become fatter (it increases insulin resistance), sicker (it decreases the inflammatory response), and dumber (it kills neural cells connected with memory in the brain). The dietary and lifestyle strategies in the Zone Lifestyle Program work together to decrease excess cortisol production by helping you reach the Anti-Inflammation Zone.

Resolution

Once the attack dogs are called off, your body still needs to remove any offending material from the battlefield. That is the job of a specialized group of white blood cells known as macrophages. Besides the debris from the alien invaders, the macrophages also digest dead cells that were under attack and any red blood cells that have leaked onto the battlefield. (It is the leakage and oxidation of hemoglobin from red blood cells that gives the purple discoloration to a bruise.) If the macrophages leave remnants behind, a constant inflammatory spark remains that can keep the inflammation process going, though at a lower intensity.

Regeneration

Once the battlefield is cleared, the vascular wall needs to be reestablished and then your body begins the regeneration of the damaged tissue. Success of the repair process is highly dependent on the type of cell that needs to be regenerated. If it's a type of cell that constantly multiplies (like a skin cell or a blood cell), then regeneration readily occurs. Cells that have a longer life span (like the endothelial cells that line the blood vessels) take longer to regenerate. Permanent cells like muscle cells (especially those of the heart) and nerve cells have extremely limited regenerative properties. Once you lose these cells to inflammatory damage, they are likely to be gone forever. This is why silent inflammation is so disastrous to the heart and the brain—organ function is permanently impaired.

Repair

The final phase of healing is the repair phase, in which new tissue is generated. This requires a careful balance of pro-inflammatory eicosanoids and anti-inflammatory eicosanoids.

Now that most of the pro-inflammatory eicosanoids are off the stage (thanks to cortisol), the real players in the repair phase are a group of anti-inflammatory eicosanoids known as lipoxins and resolvins. Lipoxins are far more powerful in reducing pro-inflammatory eicosanoids than cortisol and are far more selective because they don't shut down the "good" eicosanoids. However, another group of anti-inflammatory eicosanoids called epi-lipoxins may be even more powerful. As I discussed in the previous chapter, discoveries by Charlie Serhan of Harvard Medical School now suggest that aspirin also activates the formation of an entirely new class of eicosanoids known as aspirin-triggered lipoxins (ATLs). Thus, aspirin may work its magic not so much by inhibiting pro-inflammatory eicosanoids but perhaps by enhancing the production of powerful anti-inflammatory eicosanoids. The most powerful lipoxins produced by taking aspirin are called resolvins, which are made from long-chain omega-3 fatty acids like EPA and DHA. It is important to achieve the right balance of pro- and anti-inflammatory eicosanoids in this repair phase because this balance governs the amount of useless scar tissue that is formed. Scar tissue is repaired tissue that simply isn't put together correctly and ultimately impedes the tissue or organ function. If you have the right amount of anti-inflammatory eicosanoids, however, the repair process is orderly and the tissue is made stronger than before. In addition, the anti-inflammatory eicosanoids also cause the release of growth hormone and other hormones critical to the orderly rebuilding of new tissue. This is exactly what happens during weight training. Small micro-tears in the muscle fibers induce an initial pro-inflammatory response that finally ends in the repair phase. With the appropriate levels of anti-inflammatory eicosanoids, growth hormone, and other growth mediators, the tissue is not only repaired, but actually becomes stronger.

The healing phase of inflammation can work amazing wonders of rejuvenation to make your body stronger. Or it can fizzle out and do a half-hearted job of healing, leaving your body weaker. It all depends on the levels of anti-inflammatory eicosanoids. Being in the Anti-Inflammation Zone ensures that you have provided your immune system with all the tools it needs to dampen the pain coming from the attack phase of inflammation while enhancing the healing phase. Rather than degrading tissue and accelerating the aging process, you will constantly build new tissue. All of this slows the aging process. This is why I feel that anti-aging medicine should really be called anti-inflammation medicine.

How do you know if your body's healing processes are performing to the best of their abilities? Simply keep your SIP between 1.5 and 3. This is the key to getting inflammation to work in your favor instead of against you.

SUMMARY

Controlling both phases of inflammation is critical to maintaining wellness. The goal is to tip the balance toward cellular rejuvenation and away from the cellular degradation caused by silent inflammation. Being in the Anti-Inflammation Zone is your best indicator that you have done everything possible to achieve that goal.

The Obesity-Diabetes-Silent Inflammation Connection

Obesity is one of the biggest generators of silent inflammation. Since nearly two-thirds of Americans are now overweight, this means that the epidemic of silent inflammation is also out of control. By the same token, our diabetes epidemic has grown by 33 percent in the last decade. It should come as no surprise that all three epidemics have worsened in recent years. All three are intricately connected with a condition known as insulin resistance.

Insulin resistance occurs when your cells become less responsive to the actions of insulin, forcing your pancreas to continuously produce more insulin to drive glucose into cells. This excess insulin (produced as that response to insulin resistance) also increases the storage of body fat. So the real question behind our current obesity epidemic is what actually causes insulin resistance?

No one knows for sure, but there is a growing opinion that the molecular cause of insulin resistance may originate in the endothelial cells. Endothelial cells form a very thin barrier that separates the bloodstream from your organs. If this barrier is not working very well, you have a condition called endothelial dysfunction, which means among other things that insulin can no longer easily pass from the bloodstream through the endothelial barrier to interact with its receptors on the cell surface. It's only when insulin interacts with these receptors that the cell can take up glucose from the bloodstream. Any difficulty insulin has in getting to its receptors will keep blood glucose levels elevated. The body responds by pumping out still more insulin, now creating a condition known as hyperinsulinemia.

So now the question actually becomes, what causes endothelial dysfunction? I believe the most likely answer is silent inflammation. It is known that endothelial cell dysfunction is highly associated with increased silent inflammation. So what comes first—insulin resistance or silent inflammation? An intriguing study done at Louisiana State University recently demonstrated that consuming 1.8 grams of pure DHA per day for twelve weeks decreased the insulin resistance in overweight patients by 70 percent. To get the same amount of DHA used in this study, you would need to consume about about a tablespoon of an ultra-refined EPA/DHA concentrate per day.

To test the hypothesis that silent inflammation precedes insulin resistance, I ran a small pilot study with children who have pediatric obesity. The children were randomized into two groups. All the children had a very high SIP (about 30), as might be expected. Both groups got exactly the same dietary counseling on the Zone Diet. The only difference was that one group also got high-dose fish oil (3 grams per day of EPA and DHA). If silent inflammation was the primary cause of insulin resistance, then the group who got the Zone Diet counseling and the high-dose fish oil should have done much better in weight loss than the group that got only the Zone Diet. This is exactly what happened. As their SIPs dropped, so did their weight. This suggests that silent inflammation may be the underlying cause of insulin resistance and therefore obesity. This also means that unless you treat the underlying silent inflammation, trying to lose excess body fat is going to be very difficult, as many Americans already know so well.

OBESITY FROM A DIFFERENT VIEW

What if the epidemic rise in obesity in the last twenty years were not primarily due to the usual suspects (fast food, TV, junk food), but fueled by increased silent inflammation, which increases insulin resistance? This means that unless you reduce the underlying silent inflammation, any other approach to reduce obesity may be doomed to failure. This also means that simply restricting calories will not be enough to turn back our current obesity epidemic.

I believe that obesity starts with excess arachidonic acid (AA). You can increase AA in the bloodstream either directly by eating too much of it (it's particularly high in fatty red meats and egg yolks) or indirectly by consuming too many high glycemic-load carbohydrates, which increase insulin production, which in turn promotes increased AA production. Either way, the body goes to great lengths to take any excess AA out of the circulation and store it away in your fat depots in an effort to keep inflammation under control.

Here is where the trouble starts, because fat cells aren't simply inert balls of lard sitting on our stomach, thighs, and hips. These cells are very active glands that can secrete out large amounts of inflammation mediators if they're given the right stimulus. As your fat cells become filled with more AA, it causes an overproduction of pro-inflammatory eicosanoids in the adipose (fatty) tissue. Now you can probably guess what happens. These "bad" eicosanoids induce the formation of new inflammatory mediators that spew forth from fat cells into the surrounding circulation and generate systemic silent inflammation.

Now before you start cursing all your fat, I want to emphasize that all fat is not equal. Some types of fat are far more harmful than others. It depends on their metabolic activity. Subcutaneous fat, the fat that collects on your hips, thighs, and buttocks and makes you look like a pear, isn't that harmful. It may not look too good, but at least it won't kill you, because your body is in no rush to mobilize the AA out of these fat cells. That's why this type of fat is considered metabolically inactive. It is primarily a storage depot.

On the other hand, visceral fat can be a killer. This kind of fat collects around the abdominal organs, such as the liver, kidneys, and gallbladder and makes you look like an apple.

WHEN IS AN APPLE REALLY AN APPLE?

You may think that the easiest way to see if you have visceral fat is to look at yourself in a mirror. But this may be deceptive, because visceral fat is often found in close contact with subcutaneous fat in the abdominal region. The real indication of the amount of your abdominal fat that is actually visceral fat is measured by either your TG/HDL ratio or your fasting insulin levels. If both biomarkers are in the Anti-Inflammation Zone, then even if you look like an apple, you have relatively low levels of visceral fat.

Visceral fat is very metabolically active and causes the constant release of stored AA into the bloodstream. This is the last place you want excess AA, since it's then taken up by every one of your 60 trillion cells, making each one more likely to generate more pro-inflammatory eicosanoids, and therefore more silent inflammation throughout the body.

Visceral fat is even more insidious because it also continually releases other inflammatory mediators in addition to stored AA. Two of the worst are the pro-inflammatory cytokines, tumor necrosis factor (TNF), and interleukin-6 (IL-6). TNF is implicated in creating even more insulin resistance, whereas IL-6 triggers the liver to synthesize C-reactive protein (CRP), which can stimulate your white blood cells to begin to mount an inflammatory response to a potential infection (even though there isn't one). This means the release of even more inflammatory mediators, as discussed in chapter 13. About a third of the CRP circulating in your blood came directly from visceral fat cells. These pro-inflammatory cytokines are produced in your visceral fat as a response the increased pro-inflammatory eicosanoid production caused by increased AA levels.

This means the fatter you are (really, the more visceral fat you have), the more silent inflammation you generate. This is the smoking gun that links obesity with increased risk of heart disease, cancer, or Alzheimer's. Anything that increases silent inflammation is going to be bad for your future.

CAN YOU BE FAT AND HEALTHY?

Surprisingly, the answer is yes—but with a few caveats. You can be overweight and in a state of wellness if you keep your levels of silent inflammation under control. Since obesity generates inflammation, you may have to take more fish oil than the average person to reverse the silent inflammation induced by it. While losing weight is slow and hard, reducing silent inflammation using high-dose fish oil is rapid. How much fish oil do you need? This depends on your diet. If you are following the Zone Diet, you might need to take only 5 grams of EPA and DHA per day. If you follow the typical American (very high glycemic-load) diet, you'll need to increase your dosage of fish oil to a higher level.

Remember, all the medical complications of obesity come from the inflammation it generates. High-dose fish oil is an immediate antidote to that inflammation. Keep in mind being fat and healthy can be a dangerous game to play. It's a little like lighting a cigarette with a stick of dynamite. You can do it, but you have to be very careful. The day you stop taking adequate levels of fish oil is the day your silent inflammation will return, accelerating you toward chronic disease and faster aging. As long as you keep your SIP under control, the likelihood of maintaining your wellness is pretty good in spite of your weight.

The one-two punch of silent inflammation and increased hyperinsulinemia caused by insulin resistance if left unchecked can lead to one of the most costly of chronic diseases: diabetes.

THE DIABETES CONNECTION

Diabetes used to be a very rare disease, but times have changed. Over the last twenty years, it has become an epidemic. Let me clarify this.

Type 2 (adult-onset) diabetes has become an epidemic, while type 1 (juvenile) diabetes still remains relatively rare. Type 1 diabetes is caused by a condition in which the pancreas completely shuts down and fails to produce any insulin, causing blood sugar levels to spiral upward out of control. The more common type 2 (90 percent of all diabetics have this version) occurs when the patient develops long-term insulin resistance. As I mentioned above, insulin resistance causes the pancreas to secrete more insulin (hyperinsulinemia) in an effort to reduce blood glucose levels. Eventually, the pancreas (really the beta cells in the pancreas) just get tired and stop producing enough excess insulin. This is called beta-cell burnout. The result is that without enough insulin becoming secreted by the pancreas, blood glucose levels begin to raise to dangerous levels. The danger comes from two factors: (a) excess glucose in the blood produces free radicals (oxidative stress), and (b) excess glucose is neurotoxic to the brain. Hyperinsulinemia usually precedes the development of type 2 diabetes by about eight years, but they both come from increased insulin resistance. Starting to see the connection?

Obviously, not everyone who has insulin resistance becomes a type 2 diabetic. However, enough do—there are an estimated 16 million Americans afflicted with type 2 diabetes. This devastating disease puts a person at a two to four times greater risk of dying from heart disease and also increases the likelihood of kidney failure, blindness, impotence, and amputation. Because of these complications, type 2 diabetes is the most expensive of all chronic diseases, costing approximately $132 billion per year. As our obesity epidemic increases, so will the epidemic of type 2 diabetes. That's very bad news for the health care industry.

The good news is that taking high-dose fish oil to reduce silent inflammation (the molecular cause of insulin resistance) and following the Zone Diet will help reduce hyperinsulinemia (the consequence of insulin resistance) and begin to reverse type 2 diabetes in just six weeks.

Both of these seemingly simple solutions are fighting words to the American Diabetes Association (ADA). They've spent the last thirty years instructing diabetics to lose weight by eating less fat and consuming more carbohydrates. This has only caused a greater rise in insulin levels, leading to more weight gain and an even greater insulin output. In fact, even today the ADA still does not recognize the importance of the glycemic load as the determining factor in insulin output.

Recent research at the University of Minnesota has confirmed my contention that a low glycemic-load diet, such as the Zone Diet, is superior to the dietary recommendations of the ADA. In this study researchers put type 2 diabetics on either the Zone Diet or the ADA diet for five weeks, and then the patients were switched to the other diet for another five weeks. When the type 2 diabetics were on the Zone Diet, they had significant reductions in both blood glucose and glycosylated hemoglobin levels compared to the time they were on the ADA diet. The drop in these blood markers indicated that insulin resistance was being reduced on the Zone Diet compared to the ADA diet. To ensure that there was no confusion caused by the role of weight loss, the number of calories consumed in both diets was kept high enough to ensure that no weight loss was observed. This is another strong suggestion that insulin resistance (and therefore silent inflammation) can be reduced without losing any weight.

CAN FISH OIL REVERSE TYPE 2 DIABETES?

Published research indicates that the Zone Diet has superior effects on type 2 diabetic patients compared to the usual dietary recommendations of the ADA. But, unfortunately, that study did not include fish oil. After all, diabetes (like heart disease and depression) is virtually absent in Greenland Eskimos, who eat the most EPA and DHA of anyone in the world. Unfortunately, studies on fish oil alone and type 2 diabetes have had mixed results. A recent analysis of some twenty clinical trials with diabetics came to the conclusion that fish oil consumption has no effect—positive or negative—on blood sugar levels. Hardly a resounding triumph for fish oil. None of these studies, however, looked at the combination of the Zone Diet and fish oil. In theory, the combination of the two should be very successful.

I had the opportunity to test this hypothesis several years ago with Princeton Medical Resources, a health maintenance organization (HMO) in San Antonio. George Rapier, the owner of the HMO, approached me to see if I could help them cut health care expenses. Since type 2 diabetic patients generate the highest medical costs because of long-term complications, anything that can alleviate the condition goes right to the bottom line of the HMO.

The year before George approached me, he had brought in dietary educators trained by the ADA to counsel 400 of his more than 4,000 diabetic patients. These patients dutifully followed the recommendations outlined in their personalized meal plans provided by these ADA educators. After a year, Rapier found that his health costs for these 400 patients had increased by another $1 million!

Needless to say, George was driven to find a more effective solution. He called me after reading my first book, *The Zone,* and losing twenty-five pounds himself on the diet. He asked if I was willing to work with some of his patients but told me I had to keep the program very simple, because most of his patients had only a sixth-grade education and English was not their first language. Using only the hand-eye method that I described earlier and supplying 1.6 grams a day of EPA and DHA (I didn't have the ultra-refined EPA/DHA concentrates at that time), I put together a simple dietary education program for sixty-eight type 2 diabetic patients. After six weeks of following my dietary program, here were their results:

BLOOD TEST	START	6 WEEKS	% CHANGE	SIGNIFICANCE
Insulin	28	21	−23	< 0.0001
TG/HDL	4.2	3.1	−26	< 0.0001
HbA$_{1c}$	7.8	7.3	−7	< 0.0001
Fat Mass	72	70	−3	< 0.0001

Not only did every parameter associated with type 2 diabetes decrease, but they decreased by extraordinary amounts. The two parameters that changed the most were those markers (insulin and the TG/HDL ratio) I use to define the Anti-Inflammation Zone. Although the values were still far from optimal after six weeks, their declines were equal to that of any drug. Other markers of diabetes were similarly reduced. For example, glycosylated hemoglobin (HbA$_{1c}$) is one of the best indicators of long-term complications in type 2 diabetics. If it is below 7.3, then many of the adverse consequences (kidney failure, amputation, and blindness) simply don't occur. Finally, these diabetic patients lost excess body fat, which is exceptionally difficult because of their hyperinsulinemia.

I also want to note that the decline in each of those blood values had a very high degree of statistical significance. Statistical significance is an indication of how likely it is you will get the same results if you repeat the same experiment. The lower the number, the more likely the results can be repeated again. In this case, the statistics indicated that if the same dietary experiment were done 10,000 times, you would observe the same results 9,999 times.

As excited as I was by the results of this experiment, I know now that these results could have been even better if I had used higher levels of fish oil (about 5 grams of EPA and DHA per day). This is because insulin resistance appears to be mediated by an increase in TNF levels. The one proven way to decrease the secretion of TNF in the body is through the use of high-dose fish oil. This in turn decreases insulin resistance, which in turn lowers insulin levels. Once insulin levels are lowered, your body can finally access its own stored body fat for energy. In essence, it takes fat to burn fat, especially if that fat can reduce the release of TNF. That's what high-dose fish oil can do.

SUMMARY

If you want to reduce excess body fat or reverse type 2 diabetes, you have to reduce silent inflammation. The most important dietary tool you have for this is high-dose fish oil. The Zone Diet will also work, but at a slower pace. Combine the two and you have a powerful dietary approach to reverse the twin epidemics that threaten to destroy our health care system—obesity and diabetes.

Why Heart Disease Has Very Little to Do with Cholesterol but Everything to Do with Silent Inflammation

One of the best ways to live a longer and better life is to reduce your likelihood of dying from heart disease. If we could eliminate heart disease tomorrow, the average life expectancy of every American would increase by an estimated ten years. Although mortality from heart disease has decreased due to medical advances, the incidence of heart disease is on the rise. More of us are getting heart disease because we aren't doing enough to address the underlying cause: inflammation in the arteries. Like all silent inflammation, this arterial inflammation results from an increased production of "bad" eicosanoids. Rather than pinning your hopes on some new surgery or drug that may or may not be developed in the future, why not just avoid getting heart disease in the first place?

We are led to believe that elevated cholesterol is the cause of heart disease. As a result we have declared war on dietary cholesterol, and that has also meant a war on dietary fat. As I explained in the previous chapter, the result of that dietary approach has been an epidemic of obesity. That is why focus of the medical community has shifted to reducing blood cholesterol levels to the lowest levels possible. Not surprisingly, the most profitable drugs (statins) known to the pharmaceutical industry are the primary weapons in this continuing war. But what if cholesterol were only a minor, secondary player in heart disease?

Protecting yourself against heart disease requires far more than just simply lowering your cholesterol levels. In fact, 50 percent of the people who are hospitalized with heart attacks have normal cholesterol levels. What's more, 25 percent of people who develop premature heart attacks have no traditional risk factors at all. So if elevated cholesterol isn't the primary cause of heart disease, what is?

SILENT INFLAMMATION = BAD HEART

A heart attack is simply the death of the muscle cells in the heart due to a lack of oxygen caused by a constriction in blood flow. If this lack of oxygen is prolonged and enough heart muscle cells die, your heart attack becomes a fatal one.

There are several things that can cause the stoppage of oxygen flow to heart. A rupture could occur in a piece of unstable plaque lining the artery wall. This causes the activation of platelets, which clump together and block blood flow. You could have a spasm in the artery that blocks blood flow the to the heart. More often, it may be due to an electrical flutter, which disrupts the synchronized beating and causes the heart to stop functioning altogether. None of these heart attack causes has much to do with increased cholesterol levels, but they have everything to do with silent inflammation.

A variety of factors forge the linkage between silent inflammation and fatal heart attacks. First of all, pro-inflammatory eicosanoids inside an unstable plaque can trigger the inflammation that increases the likelihood of rupture. Often, these unstable plaques are so small that they can't be detected by conventional technology like an angiogram. When such a plaque bursts, cellular debris is released and platelets rush to the site in an attempt to repair the rupture, just as they would a wound. New blood clots formed from aggregated platelets may plug up the artery, stopping blood flow completely. This helps explain why many people do not die of heart attacks even though they have highly clogged arteries, whereas others do even though they have

CAN'T YOU JUST TAKE AN ASPIRIN A DAY?

Since inflammation is linked to heart disease, can't you just take a daily aspirin to fend it off and keep your heart healthy? After all, aspirin does a great job of reducing heart attacks. It has always been thought that aspirin works by thwarting the production of "bad" eicosanoids, such as thromboxane A_2, which sets into motion the aggregation of platelets leading to a clot.

Another reason aspirin is such a powerful weapon against heart attacks is that it may reduce the production of pro-inflammatory eicosanoids inside an existing unstable atherosclerotic plaque that would cause it to rupture in the first place. Unfortunately, aspirin can also cause death by internal bleeding. So it's by no means the ideal drug for long-term suppression of silent inflammation in the heart.

However, high-dose fish oil accomplishes the same anti-inflammatory effects of aspirin by going upstream to choke off the production of AA, which is needed to make pro-inflammatory eicosanoids in the first place. Recent studies have demonstrated that taking high-dose fish oil for only 45 days can remarkably reduce the levels of inflammation in unstable plaques, making them much less likely to rupture.

Charlie Serhan of Harvard Medical School may have found the ultimate solution to reducing inflammation in the heart. This links aspirin and fish oil and comes from his discovery of a new class of eicosanoids called aspirin-triggered epi-lipoxins. These new eicosanoids are the most powerful anti-inflammatory eicosanoids known. What's fascinating, though, is that the most powerful of these aspirin-triggered epi-lipoxins are made from EPA and DHA, the two fatty acids found in fish oil. What this means is that the more fish oil you consume, coupled with a low dose of aspirin, the greater your potential to make these newly discovered powerful anti-inflammatory epi-lipoxins. If you're at increased risk for heart disease, then taking low-dose aspirin plus high-dose fish oil may allow you to maximize production of powerful anti-inflammatory aspirin-triggered epi-lipoxins while at the same time reducing the levels of inflammation inside unstable plaques.

seemingly normal arteries. It all depends on the levels of inflammation in these small, unstable plaques.

These same pro-inflammatory eicosanoids are also the culprits behind vasospasm, the second cause of fatal heart attacks. Pro-inflammatory eicosanoids act as powerful constrictors of your arteries and can lead to a vasospasm, a potentially fatal cramp or "charley horse" that prevents blood flow to the heart.

As if all this weren't enough, lack of sufficient levels of long-chain omega-3 fatty acids in the heart muscle can also lead to a fatal heart attack caused by chaotic electric rhythms in the heart. This condition, called sudden death, accounts for more than 50 percent of all fatal heart attacks. In order to pump blood effectively, your heart muscle contracts and relaxes in a synchronized manner, which is controlled by an electrical current that depends on maintaining the levels of calcium on the outside of the heart cell membrane. The uncontrolled influx (caused by the lack of oxygen to the heart muscle cells) of these calcium ions can cause disruptions of the coordinated rhythmic contractions of the heart until it stops beating altogether. In animal studies, it has been shown that giving high doses of long-chain omega-3 fatty acids blocks the calcium channels in the heart cells and prevents this influx even if the heart cells are deprived of oxygen.

THE CHOLESTEROL MYTH

I am not saying that cholesterol has no role in heart disease, only that it is a secondary factor that plays a far lesser role in fatal heart attacks than silent inflammation. If your goal is to reduce the chances for a fatal heart attack, then it's far more important to decrease silent inflammation than to decrease cholesterol. So how did the importance of inflammation get lost, and how did hype over cholesterol get started? To answer that question, you have to go back nearly 150 years.

One of the greatest physicians in the nineteenth century was

Rudolf Virchow. Nearly 150 years ago, he stated that atherosclerosis is an inflammatory disease based on his observations of autopsies of the very rare number of people who had actually died of a heart attack. At the turn of the twentieth century, the greatest physician in America was Sir William Osler. When asked why he didn't include a chapter on heart disease in his classic textbook of medicine, he replied the disease is so rare that most physicians would never see it. However, all this began to change.

In 1913, studies by a Russian scientist demonstrated that feeding a large amount of cholesterol to rabbits induced atherosclerotic lesions. As a result of this experiment, physicians began to believe that dietary cholesterol might be the primary cause of heart disease. Unfortunately, further studies found that dietary cholesterol induced atherosclerosis in rabbits because it depressed thyroid function. If thyroid extracts were given at the same time as the dietary cholesterol, then there was no damage to the arteries. What's more, studies in primates suggested that a high-cholesterol diet only led to accelerated lesions on the arteries if the arteries were significantly inflamed in the first place. Although these findings should have put a damper on the primacy of the cholesterol connection causing heart disease, this was not the case.

The major problem of heart disease research is cause versus correlation. While you may have a *correlation* between something in the blood and heart disease, that doesn't necessarily mean that the same clinical marker is the actual *cause* of heart disease. As an example, there might be a correlation between being struck by lightning and the phase of the moon. However, this doesn't mean that the phase of the moon causes you to get hit by lighting. Today there are more than 200 risk factors that are correlated with heart disease. Does each of the risk factors cause heart disease, or are they simply a secondary occurrence once the real cause of heart disease has begun its damage? For something to truly be a cause, the amount of mortality from heart disease must increase or decrease every time that particular factor changes. On the other hand, if a risk factor has a spotty record in predicting cardiovascular mortality, then it is a secondary risk factor that comes along for the ride. Let's look at some of the cholesterol myths that have become so ingrained in our medical thinking. We have been told that one of the risk factors that causes heart disease morality is a high intake of fats. The other risk factor is supposedly high serum cholesterol.

The High-Fat Diet Myth

Epidemiological studies in the 1950s suggested that populations who ate the highest-fat diets had the highest risk of dying from heart disease. The trouble is, the researchers disregarded populations throughout the world (like the Masai in Africa, the people of Crete in the Mediterranean, and the Greenland Eskimos) who had extremely high-fat diets (much higher than the typical American's) but who had extremely low rates of heart disease. This was especially true of the Masai and Eskimos, who also eat a high-cholesterol diet. These were simply unsightly facts that were ruining a great theory. Therefore, these populations were conveniently ignored.

However, this mythology led to the endorsement of low-fat (and high glycemic-load) diets, like the USDA Food Pyramid, that have caused our current epidemic of obesity and type 2 diabetes. This in turn has increased our levels of silent inflammation in the population.

The High Serum Cholesterol Myth

Physicians used to think that we only had to worry about our total cholesterol levels. Then research found that this wasn't such a strong predictor of heart disease. The fact that the most important drug (aspirin) to prevent heart attacks had no effect on reducing cholesterol (but it does a great job of reducing inflammation) was not going to get in the way of the great story on the benefits of lowering serum cholesterol levels as much as possible. Today lowering cholesterol is the number-one priority of every cardiologist in America.

I challenge the Holy Grail of cardiology that high serum cholesterol is the cause of cardiovascular mortality for one reason only: the data. Various epidemiological studies have found that increased serum cholesterol levels occurred more often in heart disease patients. But that increase was 5 to 10 percent higher in those who developed heart disease than those who didn't. To show how small this difference is, 38 percent of the heart disease–free patients in the Framingham study had a total cholesterol level of 220 mg/dl or less, whereas 32 percent of patients with heart disease had a total cholesterol level of 220 mg/dl or less. Further analysis of the same data indicated that high total cholesterol levels after age forty-seven appeared to have no impact on cardiovascular death. The MONICA study in Europe confirmed this lack of linkage between high cholesterol and death from heart attacks. In France, subjects with cholesterol levels of around 240 mg/dl had only one-fifth the number of fatal heart attacks as subjects in Finland who had the same cholesterol levels. This is called the French Paradox. Really, though, it's only a paradox if you choose to believe that total serum cholesterol is the primary cause of death from heart disease.

As heart disease researchers found their serum cholesterol links getting weaker and weaker, they came up with more complex scenarios. Since total cholesterol was not found to be very predicative of cardiovascular death, then perhaps an individual component of total cholesterol was responsible. The "bad" cholesterol, found in the low-density lipoprotein (LDL) particles, was now the prime culprit. This launched a new war against "bad" cholesterol.

The story of "bad" cholesterol got even more complex as researchers discovered two types of LDL particles. One type consists of large, fluffy LDL particles (*good* "bad" cholesterol) that appear to have little potential to cause the development of plaques on the arteries. The other type consists of small, dense LDL particles (*bad* "bad" cholesterol) that are strongly associated with an increased risk of heart disease. So now you can have both *good* "bad" cholesterol (large fluffy LDL particles) and *bad* "bad" cholesterol (small dense LDL). Getting confused? Well, so is everyone else fighting the cholesterol wars, because we now know that the more *bad* "bad" cholesterol you have, the more likely you are to have a heart attack, while having a high level of the *good* "bad" cholesterol isn't likely to have any adverse health effects.

You very easily can identify whether you have the *bad* "bad" cholesterol or the *good* "bad" cholesterol. All you need to do is determine your ratio of triglycerides (TGs) to HDL cholesterol (TG/HDL), which would be listed on the results of your last fasting cholesterol screening. If your ratio is less than 2, you have predominantly large, fluffy LDL particles that are not going to do you much harm. If your ratio is greater than 4, you have a lot of small, dense LDL particles that can accelerate the development of atherosclerotic plaques, regardless of your total cholesterol levels or even total LDL levels. This is why the TG/HDL level is one of the blood markers I suggest to determine whether or not you are in the Anti-Inflammation Zone, whereas total cholesterol and total LDL cholesterol levels are not.

The connection between the TG/HDL ratio and heart attacks was confirmed by studies from Harvard Medical School. This research found that the higher your TG/HDL ratio, the higher your risk of having a heart attack. How much more likely? In that study, those with the highest TG/HDL ratio had sixteen times the risk compared to those with the lowest ratio. That's a huge increase in risk for the most common cause of death!

Just to put this into perspective, look at how other heart attack risk factors stack up in the chart below.

RELATIVE RISK OF HAVING A HEART ATTACK

RISK FACTOR	RELATIVE RISK (X = TIMES GREATER RISK)
Healthy with no risk factors	1 (No increase in risk)
High total cholesterol level (over 200)	2
Smoking (1 pack per day)	4
Elevated TG/HDL ratio (over 7)	16

After looking at this chart, you should be wondering why we haven't declared a national war against elevated TG/HDL levels. A high TG/HDL ratio does far more than increase your risk of heart disease. It is a marker of a metabolic syndrome, which indicates that you are developing insulin resistance. Insulin resistance leads to obesity, type 2 diabetes, and eventually to accelerated heart disease. As your TG/HDL ratio increases, this means that your insulin resistance is also increasing. The consequence of increased insulin levels means that your body is churning out far too much AA. The more AA you produce, the more silent inflammation you generate.

The importance of the TG/HDL ratio can be seen from the recently published results of the ongoing Copenhagen Male Study. Researchers tracked healthy patients who had either a low TG/HDL ratio (less than 1.7) or a high TG/HDL ratio (greater than 6) to see who would develop heart disease. They were amazed to find that the patients with the low TG/HDL ratio who smoked, didn't exercise, and had hypertension and elevated levels of LDL cholesterol had about a 50 percent lower risk of developing heart disease than those who had a far better lifestyle but a higher TG/HDL ratio. This indicates that lowering your TG/HDL ratio may have a far greater impact on whether you develop heart disease than adopting these improved lifestyle factors. Does this mean you should smoke, stay sedentary, and not worry about your blood pressure or cholesterol levels? Not at all, but it does indicate that you need to significantly improve your efforts to lower your TG/HDL ratio if your goal is to reduce heart disease.

SHOULD YOU TAKE A CHOLESTEROL-LOWERING DRUG?

It's a common scenario: You are told by your doctor that you have high cholesterol and should take a medication to lower it. You might resist at first. After all, you feel fine. But then again, you don't want to die of a sudden heart attack, and practically everyone you know is on some cholesterol-lowering drug. So, what should you do?

Before you make a decision, you need to be armed with information. Cholesterol-lowering drugs manufactured in the 1970s and

1980s were found to only modestly, if ever, reduce death from heart attacks. More ominously they often increased all-cause mortality, which of course is not a good thing. Then in 1994, a new class of cholesterol-lowering drugs, called statins, was found to be far more effective at preventing heart attacks than other cholesterol-lowering drugs. Cardiovascular researchers were certain that those wonder drugs worked their magic by lowering "bad" cholesterol levels. (As a side note, lowering insulin also lowers "bad" cholesterol levels.)

As it turns out, statins probably don't work their magic by lowering cholesterol levels. They actually have a much broader spectrum of action than anyone ever anticipated. They work as crude anti-inflammatory agents by blocking the release of C-reactive protein (CRP) from the liver. Those patients with the highest levels of CRP (a crude marker for inflammation) had the greatest decline in heart disease mortality when they took statins. Statins actually aren't very good anti-inflammatory agents, since they don't reduce pro-inflammatory cytokines such as IL-6 that cause the production of CRP (which itself is not a very good biomarker for inflammation) in the first place; they just inhibit the release of CRP from the liver. They also appear to inhibit the Rho-gene, which mediates inflammatory responses. Thus, statins work to reduce heart attacks by reducing only certain types of inflammation, whereas high-dose fish oil reduces *all* types of inflammation because it decreases AA production. The statins' ability to reduce LDL cholesterol levels may be just a secondary factor in their reduction of heart disease mortality.

What's more, statins can cause a host of side effects, including memory loss, muscle weakness, liver damage, and increased risk of nerve damage (neuropathy). In fact, half of the patients stop taking statins within a year due to these side effects. However, there is another side effect of the statins that drug companies don't like to talk about. Statins also significantly increase the production of AA. This means that long-term use of statins will ultimately increase silent inflammation. In fact, one study indicated the number of patients who developed breast cancer (another disease caused by silent inflammation) was significantly greater in patients taking statins than those who got the placebo.

This is not exactly the type of data you want to hear, especially if you are going be taking these drugs for the rest of your life.

Do I recommend statins? Not unless you have followed every course of diet and lifestyle action outlined in this book, and you are still not in the Anti-Inflammation Zone as determined by your blood chemistry. If you do take a statin, then always supplement it with high-dose fish oil to reduce the inherent increase in AA production (and therefore silent inflammation) that these drugs will cause.

THE ANTI-INFLAMMATION ZONE AND CARDIOVASCULAR MORTALITY

By now, you should understand that the heart disease risks of high-fat diets and high serum cholesterol have been overblown, and that the real risk of silent inflammation has been downplayed. If you are concerned about dying from a heart attack, your first option should be getting to the Anti-Inflammation Zone.

When I first started my research thirty years ago, I wanted to see if I could change the expression of my own genes. My genes were programmed for early death from heart disease—something that occurred in my father, my uncles, and my grandfather. Obviously, I had a very strong personal interest in learning the real cause of heart disease. I didn't buy into the cholesterol theory, but the inflammation theory made sense to me. The result was the development of the concept of the Anti-Inflammation Zone, in which inflammation could be kept under lifelong control.

The best predictors of a future heart attack come from prospective studies that follow healthy people for a number of years to determine which ones go on to develop heart disease, and then try to figure out why. Because these are expensive trials, there are very few of them. But those that exist have concluded that cholesterol levels are, in fact, a relatively poor predictor of future heart attacks. In fact, the likelihood of future heart attacks has everything to do with excess levels of pro-inflammatory eicosanoids—which are exactly the hormones that can be modified by my dietary recommendations.

When I first wrote *The Zone,* I was strongly criticized for asserting that elevated insulin levels were a major factor in heart disease. (This is despite the fact that diabetics are known to be at greatly increased risk of heart disease.) I explained in that book that the reason why elevated insulin is such a risk factor is that it increased the production of AA thereby increasing inflammation.

If reducing inflammation is so powerful in reducing our death rate from heart attacks, the solution should be simple: add more fish oil to the diet to reduce silent inflammation. The case was made for this in epidemiological studies in the late 1970s that found that Greenland Eskimos had virtually no heart disease even though they consumed a high-fat diet, rich in cholesterol. Their diet, however, was extremely rich in long-chain omega-3 fatty acids such as EPA and DHA. On the other hand, the Japanese, who consume low-fat diets, also have very low rates of heart disease. However, the fat the Japanese do consume is very rich in EPA and DHA. The common thread is that both population groups have very low SIPs. It wasn't their dietary cholesterol levels or total fat intake that made a difference in lowering their heart disease risk, but their absence of silent inflammation due to diets rich in EPA and DHA.

The most definitive proof of fish oil's benefits was found in the results of the GISSI trial in which Italian heart disease patients who had already suffered a heart attack took about 1 gram per day of ultra-refined EPA and DHA concentrates. Compared to the group taking the placebo or just vitamin E capsules, those supplementing with the fish oil over a 3.5 year period had a 45 percent reduction in their risk of having a sudden fatal heart attack (caused by an electrical disruption), a 20 percent reduction in their risk of total cardiovascular mortality, and a 10 percent reduction in overall mortality. These reductions in mortality (the only clinical end point that really counts) were equal to any statin trial. Furthermore, the divergence in death rates began to appear within three months after the beginning of the experiment.

Of course, your overall diet plays a major role in reversing heart disease risk. Powerful evidence of this comes from the Lyon Diet Heart Study, which I mentioned earlier. In this study, heart attack survivors who followed a low glycemic-load diet (with very low levels of pro-inflammatory omega-6 fatty acids) experienced a 70 percent reduction in fatal heart attacks compared to those who followed a high glycemic-load diet (with high levels of pro-inflammatory omega-6 fatty acids). More striking, not a *single* sudden death (the primary cause of cardiovascular mortality from heart disease) occurred in the group with the low glycemic-load and low omega-6 fatty acid diet.

When the researchers looked to the blood of the two groups in the Lyon Diet Heart Study to see what could explain these remarkable differences in cardiovascular mortality, they found no differences in the cholesterol levels or LDL cholesterol levels. (So much for cholesterol causing fatal heart attacks.) The primary difference between the two groups was found in their SIPs. The SIP of the individuals in the low glycemic-load diet group was 6.1 compared to 9.0 in the high glycemic-load group. Thus, it appeared as if a 30 percent reduction in the SIP resulted in a greater than 70 percent reduction in fatal heart attacks. There is no drug known to medical science that can generate these clinical results. This is why I believe the SIP is by far the most powerful predictor of future heart disease.

As dramatic as the results of the Lyon Diet Heart Study were, I believe they could have been even better if a group of patients were put on the Zone Lifestyle Program that would have enabled them to reach the Anti-Inflammation Zone. None of the patients in the study were able to reach the optimal SIP of 1.5, which is similar to that found in the Japanese, who have the lowest rates of heart disease in the world. Likewise, the TG/HDL ratio (3.4) was still elevated in both groups in the study, which indicates that insulin levels hadn't been lowered enough and that both groups were still eating diets too rich in carbohydrates.

Thus, compared to the Lyon Diet Heart Study, I believe that the combination of the Zone Diet and high-dose fish oil would have produced far superior results. This dietary program would have lowered both the TG/HDL ratio and the SIP to levels consistent with being positioned squarely in the Anti-Inflammation Zone. Based on all the available evidence we have from prospective studies, these lowered blood levels would bring your risk of fatal heart disease down to even lower levels. This is shown in the table below.

Parameter	Lyon Diet High Glycemic- Load Diet Group	Lyon Diet Low Glycemic- Load Diet Group	Parameters for Anti-Inflammation Zone
Silent Inflammation Profile (SIP)	9.1	6.1	1.5
TG/HDL ratio	3.4	3.4	1
Risk for fatal heart attacks	1.0	0.3	?

Intervention diets to reduce cardiovascular mortality, like the GISSI study and Lyon Diet Heart Study, are long and costly, which is why so few are done. I would be remiss, though, if I didn't mention another dietary intervention study with cardiovascular patients. This one used a vegetarian, high glycemic-load diet coupled with exercise and stress reduction. The Lifestyle Study divided heart disease patients into two groups, giving one group a diet that followed the guidelines of the American Heart Association and giving the other a plan for a low-fat, high-carbohydrate vegetarian diet. Below are the results after five years:

Group	Starting TG/HDL	Ending TG/HDL	Number of Fatal Heart Attacks
Intervention (Vegetarian group)	5.7	6.7	2
Control (AHA group)	4.3	4.3	1

Unlike the Lyon Diet Heart Study and the GISSI study, researchers saw an *increase* in the number of fatal heart attacks. Exercising more and practicing stress reduction almost certainly wouldn't increase the number of fatal heart attacks, but an increase in the TG/HDL ratio would. Time and time again, researchers have found that people who go on these very low-fat, high glycemic-load diets often have a dangerous increase in their triglyceride levels. This is probably why the American Heart Association considers very low-fat, very high-carbohydrate diets still to be experimental, even though they've been around for twenty years and have been recommended to tens of thousands of cardiac patients as a "proven" way to fight heart disease. I think the results of the GISSI trial and the Lyon Diet Heart Study reveal otherwise. In fact, one of the few times the American Heart Association tended to agree with me was when a position statement was issued in a 1988 issue of *Circulation* on very low-fat diets in which it was stated:

> *Very low-fat diets in the short term increase triglyceride levels and decrease HDL cholesterol levels without yielding additional decreases in LDL cholesterol levels.*
>
> *For certain persons, i.e., those with hypertriglyceridemia or hyperinsulinemia, the elderly, or the very young, the potential for elevated triglycerides, decreased HDL cholesterol levels, or nutrient inadequacy must be considered.*
>
> *Because very low-fat diets represent a radical departure from current prudent dietary guidelines, such diets must be proved both advantageous and safe before national recommendations can be issued.*

Not exactly a glowing recommendation from the American Heart Association for very low-fat, high glycemic-load diets. Although I have my disagreements with the American Heart Association's dietary guidelines in general, at least we both have the same opinion about very low-fat diets.

SUMMARY

Reaching the Anti-Inflammation Zone is your best defense against dying from a heart attack. The fastest way to get there is by following the Zone Lifestyle Program. By controlling your level of silent inflammation, you can reduce your risk of dying of heart disease to being as rare as it was at the beginning of twentieth century.

Cancer and Silent Inflammation

Although we have a far greater risk of dying from heart disease than cancer, we tend to be far more fearful of cancer—or rather, more fearful of the harrowing treatments required to manage it. After spending some $30 billion on the war against cancer, our government hasn't made any headway into finding a reliable cure for the disease or a sure-fire way to prevent it. With all the hype, the primary treatments for cancer still remain the big three: burn, cut, or poison. Although these rather barbaric approaches can potentially extend a patient's life span, they're not an ideal prescription for a good quality of life.

Researchers, though, are now pinpointing ways to reduce cancer risk. They know that eating more fruits and vegetables protects against cancer. And they know that those who take anti-inflammatory drugs on a regular basis have a reduced risk. Animal studies also suggest that high-dose fish oil appears to retard or reverse a wide variety of tumors. What clues could these observations provide to help in the prevention of cancer? I think the answer lies in the reversal of silent inflammation.

For years it has been known diets rich in fruits and vegetables tend to reduce the risk of cancer. It has always been assumed it must be the phytochemicals within these carbohydrates that are the key. But there are thousands of phytochemicals, so how do you know which one to choose? Pharmaceutical companies have tried to isolate these nutrients and put them into pills to prevent cancer. They tried and failed with vitamins, as studies found an actual increase in lung tumors from the use of beta-carotene. That's because these phytochemicals are primarily antioxidants, and therefore are not going to have a lot of potential in reducing silent inflammation.

The same epidemiological data, however, can be interpreted in another way. By eating a lot of fruits and vegetables, you are replacing high glycemic-load carbohydrates with low glycemic-load carbohydrates. This decreases the excess production of insulin. Decreased insulin production reduces not only the accumulation of excess body fat (a potent stimulator of silent inflammation), but also reduces the activity of the enzyme D5D that increases the production of AA. In essence, by eating a lot of fruits and vegetables, you get a powerful bonus—namely, decreased AA production. This translates into decreased silent inflammation.

If inflammation is the underlying cause of the progression of cancer, then anti-inflammatory drugs (regardless of their side effects) should decrease the risk of cancer. And that's exactly what you find: in colon, breast, ovarian, and other cancers, the more anti-inflammatory drugs you take, the lower your incidence of cancer.

If anti-inflammatory drugs reduce the risk of cancer, what about anti-inflammatory fish oil? Indeed, numerous animal studies have shown that high-dose fish oil does a remarkable job of slowing the rate of tumor growth. Researchers have known for years that giving animals high levels of pro-inflammatory omega-6 fatty acids (such as corn oil) would significantly increase their cancer death rates when they had tumor cells implanted in their bodies. On the other hand, when these animals were given fish oil supplementation, their implanted tumors dramatically decreased in size, and the animals experienced longer life spans. This makes perfect sense. Those getting the pro-inflammatory omega-6 fatty acids were generating more "bad" eicosanoids, while those getting fish oil were making more "good" eicosanoids. In cancer, that eicosanoid balance can spell the difference between life and death.

Another anticancer benefit that comes from fish oil is its ability to alter the genetic machinery of the cancer cell itself. It turns out that high levels of fish oil can dramatically increase the production of certain proteins that dampen down the metastatic potential of prostate cancer cells. This begins to explain why studies have found that eating fish helps slow the metastatic spread of prostate cancer in Americans, and also why the Japanese (who eat huge amounts of fish) have very low rates of prostate cancer mortality.

WHAT IS THE REAL CAUSE OF CANCER?

No one really knows what causes a normal cell to start rapidly dividing and turn cancerous. No one knows why the immune system that usually destroys these stray cancer cells sometimes fails, allowing the cells to divide and grow into tumors. One explanation may be that an immune system already on overdrive from combating increased silent inflammation may simply fail to do its job properly. Here are some the main mechanisms of cancer growth and how inflammation is involved in each of these.

Metastasis

The biggest threat caused by cancer is usually not the primary tumor but the spread or metastasis of the tumor to other parts of the body. Metastases are aided by a group of "bad" eicosanoids called hydroxylated fatty acids. These eicosanoids, derived from AA, enable tumor cells that have been shed into the bloodstream to get a foothold in a distant site in the body. One particular hydroxylated fatty acid (12-HETE) is known to cause an expansion of the endothelial cells that line the vascular system, thus allowing the cancer cell to penetrate into an organ where it can grow into a tumor that is far distant from the original primary tumor. The best way to reduce the production of these hydroxylated fatty acids is the same way you reduce all "bad" eicosanoids—lower the levels of AA in cells. This can be achieved by lowering your SIP using high-dose fish oil.

Apoptosis

We often think of cancer of cells as growing uncontrollably, but another explanation is also possible. Maybe cancer cells are simply cells that have faulty internal time clocks that normally tell them when to die. Programmed cell death, or apoptosis, is vital for our functioning. If we didn't have apoptosis, we would have no way to continually remodel our bodies by replacing old cells with new ones.

For many years, researchers thought the cancer glass was half empty, meaning they thought of cancer as an out-of-control condition that caused madly dividing malignant cells that would live forever. How could they ever stop these immortal cells that reproduced with such reckless abandon? Now many researchers are beginning to see this glass as half full. They theorize that some tumor cells may simply be healthy cells that have forgotten when to die.

Several new anticancer drugs that are now being tested are designed to induce apoptosis. The trouble is, they induce this state in both normal and malignant cells, which often means severe side effects for the patient. There is, however, one remedy that appears to induce apoptosis only in tumor cells—high-dose fish oil. Fish oil can be an extremely effective supplement to make cancer cells more susceptible to apoptosis induced by chemotherapeutic drugs or radiation, while sparing normal cells from the devastating effects of current cancer treatments.

Angiogenesis

Tumors grow by diverting nutrients from the body to themselves. They sprout new blood vessels to gain access to these nutrients, a process called angiogenesis. The Holy Grail of cancer research is to find a compound that reduces this tumor-induced angiogenesis. Research has shown that leukotrienes, among the most powerful of the "bad" pro-inflammatory eicosanoids, actually promote angiogenesis. Since leukotrienes are derived from AA you can lower your levels of these eicosanoids by improving your SIP.

Cachexia

In end-stage cancer, one of the biggest threats patients face is wasting or cachexia. This rapid weight loss usually indicates that the end is near. Cachexia is hastened by increased levels of the pro-inflammatory cytokine known as tumor necrosis factor (TNF) in the bloodstream. Since fish oil is known to depress the release of TNF, supplementing the diet with high enough levels should reduce, if not reverse, weight loss and extend a patient's life span.

In fact, that is exactly what happens. In a study, when patients with cachexia were given high levels of long-chain omega-3 fatty acids each day, they actually gained weight, whereas the control patients continued to lose weight. Subsequent studies with patients having advanced pancreatic cancer have used doses as high as 18 grams of long-chain omega-3 fatty acids per day. In both studies, patients who took the fish oil survived far beyond what was predicted for their end-stage cancers.

THE INSULIN CONNECTION

As early as 1919, physicians were aware that blood glucose levels could predict the prognosis for a cancer patient: the higher the blood glucose level, the bleaker the prognosis. As you already know, insulin resistance causes elevated blood glucose. The reason high blood glucose levels are so predictive is that cancer cells grow best in an anaerobic environment, which means they need high levels of blood glucose. Furthermore, the insulin resistance that increases blood glucose levels also increases insulin levels. This excess insulin serves as a growth factor that further promotes cell division in tumor cells. So while excess blood glucose feeds tumor cells, excess insulin encourages them to divide. Finally, excess insulin promotes the synthesis of AA, the precursor for all pro-inflammatory eicosanoids. In fact, this may explain the epidemiological studies from Italy that found that those who followed diets rich in starches (like pasta) were at increased risk of cancer compared to those who had a lower glycemic-load diet. Insulin resistance and cancer are a deadly combination—one you don't want to have if you are diagnosed with cancer.

LIVING WELL WITH CANCER IN THE ANTI-INFLAMMATION ZONE

Unfortunately, no one is ever cured of cancer, any more than they are cured of heart disease or diabetes. You simply learn to live with the condition, knowing that at any time it may recur, especially if you alter your lifestyle in a negative way.

Being in the Anti-Inflammation Zone is your best insurance policy for living well with cancer. It's your best bet for avoiding a recurrence, because it creates conditions in your body in which cancer cells can't thrive. It deprives cancer cells of vital nutrients like excess glucose and thwarts their rapid division by reducing insulin levels. Most importantly, being in the Anti-Inflammation Zone decreases AA levels thereby cutting off their supply of "bad" eicosanoids that depress the immune system. As a result, cancer cells become more visible to your normal surveillance systems, and the likelihood of their destruction is increased.

I've seen how being in the Anti-Inflammation Zone works first-hand. I'd like to recount the story of Sam, who developed a particularly aggressive brain tumor as a teenager. Brain cancer is the most difficult of all cancers to treat, because anticancer drugs have a very hard time crossing the blood-brain barrier to reach the tumor. Even though Sam's parents took him to the world's premier children's cancer center, his prognosis was grim. He would need high-risk treatments, including high-dose radiation and high-dose chemotherapy, in order to have a shot at survival.

Sam's mother asked me if there was anything else she could do. I suggested a rigorous adherence to the Zone Diet and high-dose fish oil. Sam's SIP determined the amount of fish oil he needed. To get Sam into the Anti-Inflammation Zone required, he needed about 10 grams of an ultra-refined EPA/DHA concentrate on a daily basis.

During the course of the two-year treatment program, some remarkable things happened. First, Sam would get tired after a bout of radiation or chemotherapy, but not nearly as much as other kids getting the same treatment. In fact, he was the only patient who was able to continue school through these treatments. Moreover, unlike the other kids getting this treatment, Sam's white cell counts didn't decrease. In fact, they increased. Finally, after two years of treatments, Sam was pronounced "cured." But the medical staff asked if they could do some cognitive testing on Sam. Sam and his parents wondered why, since he earned high honors in his high school courses during the treatment, but they agreed to the testing. As might be expected, Sam's cognitive abilities were excellent. But the physicians were amazed, as they explained to Sam's parents, because he was the first child ever to go through their treatment program for this type of brain tumor who did not end up having significant neurological damage after being "cured" by their treatments. By the way, Sam was accepted at one of the most competitive colleges in America.

How was Sam able to achieve this unique distinction? Unlike cancer drugs, the high levels of EPA and DHA he was taking had no trouble getting across the blood-brain barrier into the brain. Once there, the higher levels of EPA and DHA increased the apoptosis of the cancer cells when exposed to the drugs and radiation, while simultaneously protecting the normal neural cells. The rigid control of his insulin levels by the Zone Diet further enhanced the anti-inflammatory actions of the high-dose fish oil.

The reason why reaching the Anti-Inflammation Zone is so important during cancer treatment is not to replace standard therapies, but to make them more effective and less toxic.

CAN YOU PREVENT CANCER?

If high-dose fish oil can reduce the devastating side effects of traditional cancer treatments, can it also reduce the likelihood of cancer?

We know that increased levels of COX-2 enzyme (which makes pro-inflammatory eicosanoids) are strongly associated with a great number of tumors. It has been shown that the levels of EPA and DHA in cells taken from breast and prostate cancer patients are lower than in cells from control group patients. Likewise, it is known that women who eat the highest amounts of fish are the least likely to develop breast cancer. These findings suggest that cancer prevention lies in controlling silent inflammation.

If you decrease the levels of AA in the tumor cells by increasing the levels of EPA and DHA, then you can counteract the effects of the increased expression of the COX-2 enzyme. This is because you are now choking off the substrate for the COX-2 enzyme. As a result, even with increased levels of the enzyme, it will have a greatly diminished ability to make pro-inflammatory eicosanoids, such as prostaglandin E$_2$ (PGE$_2$), that are highly associated with rapid tumor growth. PGE$_2$ acts essentially like a stealthy shield that hides the identity of the cancer cell so that your immune system can't recognize it as an abnormal cell. Cutting off PGE$_2$ production means that the cancer cell can no longer hide from immune cells and is left open to attack. Reducing silent inflammation by reducing AA also means cutting off the supply of other pro-inflammatory eicosanoids, such as leukotrienes, that are important in angiogenesis for the tumor. In essence, you'll be taking away the molecular tools cancer cells use to hide from the immune system, spread to and invade other sites in the body, and divert nutrients to them.

I firmly believe that an ounce of prevention (reducing silent inflammation) is worth a pound of cure (the devastating effects of chemotherapy). Sam was lucky in his outcome because he and his family were very proactive in taking steps beyond toxic drugs and radiation. Sam understands that his unique outcome happened because he was in the Anti-Inflammation Zone. He was able to boost his body's production of anti-inflammatory eicosanoids while simultaneously lowering the production of cancer-promoting pro-inflammatory eicosanoids—something that no chemotherapy drug could do.

SUMMARY

Cancer prevention is all about reducing silent inflammation. The first step is to control insulin by eating a lot of fruits and vegetables and cutting back on high glycemic-load carbohydrates. That is a good description of the Zone Diet. Next, take adequate amounts of ultra-refined EPA/DHA concentrates until your SIP is between 1.5 and 3. If you are being treated for cancer, then these same dietary strategies are imperative to reduce the inherent toxicity of the cancer treatments.

Of course, you can choose to do nothing and hope that the standard therapies of toxic drugs and radiation will kill only the tumor cells and leave all your healthy cells intact. But given that this is a highly unrealistic expectation, why set yourself up for nasty side effects of current cancer treatment? Take the saner approach—enter the Anti-Inflammation Zone.

Brain Drain Due to Silent Inflammation

The mind is the last frontier of medical science. Your brain contains thousands of unexplained mysteries. Researchers remain humbled by its complexities as they try to pinpoint the exact areas of the brain responsible for how you speak, experience love, learn to hate, and express creativity.

Because of the complexity of neurological function, your brain is very sensitive to silent inflammation. Since the brain has no pain receptors, silent inflammation could transform into full-blown inflammation (enough to cause pain in other parts of your body), and you would still never know it. That's what makes neurological disease so terrifying. You may have no idea your brain is under inflammatory attack until it's too late, and irreversible disease has set in. The dementia caused by Alzheimer's disease, for instance, currently cannot be reversed once the damage is done. New medications may be able to slow the progression of Alzheimer's but still can't return the brain to its normal functioning state.

Your best defense against the brain drain, therefore, is a strong offense. That means keeping silent inflammation under control on a lifetime basis. High-dose fish oil is your primary anti-inflammatory "drug." Unlike pharmaceuticals that have a difficult time crossing the blood-brain barrier, the long-chain omega-3 fatty acids in fish oil don't have that problem. In fact, 60 percent of your brain's dry weight is fat, and much of this comes from DHA, a critical component necessary for nerve conduction, visual fidelity, and energy production. This is why your grandmother may have referred to fish oil as "brain food."

If fish oil is so important, then isn't it possible that a lack of fish oil in the diet will compromise your brain function? Wouldn't you be more prone to neurological disease due to silent inflammation? The answer to both questions is a resounding yes!

Previous population studies have pointed to the fact that people who live in countries where fish consumption is very high (such as Japan) have the lowest rates in the world of neurological disorders like depression. Yet, the amount of fish oil in the American diet has been steadily decreasing over the past century. It is estimated that our consumption of EPA and DHA is only 5 percent of what it was 100 years ago. During the same time period we have had a dramatic dietary increase in pro-inflammatory omega-6 fats coming from vegetable oils. This fact coupled with a dramatic increase in our insulin levels should not make it too hard to figure out why our rates of neurological disease are skyrocketing. We simply have much more silent inflammation in our brains than we had in the past.

With the recent advent of ultra-refined EPA/DHA concentrates, we now have the ability to safely raise our levels of DHA and EPA in our brain. If we can raise these levels of anti-inflammatory fatty acids high enough, we should be able to lower our risk of developing mental disorders caused by silent inflammation. More important, we may finally have the power to reverse the effects of these conditions if they've already debilitated our mental function. So, this is really the defining moment for these new purified grades of fish oil. We now finally have a product that we can take in high enough amounts to combat silent inflammation in the brain. Just like elderly people who can regain their lost muscle mass by working out with weights, I believe people with brain disorders can regain their brain function by following my dietary recommendations to reach the Anti-Inflammation Zone.

ALZHEIMER'S DISEASE

Alzheimer's disease represents the greatest fear of aging—the brain giving out before the body does. An estimated 1 to 5 percent of Americans will develop Alzheimer's disease by age 65, and by age 85 a whopping 50 percent will have it. Furthermore, it is estimated that by the year 2040 our country will have ten times more beds in nursing homes than in hospitals. If you go to a nursing home (especially one that specializes in Alzheimer's patients), you might be glimpsing your future.

Unfortunately, there are currently no drugs that can reverse mild to moderate Alzheimer's. Even those drugs touted to slow the progression of the disease aren't that effective when tested in rare independent trials not funded by drug companies. The only shot we have against Alzheimer's is our knowledge that it is an inflammatory condition.

Alzheimer's disease is thought to result from the development of amyloid plaques in the brain, similar in many ways to the plaques that clog artery walls and eventually lead to heart attacks. In fact, people who have a genetic susceptibility to heart attacks also have a far higher risk of developing Alzheimer's. Thus, using one anti-inflammatory strategy to prevent both heart disease and Alzheimer's makes sense. In fact, Hippocrates stated this some 2,300 years ago when he said, "Whatever is good for the heart is probably good for the brain."

Since reducing inflammation is good for the heart, then reducing inflammation should also be good for the brain. Evidence suggests this to be the case. Epidemiological studies have shown that those who use anti-inflammatory drugs on a regular basis have a much lower incidence of Alzheimer's disease than the general population.

Of course, I don't recommend using NSAIDs on a permanent basis because of their side effects (see chapter 12 for details), but are there dietary ways to reduce the likelihood of developing Alzheimer's? Let's look at the science. Population studies have shown that people over 85 who eat the highest amount of fish have a 40 percent lesser risk of developing Alzheimer's than non–fish eaters. Autopsy studies of patients who died from Alzheimer's reveal that the brains of these patients with the disease contained 30 percent less DHA than the brains of patients who died of other causes. In data from the landmark Framingham Heart Study, those patients who had the lowest levels of long-chain omega-3 fatty acids in their blood had a 67 percent greater likelihood of developing Alzheimer's. What's more, supplementation with DHA seems to improve the cognitive function of Alzheimer's patients, according to one intervention study. Supplementation of DHA also helped reduce the rapid development of brain lesions in a mouse model genetically engineered to develop Alzheimer's.

More ominous is that those individuals who consume the most pro-inflammatory omega-6 fatty acids (the kind found in vegetable oils) have a 250 percent increase in the development of Alzheimer's. Remember, it is the overconsumption of these fatty acids that leads to an increase in AA formation. Thus, I don't have to stretch too far to theorize that making excess levels of pro-inflammatory eicosanoids probably increases your risk of Alzheimer's. I hypothesized that the SIP in Alzheimer's patients would be greater than in age-matched normal controls. This is exactly what was found in a study by Julie Conquer at the University of Guelph in Canada. The SIP of the Alzheimer's patients was nearly twice as high as the healthy controls. Thus, the SIP can be used to predict your risk of developing Alzheimer's in the future, and the sooner you know it, the better. In fact, recently published studies have found that middle-aged men who have a high level of C-reactive protein (a cruder marker of inflammation) are at a 300 percent increased risk of developing Alzheimer's twenty-five years later.

How much EPA and DHA do you need to take to reverse the inflammation that underlies Alzheimer's? If you're healthy, just take enough (about 2.5 grams a day) to get your SIP into the optimal range of 1.5 to 3. If you already have Alzheimer's, you are going to need a lot more fish oil to reverse the inflammatory effects. My studies in more than 300 patients indicate that a daily dose of 20 grams per day (which is equivalent to 3 tablespoons of ultra-refined EPA/DHA concentrates) is necessary to reduce the SIP in Alzheimer's patients. Why so much? It appears that people with Alzheimer's have an increased beta oxidation of omega-3 fatty acids, which dramatically lowers circulating blood levels of EPA and DHA. These fatty acids are being burned up as a source of energy instead of being stored in the tissues where they can render their anti-inflammatory properties. Therefore, to reach a steady state level in the blood so that the SIP is reduced to appropriate levels, very large oral doses of EPA/DHA concentrates are required.

Another key factor for treating (and also preventing) Alzheimer's is insulin control. It has been shown that neurons that display insulin resistance are potent stimulators of amyloid plaque production. High-dose fish oil and insulin control are the two primary ways to reduce the levels of the biomarkers that define the Anti-Inflammation Zone.

In the final analysis, maintaining yourself in the Anti-Inflammation Zone for a lifetime will be your best defense against this disease. To get there you have to take high dose fish oil (at a dose determined by periodic measurements of your SIP) and control insulin to keep silent inflammation from increasing. If you have the beginnings of Alzheimer's or a strong family history, my Zone Lifestyle Program will be your best medicine, if not your only hope.

MULTIPLE SCLEROSIS

Like Alzheimer's, multiple sclerosis (MS) has a strong link to inflammation. In MS, the insulating membrane that coats nerve cells unravels due to ongoing inflammation. This makes it difficult for nerve cells to transmit their signals. Although the molecular cause of MS is unknown, scientists all agree that it's a disease primarily driven by inflammation.

Like all inflammatory conditions, MS is characterized by an overproduction of pro-inflammatory eicosanoids. The current leading treatment is weekly injections of beta-interferon, which is thought to act as an anti-inflammatory cytokine. The thought behind this drug approach is that it will inhibit the synthesis of pro-inflammatory cytokines (like gamma-interferon), which will hopefully slow the progression of the disease. Unfortunately, this extremely expensive drug approach is successful only about one-third of the time. It's used because it seems to be the only medical intervention available to MS patients.

High-dose fish oil, however, may hold far more promise as a nonpharmaceutical intervention for these patients. Long-chain omega-3 fatty acids are anti-inflammatory agents that can cross the blood-brain barrier; what's more, MS patients are known to have low levels of DHA in their brains. It is also known that long-chain omega-3 fatty acids inhibit the production of pro-inflammatory cytokines like gamma-interferon (similar to the actions of beta-interferon). This may explain why populations that consume the most fish have the lowest rates of MS.

An intervention study on MS patients, however, is the only way to prove all these theories. Such a study was performed recently in Norway in which MS patients were given high-dose fish oil supplements every day for two years and told to consume three to four fish meals per week, decrease their consumption of red meat, and eat more fruits and vegetables. (This sounds a lot like the Zone Diet.)

By the end of the first year, the patients' average SIP had decreased from 6 to 1.5 (the level found in the Japanese population) and remained at this lowered level throughout the following year. The number of MS attacks that these patients experienced decreased by 90 percent in the first year. After two years, these patients' level of disability decreased by 25 percent, which means that they actually regained a significant amount of mobility. Since MS patients usually don't get better with time, these published results are quite striking and may represent the first evidence that MS can be at least partially reversed.

ATTENTION DEFICIT DISORDER

In recent years, attention deficit disorder (ADD) has received national attention as the condition has become an epidemic in the United States, afflicting an estimated 3 to 5 percent of our children. Although there are six different types of ADD, including attention deficit/hyperactivity disorder (ADHD), I have grouped them all together as ADD. One factor common to all ADD patients is a deficiency of the neurotransmitter dopamine. Drugs such as Ritalin, which increase dopamine production, are commonly prescribed to bring these conditions under control. Since high-dose fish oil also increases dopamine levels, it would make sense that it should help alleviate ADD, without the need for drugs.

Many of my insights into ADD have come from my associations with two colleagues, Ned Hallowell, one of the most respected leaders in the treatment of ADD in children, and Dan Amen, who did pioneering work with brain scans to identify different types of ADD by determining differences in blood flow to the brain (using a specialized imaging technique called SPECT). It appears that certain areas of the brain have an altered blood flow. Here's another interesting observation: the severity of ADD is directly linked to the level of silent inflammation in the blood, as measured by the SIP. Children with ADD have a much higher SIP than children who don't. Therefore, the problem of ADD is much more complicated than simply the lack of dopamine in the brain.

Currently, the treatment of ADD has focused on drugs, such as Ritalin, that increase the levels of dopamine. But what if this apparent lack of dopamine were a secondary symptom of increased silent inflammation? It is also known from animal experiments that long-chain omega-3 fatty acids also increase dopamine levels and the number of dopamine receptors in the brain. This would indicate that ADD may be more closely connected to a nutritional deficiency (lack of dietary EPA and DHA) than any underlying medical or psychological condition. This hypothesis correlates well with animal studies that indicate after three generations of deficiencies in the intake of omega-3 fatty acids that significant behavioral and cognitive defects appear in their offspring. Today's children represent the third generation of Americans who have been exposed to a dramatic decrease of long-chain omega-3 fatty acids in their diet. Initial published studies indicate that small amounts of EPA and DHA given to children with ADD resulted in a trend toward improved behavior. In my initial pilot studies of children with ADD, I often needed to give them up to 15 grams of EPA and DHA per day to bring their SIP to a measurement of 2. Once they reach that level, their behavioral disorders become controlled to the same extent as by taking Ritalin. But unlike Ritalin, which treats only the symptoms of ADD, high-dose fish oil appears to treat the underlying cause—silent inflammation.

The reason that children with ADD need so much EPA and DHA is that they probably have the same accelerated metabolism of omega-3 fatty acids as found in Alzheimer's patients. Recent data has confirmed this hypothesis in children with ADD. So, how do you get your child to take such a high dose of fish oil on a daily basis? Simple. Make them the Big Brain Shake, as described on page 84. They'll need two shakes a day to get the necessary amount of EPA and DHA to sufficiently reduce their SIP. By using the Big Brain Shakes, you also get the additional benefit of stabilizing blood glucose levels. Other suggestions to ease the consumption of fish oil are on pages 83–84. One major caveat: Once you reduce the fish oil intake, the SIP will probably increase again, and all the behavioral benefits quickly erode.

PARKINSON'S DISEASE

Parkinson's disease has similarities to both Alzheimer's and ADD. It is an inflammatory neurological condition in a specialized part of the brain (substantia nigra) that is characterized by the loss of dopamine. Parkinson's is one of the most feared neurological diseases, because you retain all of your mental faculties inside a body that no longer responds to your commands. In other words, your mind is trapped in an increasingly dysfunctional body.

Unfortunately, simply replacing dopamine in the brain by giving oral doses of dopamine is not as easy as you might think. Dr. Oliver Sacks's initial exciting results of giving dietary dopamine to his patients (who had extreme Parkinson-like symptoms, but not true Parkinson's disease) were recounted in the book (and movie) *Awakenings*. In a matter of weeks, people who had been immobile and unable to speak—trapped within frozen bodies like a living tomb—were able to move again and reenter the world. The side effects of this drug soon made it an unlikely choice for long-term chronic treatment. These side effects included uncontrolled tremors and new neurological problems.

Today, we hear of potential new treatments like the implantation of stem cells in the brain that, in theory, will grow into new nerve cells (and hopefully not become cancer cells). These advances, however, may be decades away even if they prove to be useful. I believe that a safer and potentially more successful approach is already at hand: the reduction of silent inflammation in the brain.

My optimism comes from the results that I have seen over the past three years in several patients. One particularly inspiring story was a fifty-five-year-old world-class swimmer who came to me after being diagnosed with Parkinson's. He had set numerous world records in master's competitions and wasn't ready to give in to his disease. I immediately put him on a regimen of high-dose fish oil (using a daily dose of about 15 grams of EPA and DHA) and strict adherence to the Zone Diet. He is now swimming faster than he was three years earlier. Recently, he went to Utah to take skiing lessons for the first time in his life and the instructor told him that he had never seen such balance in a beginning skier. Not bad for a Parkinson's patient.

DEPRESSION

Clinical depression is a disabling condition in which you lose pleasure in all things that brought you enjoyment in the past. In fact, it becomes difficult to conjure up previously happy times. Any motivation for the future, let alone the next day, evaporates.

Depression has increased significantly in the past century, with nearly 20 million people in the United States now affected by it. The increase in its incidence correlates very strikingly with our decreasing intake of fish and fish oil in the same time period (much like the increased incidence of ADD).

Psychiatric researchers learned many years ago that depression is often associated with a lack of the neurotransmitter serotonin. In fact, drug companies have made billions from the development of drugs to boost serotonin levels, such as Prozac, Paxil, and Zoloft, all of which have become household names. More recent research has found that even nondepressed people experience an improvement in their moods when they take one of these drugs.

You probably wouldn't think of depression as an inflammatory disease, yet the SIP actually corresponds to the severity of the depression. Those who have higher levels of silent inflammation have more severe forms of depression. Why? One surprising benefit of high-dose fish oil is that it increases serotonin levels, just as it increases dopamine levels. This is confirmed by epidemiological evidence that shows that populations who eat a lot of fish (Greenland Eskimos and the Japanese) have very low rates of depression. In fact, the rates of depression in Japan are just a fraction of the rates in America and other countries where fish consumption is minimal. In fact, New Zealanders, who eat the least amount of fish in the industrialized world, have fifty times the rate of depression as the Japanese. (What's more, they eat very large amounts of pro-inflammatory omega-6 fatty acids.) In Greenland, Eskimos (who consume some 7 to 10 grams per day of long-chain omega-3 fatty acids) have virtually no depression even though their living conditions might seem pretty depressing, with only an hour or two of sunlight a day during the winter months. Finally, clinical studies in Europe indicate that the lower the levels of omega-3 fatty acids in the blood, the greater the incidence of depression.

One reason that increased consumption of omega-3 fatty acids would improve depression is that it reduces AA levels. This leads to a reduction in the production of pro-inflammatory eicosanoids, such as PGE$_2$, which is known to be present in much higher levels in the spinal fluid of depressed patients compared to healthy control patients.

All of these suggestive bits of research are just clues. But an intervention study conducted by Andrew Stoll and his colleagues at Harvard Medical School has provided some hard-and-fast evidence. In this experiment, one group of patients with bipolar depression took approximately 10 grams per day of EPA and DHA (approximately 4 teaspoons of an ultra-refined EPA/DHA concentrate). The other group of patients took a placebo containing olive oil. Four months into the nine-month-long trial, the researchers ended the trial early because the divergence between the fish oil group and the control group was so great that they felt it was unethical to continue the study. Those in the high-dose fish oil group had a significant stabilization in their symptoms, while those in the olive oil control group had a significant worsening of their symptoms. Similar studies have confirmed the benefits of using fish oil in clinically depressed patients (who don't have bipolar depression) with the mood-lifting benefits coming as early as three weeks.

As dramatic as these result were, I believe they could have been even better if the Harvard researchers had brought these patients' insulin levels under control (using the Zone Diet) while titrating with even higher levels of fish oil using the SIP to indicate when they had reached the Anti-Inflammation Zone. A lower level of insulin would have further decreased the production of AA and thus enhanced the benefits of high-dose fish oil supplementation.

SCHIZOPHRENIA

Characterized by hallucinations, delusions, inner voices, and highly abnormal behavior, schizophrenia has been feared through the ages. With the advent of new drugs, schizophrenia now appears to be a "controllable" disease. The drugs, however, don't work in all patients, and many patients refuse to take their medications because of highly unpleasant side effects, such as a flattening of the personality and the loss of creative thought.

The cause of schizophrenia remains unknown, and even the understanding of how the drugs work to alleviate it remains murky. What is clear is that schizophrenics have very low levels of omega-3 fatty acids in their bloodstream compared to healthy individuals. Early attempts to improve schizophrenia by supplementation with omega-3 fatty acids alone have been mixed. EPA supplementation seemed to have a beneficial effect, but DHA supplementation was relatively ineffective. This illustrates why you have to use a combination of both to treat neurological disease. EPA has anti-inflammatory properties, and DHA provides the structural properties necessary for optimal brain function. Using one without the other for treating neurological disorders is a nutritional recipe for failure.

Of course, the other question is whether these researchers administered high enough doses of the EPA and DHA to see consistent results. All of the published studies in schizophrenia (like virtually all intervention studies using fish oil) are based on guessing at a dose of fish oil as opposed to titrating the doses of EPA and DHA upward until you reach an appropriate level of the SIP as measured by the blood.

AUTISM

As might be expected, those with autism tend to have the same decreased EPA and DHA levels and increased SIP as observed with other neurological conditions. To date, no intervention studies have been performed to see whether high-dose fish oil supplementation can bring about behavioral improvements. Given the link between brain disorders, inflammation, and low omega-3 levels, I would theorize that these children could benefit from supplementation. They would, however, need a high dosage of EPA and DHA (probably similar to children with ADD) to reduce their SIP to a level in which positive behavioral changes could be seen. Again, this would require periodic monitoring of the blood to adjust the dose as needed.

VIOLENT BEHAVIOR

Although not officially considered a mental disease, many people have a tendency to use violence to solve problems in their daily life. Violent behavior may have an underlying biochemical basis that can be corrected by a reduction in the SIP. For example, animals that demonstrate abnormal aggression patterns usually have low blood levels of DHA. Studies have also found that violent prison inmates have lower levels of DHA in their blood than nonviolent prison inmates. When prison inmates are given supplements of fish oil, violence decreases.

It's now well documented that violence (and even violent video games) increases the levels of dopamine. Therefore, people may have a tendency to use violence as a form of self-medication to increase depressed levels of dopamine. Other studies have demonstrated that low levels of serotonin may also contribute to violent behavior since serotonin acts like a "morality" hormone stopping us from doing impulsive acts. If low levels of neurotransmitters (such as serotonin and/or dopamine) play a potent role in violent behavior, perhaps supplementation with high-dose fish oil (which can raise both) may play a critical role in behavior modification.

ALCOHOLISM

Alcoholism is a disease with a strong genetic component and a strong link to depression and other mood disorders. Those who abuse alcohol often find that their drive for the substance far outweighs the negative social consequences of its use.

Obviously, not everyone who drinks becomes an alcoholic, but alcoholics often have lower levels of omega-3 fatty acids in their blood compared to nonalcoholics. Alcohol also depletes DHA in the brain. By the same token, alcohol consumed by a pregnant woman depletes DHA in the fetal brain, which can lead to fetal alcohol syndrome and permanent brain damage.

Alcoholics also have lower levels of GLA, the building block of "good" eicosanoids, in their bloodstream. This would strongly suggest that supplementation with high-dose fish oil should be coupled with small amounts of GLA (probably about 10 mg per day), which should have significant benefits in reducing cravings for alcohol.

As important as high-dose fish oil (plus GLA) is for treatment of alcoholism, consistent insulin control is just as vital. This is clear if you ever go to an Alcoholics Anonymous meeting and see a table filled with doughnuts. Sugary carbohydrates are just another form of self-medication to help maintain blood sugar levels. Without insulin control, supplementation with high-dose fish oil will have little lasting effect in treating alcoholism. Following all the components of the Zone Lifestyle Program will provide the recovering alcoholic with the hormonal tools necessary to overcome their poor genes.

SUMMARY

Reaching the Anti-Inflammation Zone is the best way to ensure that your brain is not under constant inflammatory attack. Since you won't have any outward signs of "pain in the brain," you won't know you're under the brain drain until it's too late. That's why you need to get a measurement of your SIP to see where you are, and to do periodic measurements to ensure that you're staying in the Anti-Inflammation Zone. It's your best shot at avoiding those diseases you fear most—the ones that not only drain your brain, but also drain life of its maximum potential.

Screaming Pain

Throughout this book, I talk about silent inflammation and its impact on chronic disease. Silent inflammation, however, is still inflammation. It's just below the perception of pain. What about when inflammation becomes severe enough to pass the pain threshold? It's at this point that you have screaming pain, the kind of classic inflammation that physicians have battled ever since the beginning of modern medicine more than 2,000 years ago.

Screaming pain caused by inflammation can encompass a variety of different medical conditions. In general, if a condition ends with "itis" it simply means that inflammation is involved. Here are a few examples:

Medical Description	Site of Inflammation
Arthritis	Joints
Encephalitis	Brain
Pancreatitis	Pancreas
Hepatitis	Liver
Meningitis	Brain
Bronchitis	Lungs
Colitis	Colon
Gastritis	Stomach

There are, however, a number of other inflammatory conditions that can also cause screaming pain, including

Fibromyalgia

Chronic fatigue syndrome

Crohn's disease

End-stage cancer

Of course, those diseases caused by silent inflammation (heart disease, Alzheimer's, diabetes, cancer, and so on) that I've already discussed can all develop into screaming pain if they cause enough organ damage. At this point the damage caused by silent inflammation has passed the threshold where you register pain, and now finally has your attention.

As you now know, the underlying cause of pain is ultimately an overproduction of pro-inflammatory eicosanoids. Thus, it's reasonable to think that reaching the Anti-Inflammation Zone should be your first choice against chronic screaming pain. And this means finding the optimal dose of high-dose fish oil.

You might think that my continued touting of high-dose fish oil as a universal medical treatment sounds suspiciously like the snake-oil salesmen of the turn of the twentieth century. But once you understand that virtually every chronic disease, including screaming pain, is caused by an overproduction of pro-inflammatory eicosanoids, you'll realize that the universal need for high-dose fish oil to help you reach the Anti-Inflammation Zone makes perfect medical sense.

One of the major challenges in the treatment of pain through the centuries is that there's been no physiologic way to measure its severity. Doctors rely only on their patients' reporting of symptoms. Without any clinical way to measure a treatment's effectiveness, pain management often borders on voodoo.

Now the SIP provides the necessary information on the underlying cause of pain—overproduction of pro-inflammatory eicosanoids.

WHAT'S WRONG WITH SNAKE OIL ANYWAY?

The original snake oil was actually grounded in sound science. Derived from sea snakes, this medicinal oil was brought to America by Chinese immigrants in the late nineteenth century. Sea snakes feed exclusively upon fish. As a consequence, the extracted oil from these sea snakes was very rich in EPA and DHA. In fact, authentic sea snake oil contains a higher concentration of EPA and DHA than cod liver oil does. Because of its anti-inflammatory properties, sea snake oil may have been among the best "drugs" of its time. Its negative reputation came about when the public was sold adulterated products that contained no EPA or DHA but tasted just as bad. (Sounds a little like the early days of the health food industry.) Ultra-refined EPA/DHA concentrates should be considered the twenty-first-century version of authentic sea snake oil.

If your SIP is not being reduced by your doctor's anti-inflammatory pain treatments, it means that you are simply treating the symptoms of screaming pain, not the cause. As a result, you'll probably wind up with screaming pain as a chronic companion, and you'll have to live with using ever more costly anti-inflammatory drugs with their associated side effects.

THE PROBLEM WITH ANTI-INFLAMMATORY DRUGS

Although it seems to make perfect sense to treat screaming pain at its source (excess levels of AA), the drug industry has focused all of its attention instead on reducing the collateral damage that comes from excess AA. In particular, they develop drugs that inhibit the enzymes that make pro-inflammatory eicosanoids derived from AA. This is like calling for the fire truck after the house has burned down. As I mentioned in an earlier chapter, this approach is known as *going downstream*. This is how aspirin and other nonsteroidal anti-inflammatory drugs (NSAIDs) work.

The most powerful pain medications, however, are corticosteroids. They treat pain by *going upstream* to prevent the release of AA from the membranes. Unfortunately, corticosteroids also inhibit the release of both DGLA and EPA. Although corticosteroids have immediate pain-alleviating effects, they knock out all eicosanoids ("good" and "bad") without any discrimination. This is why extended use of corticosteroids can lead to severe side effects such as immune system depression, cognitive impairment, and insulin resistance. Because of these side effects, corticosteroids are currently the drugs of last resort for treating screaming pain.

Let's say, though, that you could go even farther upstream to treat screaming pain, but without any of the harmful side effects of corticosteroids. You do this by actually lowering the levels of AA in the membrane without affecting the levels of DGLA or EPA. Now you reduce the production of pro-inflammatory eicosanoids without inhibiting the powerful anti-inflammatory eicosanoids. This would give you an exceptionally powerful weapon for treating not only screaming pain, but also virtually every disease condition that has an inflammatory component. Herein lies the power of ultra-refined EPA/DHA concentrates: they work in concert with every anti-inflammatory drug because they go upstream while drugs go downstream. Using ultra-refined EPA/DHA concentrates simply represents a far more elegant method to treat both screaming pain and chronic disease. But the big drug companies are very nervous about ultra-refined EPA/DHA concentrates for two reasons. First, EPA/DHA concentrates represent a far more rational way to treat inflammation than current drugs. The second reason is that EPA/DHA concentrates can't be patented.

Reaching the Anti-Inflammation Zone is a necessary first step in treating screaming pain. Once you are there, you will have reduced the levels of AA in each of your 60 trillion cells and in the process choked off the raw material required to make pro-inflammatory eicosanoids. Let's look at some of the screaming pain conditions that high-dose fish oil has been shown to significantly improve.

ARTHRITIS

The first published journal article on the benefits of high-dose fish oil as a treatment for arthritis appeared in 1775. The oil used in that study was a very crude form of cod liver oil. Patients who could stomach the horrific-tasting oil, however, enjoyed spectacular pain relief. Others found the oil too putrid to stomach, so they turned to more pleasant tasting (but far less effective) anti-inflammatory elixirs, such as alcohol (remember it also has some anti-inflammatory properties), to manage their arthritis.

Now more than two centuries later, fish oil has finally returned to the arthritis scene. In the 1980s, positive research findings ushered in claims that fish oil was a "new" miracle cure for arthritis. Since fish oil was now more refined and in soft gelatin capsules, it was far easier to swallow than in the past. Early studies used only 3 to 4 grams of long-chain omega-3 fatty acids, so the results were positive, but not spectacular. There appear to be two reasons for this. First, the dose was too low to significantly alter AA levels. Second, there is high variability between the oral dose given and the actual amount that ends up in the bloodstream. This is why the SIP is so important in guiding you to the right dosage.

AUTOIMMUNE DISORDERS

Autoimmune disorders, in which the immune system attacks the body as if it were a foreign invader, can also be alleviated with high-dose fish oil. MS, for example, responds well to high-dose fish oil, as I described in chapter 17. Lupus, a life-threatening condition that can cause kidney failure and many other problems, can also be more effectively managed with high-dose fish oil supplementation. When mice that had been specially bred to develop lupus were supplemented with high-dose fish oil, they lived much longer than they normally would have. More exciting was that injections of anti-inflammatory eicosanoids completely halted the progression of the disease in these animals, even after the disease was well established.

IgA nephropathy is another autoimmune disease in which the immune system attacks the kidneys. Long-term studies in patients using high-dose fish oil have shown a dramatic reduction in the development of kidney failure in these patients compared to those who took a placebo. Remember that fish oil not only acts as a modulator of pro-inflammatory eicosanoids but also inhibits the release of various inflammatory cytokines, such as IL-6 and tumor necrosis factor (TNF). The ability of high-dose fish oil to reduce a broad spectrum of these inflammatory mediators (eicosanoids and cytokines) is what makes it the first line of treatment for screaming pain.

END-STAGE CANCER PAIN

Although cancer is ultimately caused by silent inflammation, in the final stages it is characterized by intense screaming pain. The pain is usually so extreme that patients need to be put on powerful narcotic drugs that put them into hazy mental states and make it difficult for them to connect with loved ones near the time of death. If given the choice, most patients would prefer to die in their own homes with their dignity and mental facilities intact, surrounded by their loved ones. Instead, they often are left to die in a sterile hospital and forced into a drug stupor to dull the pain.

This was the exact dilemma faced by Akira, the father of a close friend of mine. Akira was eighty-five when he was diagnosed with nontreatable pancreatic cancer. His HMO told him the only treatment that could be provided was heavy doses of narcotics to ease the oncoming pain. Rather than ending his life that way, he decided to try an alternative route. He started taking very high-dose fish oil (about 30 grams of EPA and DHA per day). Each week the nurse from the HMO would come by asking if he wanted his narcotics because his pain must be so intense. Although he was getting weaker with fatigue, he had very little pain. When he did die, he was in full command of his mental abilities and was able to be surrounded by his family in his own home and without pain. That is the way life should end.

As I discussed earlier, wasting (cachexia) is another manifestation of screaming pain in end-stage cancer patients. Very high-dose fish oil (about 18 grams per day) is also the only known treatment to reduce wasting. It works by lowering the production of the pro-inflammatory cytokine called tumor necrosis factor (TNF). This is the same pro-inflammatory cytokine reduced by injections of the drug Enbreal. This reduction in TNF (and corresponding decrease in pain) has made Enbreal the hottest selling drug (more than $500 million in 2003) for the treatment of rheumatoid arthritis. Too bad these patients don't realize that high-dose fish oil is cheaper and a lot easier to take (using the Big Brain Shake) than injections of Enbreal. Of course, it is highly unlikely that the drug companies are going to tell them.

ATHLETIC PAIN

Elite athletes are often racked with screaming pain because of the demands of intense training and competition. This is why the most widely prescribed drugs in sports medicine are anti-inflammatory drugs. Elite athletes can't train without them.

One such case was of a top swimmer in Italy, Lorenzo Vismara. At twenty-six, he had constant inflammatory injuries, and his coaches had gone to every sports medicine specialist in Europe looking for answers but had almost given up. In essence, Lorenzo was told that his days on the national team were numbered.

In desperation, the coaches turned to an Italian colleague of mine, Dr. Riccardo Pina, for one last try. Dr. Pina quickly analyzed the problem and pinpointed Lorenzo's diet as the culprit. Like many elite athletes, Lorenzo thought that he had a blast furnace for a stomach and could eat anything he liked, since he would burn it off later through his swimming.

It turns out that Lorenzo's high glycemic-load diet had been fueling silent inflammation, which had broken through into full-fledged screaming pain. Immediately, Lorenzo was put on the Zone Diet (Italian-style, of course) and high-dose fish oil (7.5 grams of EPA and DHA per day). After a month, both his SIP and his athletic performance had begun to improve. A year later, Lorenzo set seven Italian national records in a single swim meet. Not bad for someone who had almost been dropped from the national team just a year earlier.

As a side note to this story, the Italian national basketball team also went to Dr. Pina for help. They were predicted to finish last in the European qualifying championships for the 2004 Olympics, and therefore had nothing to lose. The team adopted the same dietary program as Lorenzo. Six months later, they qualified for the Olympics by finishing third in the European championships. Then they soundly beat the American team composed of NBA All-Stars by more than twenty points in a pre-Olympic exhibition match. They wound up taking a silver medal at the 2004 Athens Olympics, much to shock of the entire international basketball community. Instead of talking about being in "the zone," athletes (especially those racked by screaming pain) should really aim at getting into the Anti-Inflammation Zone.

MY PRESCRIPTION FOR SCREAMING PAIN

Screaming pain demands immediate attention, and you need a two-fold approach. First, use an over-the-counter anti-inflammatory drug such as aspirin or NSAIDs to get the fastest possible action. They do work; it's using them long-term that causes all the problems. But the second approach is much more important: start moving yourself aggressively toward the Anti-Inflammation Zone. I would suggest starting with a daily dose of about 7.5 grams per day of EPA and DHA (this is equivalent to 1 tablespoon of an ultra-refined EPA/DHA concentrate) to reduce the levels of AA in your membranes. Although it would be ideal to take an SIP at this time, you want to treat the pain. Even at this dosage of fish oil it will take about thirty days to see a reduction in levels of AA. After thirty days, gradually reduce your dose of the anti-inflammatory drug while keeping the same dose of the fish oil. Then after another two weeks, start reducing the dosage of the fish oil until the pain returns. In an ideal world, the fish oil alone should be able to handle the pain, but in the real world you may need combination of a low-dose anti-inflammatory drug with high-dose fish oil to do the job. You should consider taking your SIP every 6 months to make sure you are taking adequate levels of EPA and DHA to keep AA levels under control.

SUMMARY

Chronic pain is disabling and robs life of much of its pleasure. The root cause is surplus AA that leads to excess production of pro-inflammatory eicosanoids. Rather than taking anti-inflammatory drugs on a long-term basis that work by going downstream to try to solve the problem, think about going upstream to attack the root cause (excess AA). Your body will be eternally grateful if you do.

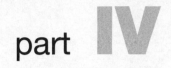

What Will Our Future Be?

Who Is to Blame for the Epidemic of Silent Inflammation?

Today, Americans spend more money on health care than anyone in the world, and our results are pretty dismal. By virtually every marker of national wellness, America ranks relatively low compared to other developed countries of the world. I believe much of this is due to the epidemic increase of silent inflammation in our society. The inevitable question is, who is to blame for this dramatic increase in silent inflammation and its negative impact on our wellness?

TECHNOLOGY

Ironically, the ultimate answer may be technology. We have become addicted to technology. Technology does increase productivity, but it also compresses time for simple human endeavors, such as preparing hormonally balanced meals and having the time to eat them at a leisurely pace. We've become a fast-food generation, and I'm not just talking about McDonald's and Pizza Hut. It is the same technology that has given us instant oatmeal that cooks in 1 minute instead of 30. I'm talking about breakfast cereals, premade sandwiches for lunch, and frozen dinners that can be microwaved in seconds. Real cooking with raw ingredients has become a lost art in America, because we have simply run out of time.

As a result, a growing number of Americans eat outside the home because it simply takes too long a time to prepare food. Fast-food restaurants exist because they prepare food fast, but other restaurants are not far behind in terms of speed. As a result, more than 50 percent of our meals are eaten outside the home. All restaurants have an overwhelming urge to please you so that you will visit them again. The easiest way to give you a lot of food is to use the most inexpensive ingredients possible. That means a lot of grains and starches and extra fat (primarily rich in pro-inflammatory omega-6 fatty acids) to make the food taste better. We have become victims of our success in the technology of agribusiness. We have the cheapest food in the world today, and as a result we eat out more often and eat more of it.

OUR GENES

New and changing technology constantly increases our productivity. On the other hand, as I discussed in chapter 2, our genes are constant, rooted in our evolutionary past. We now realize how finely tuned and tightly intertwined our genes are with our hormonal systems. They work in concert to not only control the flow of storage of fat in our bodies but also to maintain the appropriate levels of inflammatory responses. These systems evolved while humans were consuming a low glycemic-load diet with adequate protein and long-chain omega-3 fats (a Paleolithic diet) that was relatively constant over time. But this tight linkage between hormones and diet has been sabotaged by today's dietary changes.

Remember, our survival as a species was highly predicated on our ability to store excess calories as fat to be used for a hungry day and to mount inflammatory attacks against alien microbial invaders. That was a great advantage during times of famine and no public health practices to speak of, but the same genes now conspire against us in an environment of the continual oversupply of calories (primarily composed of inexpensive high glycemic-load carbohydrates) and increasing levels of pro-inflammatory omega-6 fatty acids in our food supply. Together they have made inflammatory diets the norm in America.

GOVERNMENT

Blaming time compression caused by technology and our genes may be a little obscure for the media, but pointing a finger at the government is easy. The entire infrastructure of the American agribusiness community is based on grain and starch production. The grain lobbies are among the most powerful in the government. The Department of Agriculture is devoted to keeping those lobbies happy, and is far less interested in the impact of their policies on our nation's health. That is why asking the USDA to develop the Food Pyramid was like asking the fox to guard the henhouse.

The problem started with subsidies to farmers. These were begun in the Depression to protect the family farm because a significant part of our population worked there. Today, these subsidies are nearly $20 billion per year even though today less than 1 percent of Americans work on farms. This is because the technological advances of giant agribusiness corporations have made them extraneous. As a result, there aren't as many votes coming from farms as in the past; they have been replaced by corporate contributions, which are the mother's milk of politics. These government subsidies continue even though we produce twice as much food as we should be consuming. Why do these subsidies continue if we are producing too much food? The two most powerful agricultural lobbies (and hence the beneficiaries of these subsidies) come from the corn and wheat lobbies. The vast majority of the corn that's grown goes to feeding cattle and producing corn syrup for sweeteners. Just for good measure (even though it is another boondoggle), excess corn is being converted into ethanol for automobiles. The wheat lobby is just as powerful, especially considering that animals (the primary beneficiaries of corn subsidies) will not eat wheat. They will eat corn, oats, and a lot of other grains, but not wheat. In fact, the primary use for wheat is for humans, but in the form of high glycemic-load foods such as bread, breakfast cereals, pasta, and bagels. Therefore, the only way to unload the excess wheat we produce is to get humans to eat more of the products that come from it. This is the other mission of the USDA: to make sure that Americans eat excess commodities. Therefore, no one should be too surprised when the USDA eagerly promotes the Food Pyramid consisting primarily of grains and starches such as wheat and corn.

While the wheat and corn products are living high on the hog of government largesse, less than 1 percent of all government subsidies go to fruit and vegetable production. In fact, it is estimated that even if Americans actually ate the meager amounts of fruits and vegetables recommended by the Food Pyramid, the current acreage would have to be doubled from that used in current production. This extra acreage would most likely have to come from that currently used for corn and wheat production—a highly unlikely situation.

Another destination of USDA subsidies is the soybean producers, primarily to entice them to produce more soybean oil, which is rich in pro-inflammatory omega-6 fatty acids. If there were a formula to create an epidemic of silent inflammation in America, then supporting the excessive production of both high glycemic-load carbohydrates and pro-inflammatory omega-6 fatty acids would be a surefire winner. But the USDA is not alone. They have an ideal partner in the processed food industry.

PROCESSED FOOD MANUFACTURING

Subsidies from the USDA have made vegetable oils rich in omega-6 fatty acids and refined grain products (flours and sweeteners) from wheat and corn the cheapest food commodities in the world in terms of price per calorie. As a result, the processed food industry has used every trick in the book to incorporate these cheap commodities into processed foods that not only have a lengthy shelf life, but also have much higher profit margins. Today, a large supermarket may contain up to 50,000 items, much of it processed foods made from refined grains and cheap fats. The annual sales of such processed foods are about $175 billion per year. This number is frighteningly close to the $160 billion per year spent on prescription drugs in America.

The processed food industry in the United States is the most technologically advanced in the world, as it can make virtually anything out of cheap refined grains and vegetable oils. More important, the processed food industry also knows how to make them taste great. There is another dilemma with processed food—palatability versus satiation. Foods that are very palatable induce hunger (because they are rich in high glycemic-load carbohydrates). Foods that induce satiety (control of hunger) are not very palatable. A candy bar is very palatable, but it doesn't control your hunger very well. A plate of broccoli is very satiating, but not very palatable. Human nature drives us toward palatability, and the food industry has the rights tools (thanks to the subsidies from the USDA) to make exactly what we like to eat. But just to leave no stone unturned, the food industry spends about $33 billion per year in advertising (one-third on advertising to children) to let you know where you can find the cheapest, most palatable foods in the world.

This leads to the real problem of cheap food. For people in lower socioeconomic groups, the best economic decision is to buy food products with the greatest number of calories for the least amount of money. In the old days, it used to be rice, bread, and potatoes. Now it is processed food composed of refined grains, sugars, and vegetable oils. In fact, the cost of fresh fruits and vegetables is 100 to 400 times greater per calorie than refined grains, sugars, and vegetable oils. Asking the poor to buy more fresh fruits and vegetables to lower the glycemic load of their diets is, according to Adam Drewnowski of the University of Washington, the equivalent of "economic elitism." It's simply not going to happen. Why? The USDA food subsidies keep the real prices of grains and starches and vegetable oil incredibly low, and the processed food industry transforms these commodities into extremely palatable, inexpensive foods.

Spokepersons for the processed food industry have also taken a lesson from the tobacco industry, stating that eating their products is purely a personal responsibility. If you really want to lose weight, then you should "eat less and exercise more." What they don't tell you is that you would have to walk for 6 hours to burn off the calories in one supersize McDonald's Big Mac value meal. And if Americans really did partake in the other part of that mantra to "eat less," then very soon the entire American agribusiness industry (as well as a significant portion of the processed food, grocery, and restaurant industries) would collapse because they need as many people as possible eating as much food as possible to make profits.

Are the USDA and the entire food industry the only organizations responsible for current epidemic of silent inflammation? There's still another unlikely suspect: the American medical establishment.

"I THOUGHT IT WAS GOOD FOR YOU"

The road to hell is paved with good intentions. Unfortunately, the good intentions of the medical establishment to fight heart disease were ultimately based on bad science, and indirectly led to our epidemic of silent inflammation. Beginning in the 1950s an increasing stream of medical researchers called for a war against fat because it contains cholesterol. Dietary cholesterol was seen as the causative agent of heart disease (which it is not). The solution was to remove many sources of cholesterol (especially animal protein) from the diet and replace them with fat-free carbohydrates (such as grains and starches). If you were going to add any fat to the diet, you had to make sure it was omega-6 fat, since it appeared to lower cholesterol.

In hindsight, these dietary recommendations endorsed by the medical establishment were a surefire way to set the stage for the epidemic increase in silent inflammation. Nonetheless, this call for action from medical researchers (who knew very little of the hormonal consequences of food) was quickly taken up by a new generation of nutritionists (who knew absolutely nothing of the hormonal consequences of food). They quickly mobilized to spread the word that fat was bad and fat-free grains and starchy carbohydrates were next to godliness. They never understood that the more high glyccmic-load carbohydrates you eat, the hungrier you become. And with increased hunger comes increased calorie consumption, primarily from more fat-free carbohydrates. This is why in the past thirty years the average calorie consumption has increased by some 300 calories per day. We are not more active, but simply more hungry due to increased insulin levels.

Although the medical establishment was convinced that dietary fat and cholesterol caused heart disease, one clinical trial after another found virtually no evidence that eating less fat (or cholesterol) had any impact on heart disease. To line up political support (since there was little, if any, scientific support) for the war on fat, the government decided to arrange a "consensus" conference on dietary fat and cholesterol in the late 1980s. Government organizers invited a disproportionate number of academic experts who agreed with their position that dietary fat and cholesterol caused heart disease, and, of course, a few who didn't. Everyone gave his or her viewpoint, and then they voted. Not surprisingly, the conference issued the statement that if you lowered your intake of dietary cholesterol and fat, you would reduce the risk of having a heart attack.

The fact that there was no scientific study to support that statement did not deter the massive public health campaign to change the dietary habits of Americans. The USDA used this conference as a basis to validate their famous Food Pyramid, which is now becoming more recognized as faulty and misleading. As Walter Willett, chairman of the Department of Public Health at Harvard Medical School, has said about the USDA's recommendations in his book *Eat, Drink, and Be Healthy:* "The USDA Pyramid is wrong. It was built on shaky scientific ground. . . . the USDA Pyramid offers wishy-washy, scientifically unfounded advice . . . nor has it ever been tested to see if it really works."

This is not exactly a resounding endorsement of the USDA Food Pyramid from Harvard. Looking back in hindsight, the USDA Food Pyramid may rank pretty close to the bottom as the worst government program ever conceived and implemented. This war on dietary fat and cholesterol was launched with great fanfare by the medical establishment and continues today. The weapons of that war against cholesterol were provided by the government (cheap fat-free high glycemic-load carbohydrates and pro-inflammatory omega-6 fatty acids). Little did anyone suspect that this war based on good intentions would undermine the health of millions of Americans by unleashing a new and frightening epidemic of silent inflammation that is fueled by obesity.

The newest version of the USDA Food Pyramid, scheduled for release in 2005, still ignores the role of the glycemic load in the diet, but at least it recommends more fruits and vegetables. But the new guidelines are so loose that they don't provide any useful information to reverse our twin epidemics of obesity and silent inflammation. It's basically business as usual for agribusiness and processed food manufacturing industries. Any major change in the status quo would cause a political shake-up and decreased political contributions from the agricultural industry. Of course, no one in government wants that to happen.

NOT LISTENING TO YOUR GRANDMOTHER

There is one final player in our drama of who is to blame for the epidemic of silent inflammation—us and our failure to heed our grandmothers' advice on fish oil. Standard issue to virtually every child two generations ago was a daily dose of a tablespoon of cod liver oil. Although it still ranks as one of most digusting foods of all time, this dosage did provide about 2.5 grams of EPA and DHA, which provide significant anti-inflammatory properties. The day that parents in America stopped giving their children high-dose fish oil may have been the greatest public health disaster of the twentieth century. Our epidemic of silent inflammation is the result.

THE EXPORTING OF SILENT INFLAMMATION

Many trends start in the United States and then cover the globe. Our epidemic of silent inflammation is just another one of them. We exported Big Macs and Coca-Cola, and now the USDA Food Pyramid. Virtually every government in the world has adopted it as the standard on which their national dietary recommendations are based. Not surprisingly, obesity has become a worldwide problem, with more people overweight today than malnourished. The same trends I outlined that are currently at work in America (time compression due to technology, the availability of cheap food ingredients, and the desire for palatability) have come together to export our epidemic of silent inflammation to Europe and are emerging in middle classes of the Far East, Latin America, and India. In fact, Italian children are now the fattest in Europe, whereas only a few short years ago, they were among the leanest. With this increase in body weight comes the corresponding increase in silent inflammation and acceleration of the development of chronic disease such as type 2 diabetes. In fact, today there are more type 2 diabetics in either India or China than there are in the United States. If the epidemic of type 2 diabetes threatens to destroy the U.S. health care system because of its cost, what will be the impact of that disease on the Chinese and Indian health care systems, which have a far lower capacity to pay for the overwhelming health burden (blindness, amputation, heart disease, and kidney failure) induced by type 2 diabetes?

Am I pessimistic? Not really. You can't solve a problem unless you know what actually causes it. Pointing the finger of guilt at the government, agribusiness, fast-food restaurants, or the processed food manufacturing industry is easy to do, but misses the mark. The real problem is our lack of knowledge of how to take control of our hormones. Ultimately, you have to decide to change your future by controlling your hormones to get into the Anti-Inflammation Zone. But this requires understanding the hormonal consequences of your food choices.

The final chapter of this book summarizes the steps our society needs to take to get rid of this epidemic of silent inflammation and the consequences that will occur if we don't.

Avoiding the Coming Collapse of the Health Care System

Despite all the advances in modern medicine, we seem powerless to turn back the epidemic of silent inflammation that threatens to destroy our current health care system. In essence, the wellness of Americans is rapidly eroding.

Our diets have changed so rapidly that their hormonal consequences are now overwhelming our genes. Because we have ignored the hormonal consequences of our diet, the greatest threat to America is the potential collapse of our health care system—and it looms just ahead. The first signs of that collapse are now appearing, with the rapid increases in health care insurance and the growing number of people who can't pay for it.

The number-one chronic disease that will accelerate this collapse is the growing epidemic of type 2 diabetes. This is the most expensive of all diseases, because patients often become severely debilitated, though they can live for years with this debilitation. It is the number-one cause of blindness, the primary cause of amputation, a major trigger of heart disease, and a common cause of kidney failure. It costs more than $200,000 per year to keep a single kidney dialysis patient alive. Overall, this condition now costs our country $132 billion a year.

Currently, about 7 percent of adult Americans have type 2 diabetes, and I estimate once that figure reaches 10 percent of the adult population, we will be unable to pay for the resulting health care costs, regardless of our economic strength. The only question is how long it will be before we reach that magic 10 percent figure. It might be as early as five years from now, maybe fifteen years at the most. It doesn't matter if we have universal health insurance, private insurance, or no health insurance at all. The American health care system will simply go bankrupt. But whenever that time comes, everyone in America will be asking, What happened? By the time the epidemic of silent inflammation takes its full toll, it will be too late. Type 2 diabetes will be only the first in a line of many other chronic diseases, such as heart disease, cancer, and Alzheimer's, that will begin to strike at an earlier age and affect an even greater percentage of our population. If type 2 diabetes is not the crushing blow to our health care system, then these other diseases fueled by silent inflammation will soon finish the job.

Paying for health insurance is the new major battleground for American workers and employers. We live in the richest country in the world, and yet more than 40 million people are not insured. Why is health insurance so expensive? Simply ask the HMOs. Nearly 80 percent of the costs for an average HMO goes to pay for disease conditions strongly associated with silent inflammation. The longer silent inflammation is left untreated, the more damage accumulates. This is why health insurance costs are so rapidly rising, and we are increasingly unable to pay for them. The truth is, employers are already resisting the increased rates by reducing their hiring of new employees.

Although the future looks bleak, we can change it if we immediately begin to take the steps needed to reverse silent inflammation. This will require realistic approaches for individuals, not meaningless political slogans. The steps I discuss below will also address pediatric and adolescent obesity, the fastest-growing segment of our obesity epidemic. It is now estimated that one-third of the children born after 2000 will develop type 2 diabetes at some point in their lives. They will be more likely to develop heart disease, cancer, and neurological disorders at a relatively early age. I fear that unless we take these steps, the next generation of Americans may be the first in recorded history whose actual life span is shorter than their parents.

That's the bad news. If we do nothing, the future is clear. It's bleak, very bleak. Therefore, we might ask: What are insurance companies, corporations, and the government doing about this impeding collapse of our health care system?

INSURANCE COMPANIES

Insurance companies should be at the forefront of the battle against silent inflammation, since they ultimately pay for its consequences. That makes sense until you realize that insurance companies are simply bookies. As long as they get their spread, they are willing to take your money. Here is where health insurance is really a sucker's bet. In essence, you give money to the insurance company fearing that you will get sick. They take your money betting that you won't get sick. Like any good bookie, they simply figure the odds so no matter what the outcome, they make a profit. They have no real interest in promoting the reduction of silent inflammation, since you will keep paying for the health insurance regardless of the cost. If the population gets sicker, they simply raise rates to cover the increased cost. If you can't pay for the increased premiums, it's your problem.

While it's easy to be cynical about insurance companies, I think they would change their tune if they were convinced that they could make more money by maintaining your wellness than by treating the symptoms of disease. This could be done by capitation, in which the physician gets paid for keeping his patients well as determined by an inexpensive blood test like the TG/HDL ratio. If the patients keep the TG/HDL under a certain level (such as 2), the physician would get a bonus. If it is over that for his patients, he gets paid as usual for treating the symptoms of chronic disease. This provides physicians with a real incentive to educate their patients on how diet and high-dose fish oil can quickly alter that ratio. The clinical data are quite clear: once TG/HDL drops, good things happen. Unfortunately, it may take decades for insurers to come to this conclusion—but we can still hope.

SELF-INSURED CORPORATIONS

Many corporations insure their employees themselves. But they've found that rising health care costs take a toll on corporate earnings. Here, though, the future may be a little brighter. Frankly, there has been little economic incentive for corporations to promote wellness. This is because if the employees go somewhere elsewhere in a few years, their next employer gets all the potential health benefits without paying for them, and the original corporation has nothing to show for its expenditures. However, if employers could be convinced that a true wellness program brings an immediate increase in employee productivity, then they would see an improvement in their bottom line and would have a financial incentive to enact changes.

This is exactly the benefit that the Zone Diet provides to employers. Within seven days, companies can start seeing significant increases in employee productivity. At most companies, employee productivity virtually shuts down between 2 and 3 in the afternoon as blood sugar levels fall due to a high-glycemic meal at lunch. It actually becomes cheaper to provide subsidized meals to stabilize their employees' blood glucose so that they are more productive throughout the day. Crude implementation of this concept is found in some computer companies and Wall Street brokerage houses. The computer companies give their employees free sugar-laden soft drinks throughout the day to artificially maintain blood glucose levels. The Wall Street brokerage houses constantly pass free food carts among their traders to accomplish the same goal. The fact that both types of employees are being burned out because of increased levels of silent inflammation is of little concern to the corporation as long as they're getting greater productivity. On the other hand, the cost of providing Zone meals and snacks would be about the same, but would reverse silent inflammation instead of increasing it. Other corporations with in-house cafeterias could provide subsidized Zone meals or allow their employees to pay full price for a typical high glycemic-load meal. This is not a difficult choice for the employee to make. The employer would get real-time increases in productivity, and any reduction in future health care costs is the icing, not the cake. This is something that should appeal to the chief financial officer, because it doesn't cost much compared to increased productivity. With new markers of wellness (such as the SIP and the more inexpensive TG/HDL ratio), the actual return on investment of corporate wellness programs (including subsidized meals) can be finally validated and audited. Rather than simply installing more jogging trails or putting in more gyms, corporations could tell by the blood of the employees whether or not their investment in wellness is actually working. If the blood parameters that determine wellness (and primarily the extent of silent inflammation) aren't improving, then they can simply stop the expenditures and focus on those activities that actually increase wellness (and productivity). Unfortunately, it will take time for even the most innovative corporations to integrate this type of thinking into their existing wellness programs, even if the financial logic is overwhelming.

GOVERNMENT

As I pointed out earlier, a major factor in the silent inflammation epidemic has been government subsidies provided to grain farmers and soybean producers. Of course, the government could start giving major subsidies to fruit and vegetable producers to level the playing field, but that approach is unlikely with our growing deficits. An even less likely scenario is to reduce current subsidiaries to the wheat and corn producers. It is all about political contributors and powerful lobbies. This is why the government is very willing to increase Medicare coverage for drugs that only treat the symptoms of chronic diseases that result from silent inflammation, but is unlikely to address the underlying problem of subsidizing an industry (agribusiness) that is overproducing the commodities used to fuel silent inflammation. Even more ominous is that we are only a few years away from the time that the first baby boomers can access all the benefits of Medicare. That will quickly become a time of financial reckoning as the government simply doesn't have the money to pay these coming medical bills.

PROCESSED FOOD MANUFACTURING COMPANIES

I feel the most likely institution to help reverse the epidemic of silent inflammation will ultimately be the processed food manufacturing sector. These are exactly the people who got us into this epidemic of silent inflammation in the first place, and surprisingly, they are the most likely to lead us out. As I stated in the last chapter, the processed food companies have mastered the art of taking cheap commodities (thanks to government subsidies) and have turned out low-price processed foods with great taste but little satiation. But the technology is there to also produce great tasting, inexpensive processed foods that have both palatability and satiation if you are able to add more protein (soy and dairy are the most likely choices) without compromising taste. If you can, then you immediately cut the Gordian knot of hunger by this improved balance of protein to carbohydrate. If you aren't hungry between meals, then you don't consume as many calories. With decreased calorie consumption comes weight loss and the reduction of the primary generator of silent inflammation: excess body fat. In essence, you want to make the most healthful, hormonally correct junk foods known to science. Such a strategy would reach all levels of our society. It is a strategy that is ideally suited for our increasing time compression due to technology, and one that relies upon cheap agricultural commodities to construct foods that will provide both palatibility and satiation at a very affordable price.

Telling people to "eat less and exercise more" has not and will not work. Telling people to eat more fresh fruits and vegetables is nice, but it is possible only for those in the higher economic brackets. Having broad access to healthful junk foods (nutrition bars, ice cream, milkshakes, corn chips, pizza dough, and so on) may be our only way out of the coming health care collapse. I know it can be done, because I have developed prototypes of all of these in my laboratory that are virtually indistinguishable from today's typical junk food. It is a bold approach that is certain to raise the ire of the nutritional community, but as I see it, is may be our only institutional hope. The only question is whether or not the giant corporations in the processed food industry can make money selling healthful junk food. If they can, the epidemic of silent inflammation may be quickly turned around.

INDIVIDUAL RESPONSIBILITY

The good news is you don't have to wait for institutions and other powerful forces in corporate America to reverse silent inflammation. You have the power today to begin to change your future by reducing the levels of silent inflammation in your body. The payoff is almost immediate, and in many cases nearly miraculous.

Ultimately, maintaining wellness by reducing silent inflammation is your own personal responsibility. However, in a time-compressed society you have to develop a plan to get the maximum results in the least amount of time. That plan is encompassed in the Zone Lifestyle Program, which brings you into the Anti-Inflammation Zone with the least amount of effort.

If you are willing to spend only fifteen seconds a day to reduce silent inflammation, then taking enough fish oil will be your best time investment. Nothing works faster and quicker than high-dose fish oil. Here's one government subsidy that would immediately improve the wellness of every American without causing a political storm in the agricultural industry: giving free fish oil to everyone who wanted it. This is not as far-fetched as you might think, since it is currently being done in Italy and Finland. Both countries have a nationalized health care program, and they have put ultra-refined EPA/DHA concentrates on the approved pharmacy drug list so that every citizen in those countries has their fish oil provided free of charge.

If you are willing to commit to more effort, then following the Zone Diet is just as critical for reversing silent inflammation, because it is your ticket to losing excess body fat at the quickest possible rate. Let's face it, losing weight is hard, and keeping it off is almost impossible given the ongoing temptations of carbohydrate-rich offerings from the processed food manufacturers. But you have to eat, so you might as well eat smart.

There is no question that you can lose weight on any diet as long as you restrict calories. But eventually either increased hunger due to increased insulin (on a high-carbohydrate diet) or increased cortisol production (on a low-carbohydrate diet) will be your hormonal undoing. That is why a recent one-year clinical study at Tufts Medical School has shown that dieters are able to stick to the Zone Diet more easily than to either high- or low-carbohydrate diets. It is all about your ability to control hunger between meals. If you aren't hungry, you don't need much willpower to cut back on calories. On the other hand, if you are constantly hungry, you'll need tremendous willpower, or you'll eat excess calories. As most Americans know, the latter possibility is the more likely outcome.

Finally, there is the role of exercise and meditation in reducing silent inflammation. Both require more time commitment, and they will not have the same relative impact on reducing silent inflammation as high-dose fish oil and the Zone Diet. Nonetheless, if used correctly they are powerful secondary components to keep you in the Anti-Inflammation Zone once you have reached it by diet.

Controlling silent inflammation is a lifetime struggle. Remember, the barbarians are at the gate just waiting for the opportunity to lay waste to your future. Your first line of defense against silent inflammation is losing excess body fat. Yes, it's hard. That's why you have to realize the genes of your Paleolithic ancestors are the same ones you carry today. You can't change your genes, but you can follow the Zone Lifestyle Program that makes those genes work for you, not against you.

But don't take my word on it. Your blood will tell you if you're in the Anti-Inflammation Zone, and therefore in a state of wellness. Just keep adjusting your diet and lifestyle until your blood says you are there. Once you are, try to maintain that same lifestyle for a lifetime. If not, silent inflammation will be your constant companion.

In the final analysis, all you have to do is to follow the simple prescriptions in this book and begin to move yourself back to a state of wellness by reducing silent inflammation. All revolutions usually begin with the individual. The wellness revolution is no different.

Continuing Support

The scientific data that supports the Zone is constantly expanding. This is why I maintain several websites to help keep you at the cutting edge of dietary hormonal control theory.

- If you are looking for Zone functional foods and ultra-refined EPA/DHA concentrates that have been clinically tested you should visit www.zonelabsinc.com or call Zone Labs Inc. directly at 1-800-404-8171

- If you are looking for help in constructing Zone meals and snacks, I would suggest visiting www.zonediet.com.

- To gain a deeper insight into my Zone technology along with helpful, practical hints, I would advise you to go to my website, www.drsears.com, which contains a tremendous set of past archives to allow you to go to any depth on the science behind the Zone.

- If you are interested in learning more about the clinical trials that are currently underway to investigate how the diet can affect silent inflammation, I suggest that you go to www.inflammationresearchfoundation.org. This is the website of my nonprofit foundation, which is conducting a wide number of clinical trials on the role of diet to reduce inflammation in chronic conditions such as obesity, type 2 diabetes, heart disease, neurological disorders, cancer, and other inflammatory conditions.

Of course, you can always call my staff at 1-800-404-8171 to help answer your questions about the role of diet in reducing silent inflammation.

Appendix B

Favorable and Unfavorable Carbohydrates

There is no such thing as a forbidden carbohydrate on the Zone Diet, but there are choices that you have to make that will determine your ability to control insulin, and thus silent inflammation. The choices are based on the glycemic load of that carbohydrate. The higher the glycemic load of a meal, the more insulin that will be produced. The terms *Favorable* and *Unfavorable* simply represent the glycemic load of a carbohydrate. A typical serving size of a Favorable carbohydrate has a low glycemic load, whereas the same serving size of an Unfavorable carbohydrate has a high glycemic load.

To make a Zone meal, start by having some low-fat protein that is the size and thickness of the palm of your hand. Then add an adequate amount of Favorable carbohydrates that are no greater than twice the volume of low-fat protein. By making most of your carbohydrates at a meal come from Favorable carbohydrates, you will reduce insulin secretion. Try to always make sure that at least two-thirds of the carbohydrates on your plate are from the Favorable list.

Finally, add a dash (that's a small amount) of monounsaturated fat, such as olive oil, slivered almonds, or avocado, to complete your Zone meal.

Favorable	Unfavorable
Nonstarchy vegetables	Grains
Fruits	Starches
	Fruit juices
	Bread, cereals, pasta
	Processed (i.e., junk) foods

Zone Carbohydrate Blocks

You can further quantify Favorable and Unfavorable carbohydrates using Zone Carbohydrate Blocks. One Carbohydrate Block is defined as 9 grams of insulin-stimulating carbohydrate (total carbohydrates minus fiber). Favorable carbohydrates are those that have a low glycemic load, whereas Unfavorable carbohydrates have a high glycemic load. The Zone Carbohydrate Block method simply allows you to quantify the total amount of carbohydrates at a meal with greater precision.

To construct a Zone meal, you start by adding some low-fat protein to your plate that is no bigger or thicker than the palm of your hand. The typical female will require about 3 ounces of protein, whereas the average male will require about 4 ounces of protein. Then add the appropriate amount of Zone Carbohydrates Blocks. An average female would need about 3 Zone Carbohydrate Blocks at the meal, whereas the average male would require 4 Zone Carbohydrate Blocks at a meal. Always try to make sure that more than two-thirds of your carbohydrates come from the Favorable carbohydrate list. If you do, you will have a very bountiful plate at each meal.

Finally, add a dash (that's a small amount) of monounsaturated fat, such as olive oil, slivered almonds, or avocado, to complete your Zone meal.

FAVORABLE CARBOHYDRATES

Cooked Vegetables	Amount for 1 Zone Carbohydrate Block
Artichokes	4 large
Artichoke hearts	1 cup
Asparagus	12 spears
Beans, green or wax	1½ cups
Beans, black	¼ cup
Bok choy	3 cups
Broccoli	4 cups
Brussels sprouts	1½ cups
Cabbage	3 cups
Carrots, sliced	1 cup
Cauliflower	4 cups
Chickpeas	¼ cup
Collard greens, chopped	2 cups
Eggplant	1½ cups
Kale	2 cups
Kidney beans	¼ cup
Leeks	1 cup
Lentils	¼ cup
Mushrooms, boiled	2 cups
Okra, sliced	1 cup
Onions, chopped and boiled	½ cup
Sauerkraut	1 cup
Spaghetti squash	1 cup
Spinach, chopped	4 cups
Swiss chard, chopped	2½ cups
Turnip, mashed	1½ cups
Turnip greens, chopped	4 cups
Yellow squash, sliced	2 cups
Zucchini, sliced	2 cups

Raw Vegetables	Amount for 1 Zone Carbohydrate Block
Alfalfa sprouts	10 cups
Bamboo shoots	4 cups
Bean sprouts	3 cups
Broccoli florets	4 cups
Cabbage, shredded	4 cups
Carrots, shredded	1 cup
Cauliflower florets	4 cups
Celery, sliced	2 cups
Cucumber	1½ medium
Cucumber, sliced	4 cups
Endive, chopped	10 cups
Escarole, chopped	10 cups
Green or red bell peppers	2
Green or red bell peppers, chopped	2 cups
Hummus	¼ cup
Jalapeño peppers	2 cups
Lettuce, iceberg (6-inch diameter)	2 heads
Lettuce, romaine, chopped	10 cups
Mushrooms, chopped	4 cups
Onions, chopped	1½ cups
Radishes, sliced	4 cups
Salsa	½ cup
Snow peas	1½ cups
Spinach, chopped	10 cups
Tomato	2
Tomato, cherry	2 cups
Tomato, chopped	1½ cups
Water chestnuts	½ cup
Watercress	10 cups

Fruits	Amount for 1 Zone Carbohydrate Block
Apple	½ apple
Applesauce, unsweetened	⅓ cup
Apricots	3
Blackberries	¾ cup
Boysenberries	½ cup
Cherries	8
Fruit cocktail, light	⅓ cup
Grapes	½ cup
Grapefruit	½
Kiwi	1
Lemon	1
Lime	1
Nectarine, medium	½
Orange	½
Orange, mandarin, canned in water	⅓ cup
Peach	1
Peaches, canned in water, sliced	½ cup
Pear	½
Plum	1
Raspberries	1 cup
Strawberries, diced fine	1 cup
Tangerine	1

Grains	Amount for 1 Zone Carbohydrate Block
Barley, dry	¼ cup
Oatmeal, slow-cooking, cooked	⅓ cup
Oatmeal, slow-cooking, dry	½ oz.

Dairy	Amount for 1 Zone Carbohydrate Block
Milk (low-fat)	1 cup
Milk, soy	1 cup
Yogurt, plain	½ cup

Unfavorable Carbohydrates

Cooked Vegetables	Amount for 1 Zone Carbohydrate Block
Acorn squash	½ cup
Beans, baked	¼ cup
Beans, refried	¼ cup
Beets, sliced	½ cup
Butternut squash	½ cup
Corn	¼ cup
French fries	5
Lima beans	¼ cup
Parsnips	⅓ cup
Peas	½ cup
Pinto beans	¼ cup
Potato, baked	¼
Potato, boiled	⅓ cup
Potato, mashed	¼ cup
Sweet potato, baked	⅓ cup
Sweet potato, mashed	¼ cup

Fruits	Amount for 1 Zone Carbohydrate Block
Banana	⅓
Cantaloupe	¼
Cantaloupe, cubed	¾ cup
Cranberries	¾ cup
Cranberry sauce	3 teaspoons
Fig	1
Guava	½
Honeydrew melon, cubed	⅔ cup
Kumquat	3
Mango, sliced	⅓ cup
Papaya, cubed	¾ cup
Pineapple, diced	½ cup
Prunes, dried	2
Raisins	1 tablespoon
Watermelon, cubed	¾ cup

Fruit Juices	Amount for 1 Zone Carbohydrate Block
Apple	⅓ cup
Apple cider	⅓ cup
Cranberry	¼ cup
Fruit punch	¼ cup
Grape	¼ cup
Grapefruit	⅓ cup
Lemonade, unsweetened	⅓ cup
Lime	⅓ cup
Orange	⅓ cup
Pineapple	¼ cup
Tomato	1 cup
V-8	¾ cup

Grains, Cereals, and Breads	Amount for 1 Zone Carbohydrate Block
Bagel, small	¼
Biscuit	½
Bread crumbs	½ oz.
Bread, whole-grain or white	½ slice
Breadstick, hard	1
Breadstick, soft	½
Breakfast cereal, dry	½ oz.
Buckwheat, dry	½ oz.
Bulgur wheat, dry	½ oz.
Cornbread	1 4-inch square
Cornstarch	4 teaspoons
Couscous, dry	½ oz.
Cracker, graham	1½
Cracker, saltine	4
Cracker, Triscuit	3
Croissant, plain	¼
English muffin	¼
Granola	½ oz.
Grits, cooked	⅓ cup

Melba toast	½ oz.
Millet, dry	½ oz.
Muffin, blueberry mini	½
Noodles, egg, cooked	¼ cup
Pancake, 4-inch	1
Pasta, cooked	¼ cup
Pita bread	½ pocket
Pita bread, mini	1 pocket
Popcorn, popped	2 cups
Rice, brown, cooked	⅕ cup
Rice, white, cooked	⅕ cup
Rice cake	1
Roll, bulkie	¼
Roll, small dinner	½
Roll, hamburger	½
Taco shell	1
Tortilla, 6-inch corn	1
Tortilla, 8-inch flour	½
Waffle	½

Alcohol	Amount for 1 Zone Carbohydrate Block
Beer, light	6 oz.
Beer, regular	4 oz.
Distilled spirits	1 oz.
Wine	4 oz.

Miscellaneous	Amount for 1 Zone Carbohydrate Block
Barbeque sauce	2 tablespoons
Cake	⅓ slice
Candy bar	¼
Catsup	2 tablespoons
Cocktail sauce	2 tablespoons
Cookie, small	1
Frozen tofu	⅙ cup
Honey	½ tablespoon

Ice cream, regular	¼ cup
Ice cream, premium	⅛ cup
Jam or jelly	2 tablespoons
Molasses, light	½ teaspoon
Plum sauce	1½ tablespoons
Potato chips	½ oz.
Pretzels	½ oz.
Sugar, brown	2 teaspoons
Sugar, cube	3
Sugar, granulated	2 teaspooons
Sugar, confectioners'	1 tablespoon
Syrup, maple	2 teaspoons
Syrup, pancake	2 teaspoons
Teriyaki sauce	1 tablespoon
Tortilla chips	½ oz.

Appendix D

Zone Points

Zone Points are another way to determine the glycemic load of each meal. Zone Points represent the relative glycemic load for a standard serving size of carbohydrate.

To construct a Zone meal, start by having an appropriate amount of low-fat protein that is the size and thickness of the palm of your hand. This is about 3 ounces of low-fat protein for the typical female, and about 4 ounces of low-fat protein for the typical male. Then add enough carbohydrates to balance out the protein. The typical female should consume about 15 Zone Points per meal, whereas the average male should consume 20 Zone Points per meal. As with the Zone Carbohydrate Blocks, try to make at least two-thirds of your carbohydrates come from Favorable carbohydrates at each meal. You can also see by using the Zone Points system that Favorable carbohydrates make very bountiful meals, whereas using Unfavorable carbohydrates will leave a lot of empty space on your plate. The secret is knowing when to stop adding carbohydrates to the meal.

Finally, add a dash (that's a small amount) of monounsaturated fat, such as olive oil, slivered almonds, or avocado, to complete your Zone meal.

Favorable Carbohydrates

Cooked Vegetables	Serving Size	Zone Points
Artichokes	½ cup	3
Artichoke hearts	½ cup	2
Asparagus	1 cup	3
Beans, green or wax	½ cup	3
Beans, black	½ cup	6
Bok choy	½ cup	1
Broccoli	1 cup	1
Brussels sprouts	½ cup	1
Cabbage	1 cup	1
Carrots, sliced	1 cup	4
Cauliflower	1 cup	1
Chickpeas	½ cup	6
Collard greens, chopped	1 cup	1
Eggplant	½ cup	3
Kale	1 cup	2
Kidney beans	½ cup	6
Leeks	½ cup	2
Lentils	½ cup	6
Mushrooms, boiled	½ cup	1
Okra, sliced	½ cup	2
Onions, chopped and boiled	½ cup	3
Sauerkraut	½ cup	2
Spaghetti squash	½ cup	2
Spinach, chopped	½ cup	1
Swiss chard, chopped	1 cup	1
Turnip, mashed	½ cup	1
Turnip greens, chopped	1 cup	1
Yellow squash, sliced	½ cup	1
Zucchini, sliced	½ cup	1

Raw Vegetables	Serving Size	Zone Points
Alfalfa sprouts	1 cup	1
Bamboo shoots	1 cup	1
Bean sprouts	1 cup	1
Broccoli florets	1 cup	1
Cabbage, shredded	1 cup	1
Carrots, shredded	1 cup	4
Cauliflower florets	1 cup	1
Celery, sliced	½ cup	1
Chickpeas	½ cup	6
Cucumber	1 medium	2
Cucumber, sliced	1 cup	1
Endive, chopped	1 cup	1
Escarole, chopped	1 cup	1
Green or red bell peppers	1	2
Green or red bell peppers, chopped	1 cup	1
Hummus	½ cup	3
Jalapeño peppers	½ cup	1
Lettuce, iceberg (6-inch diameter).	1 cup	1
Lettuce, romaine, chopped	1 cup	1
Mushrooms, chopped	1 cup	1
Onions, chopped	½ cup	1
Radishes, sliced	1 cup	1
Salsa	½ cup	3
Snow peas	½ cup	1
Spinach, chopped	1 cup	1
Tomato	1	1
Tomato, cherry	½ cup	1
Tomato, chopped	½ cup	1
Water chestnuts	½ cup	3
Watercress	1 cup	1

Fruits	Serving Size	Zone Points
Apple	1 apple	10
Applesauce, unsweetened	½ cup	8
Apricots	4	9
Blackberries	¾ cup	3
Blueberries	¾ cup	5
Boysenberries	¾ cup	5
Cherries	12	8
Fruit cocktail, light	½ cup	8
Grapes	½ cup	5
Grapefruit	½	5
Kiwi	1	5
Lemon	1	5
Lime	1	5
Nectarine, medium	1	10
Orange	1	10
Orange, mandarin, canned in water	¾ cup	11
Peach	1	5
Peaches, canned in water	½ cup	5
Pear	1	10
Plum	1	5
Raspberries	1 cup	5
Strawberries, diced fine	1 cup	3
Tangerine	1	5

Grains	Serving Size	Zone Points
Barley, dry	½ cup	20
Oatmeal, slow-cooking, cooked	½ cup	8
Oatmeal, slow-cooking, dry	½ cup	20

Dairy	Serving Size	Zone Points
Milk (low-fat)	1 cup	5
Milk, soy	1 cup	5
Yogurt, plain	1 cup	5

Unfavorable Carbohydrates

Cooked Vegetables	Serving Size	Zone Points
Acorn squash	½ cup	7
Beans, baked	½ cup	14
Beans, refried	½ cup	14
Beets, sliced	½ cup	7
Butternut squash	½ cup	7
Corn	½ cup	14
French fries	20	28
Lima beans	½ cup	14
Parsnips	½ cup	11
Peas	½ cup	7
Pinto beans	½ cup	14
Potato, baked	½ cup	14
Potato, boiled	½ cup	11
Potato, mashed	½ cup	14
Sweet potato, baked	½ cup	11
Sweet potato, mashed	½ cup	14

Fruits	Serving Size	Zone Points
Banana	1	21
Cantaloupe	⅛	9
Cantaloupe, cubed	½ cup	6
Cranberries	½ cup	6
Cranberry sauce	¼ cup	21
Fig	1	7
Guava	½ cup	7
Honeydrew melon, cubed	1 cup	11
Kumquat	1	2
Mango, sliced	½ cup	11
Papaya, cubed	1 cup	9
Pineapple, diced	½ cup	7
Prunes, dried	½ cup	25
Raisins	2 tablespoons	14
Watermelon, cubed	1 cup	11

Fruit Juices	Serving Size	Zone Points
Apple	½ cup	11
Apple cider	½ cup	11
Cranberry	½ cup	14
Fruit punch	½ cup	14
Grape	½ cup	14
Grapefruit	½ cup	11
Lemonade, unsweetened	½ cup	11
Lime	½ cup	11
Orange	½ cup	11
Pineapple	½ cup	14
Tomato	½ cup	4
V-8	½ cup	5

Grains, Cereals, and Breads	Serving Size	Zone Points
Bagel, small	½	14
Biscuit	1	14
Bread crumbs	1 oz.	14
Bread, whole-grain or white	1 slice	14
Breadstick, hard	2	14
Breadstick, soft	1	14
Breakfast cereal, dry	1 oz.	14
Buckwheat, dry	1 oz.	14
Bulgur wheat, dry	1 oz.	14
Cornbread	2 oz.	14
Cornstarch	4 teaspoons	7
Couscous, dry	1 oz.	14
Cracker, graham	3	14
Cracker, saltine	6	11
Cracker, Triscuit	5	14
Croissant, plain	1	28
English muffin	1	28
Granola	¼ cup	14
Grits, cooked	½ cup	11

Melba toast	4 slices	14
Millet, dry	1 oz.	14
Muffin, blueberry mini	1	14
Noodles, egg, cooked	½ cup	14
Pancake, 4-inch	2	14
Pasta, cooked	½ cup	14
Pita bread	1 pocket	14
Pita bread, mini	1 pocket	7
Popcorn, popped	3 cups	11
Rice, brown, cooked	½ cup	18
Rice, white, cooked	½ cup	18
Rice cake	2	14
Roll, bulkie	½	14
Roll, small dinner	1	14
Roll, hamburger	1	14
Taco shell	2	14
Tortilla, 6-inch corn	1	7
Tortilla, 8-inch flour	1	14
Waffle	1	14

Alcohol	Serving Size	Zone Points
Beer, light	12 oz.	14
Beer, regular	12 oz.	21
Distilled spirits	1 oz.	7
Wine	4 oz.	7

Miscellaneous	Serving Size	Zone Points
Barbeque sauce	2 tablespoons	7
Cake	1 slice	21
Candy bar	1	28
Catsup	1 tablespoon	4
Cocktail sauce	1 tablespoon	4
Cookie, small	2	14
Frozen tofu	½ cup	21
Honey	1 tablespoon	14

Ice cream, regular	½ cup	14
Ice cream, premium	½ cup	21
Jam or jelly	1 tablespoon	4
Molasses, light	1 teaspoon	14
Plum sauce	4 teaspoons	7
Potato chips	1 oz.	14
Pretzels	1 oz.	14
Sugar, brown	1 tablespoon	11
Sugar, cube	1	2
Sugar, granulated	1 tablespoon	11
Sugar, confectioners'	1 tablespoon	7
Syrup, maple	1 tablespoon	11
Syrup, pancake	1 tablespoon	11
Teriyaki sauce	1 tablespoon	7
Tortilla chips	1 oz.	14

Appendix E

Body Fat Calculations

A rapid way to determine your percentage of body fat is simply to use a tape measure. You should make all measurements on bare skin (not through clothing), and make sure that the tape fits snugly but does not compress the skin and underlying tissue. Take all measurements three times and calculate the average. All measurements should be in inches.

CALCULATING BODY-FAT PERCENTAGES FOR FEMALES

There are five steps you must take to calculate your percentage of body fat:

1. While keeping the tape level, measure your hips at their widest point, and your waist at the umbilicus (i.e., belly button). It is critical that you measure at the belly button and not at the narrowest point of your waist. Take each of these measurements three times and compute the average.
2. Measure your height in inches without shoes.
3. Record your height, waist, and hip measurements on the accompanying worksheet.
4. Find each of these measurements in the appropriate column in the accompanying tables and record the constants on the worksheet.
5. Add constants A and B, then subtract constant C for this sum and round to the nearest whole number. That figure is your percentage of body fat.

Conversion Constants for Calculation of Percentage of Body Fat in Females

Hips		Abdomen		Height	
Inches	Constant A	Inches	Constant B	Inches	Constant C
30	33.48	20	14.22	55	33.52
30.5	33.83	20.5	14.40	55.5	33.67
31	34.87	21.0	14.93	56	34.13
31.5	35.22	21.5	15.11	56.5	34.28
32	36.27	22	15.64	57	34.74
32.5	36.62	22.5	15.82	57.5	34.89
33	37.67	23	16.35	58	35.35
33.5	38.02	23.5	16.53	58.5	35.50
34	39.06	24	17.06	59	35.96
34.5	39.41	24.5	17.24	59.5	36.11
35	40.46	25	17.78	60	36.57
35.5	40.81	25.5	17.96	60.5	36.72
36	41.86	26	18.49	61	37.18
36.5	42.21	26.5	18.67	61.5	37.33
37	43.25	27	19.20	62	37.79
37.5	43.60	27.5	19.38	62.5	37.94
38	44.65	28	19.91	63	38.40
38.5	45.32	28.5	20.27	63.5	38.70
39	46.05	29	20.62	64	39.01
39.5	46.40	29.5	20.80	64.5	39.16
40	47.44	30	21.33	65	39.62
40.5	47.79	30.5	21.51	65.5	39.77
41	48.84	31	22.04	66	40.23
41.5	49.19	31.5	22.22	66.5	40.38
42	50.24	32	22.75	67	40.84
42.5	50.59	32.5	22.93	67.5	40.99
43	51.64	33	23.46	68	41.45
43.5	51.99	33.5	23.64	68.5	41.60
44	53.03	34	24.18	69	42.06
44.5	53.41	34.5	24.36	69.5	42.21

Hips		Abdomen		Height	
Inches	Constant A	Inches	Constant B	Inches	Constant C
45	54.53	35	24.89	70	42.67
45.5	54.86	35.5	25.07	70.5	42.82
46	55.83	36	25.60	71	43.28
46.5	56.18	36.5	25.78	71.5	43.43
47	57.22	37	26.31	72	43.89
47.5	57.57	37.5	26.49	72.5	44.04
48	58.62	38	27.02	73	44.50
48.5	58.97	38.5	27.20	73.5	44.65
49	60.02	39	27.73	74	45.11
49.5	60.37	39.5	27.91	74.5	45.26
50	61.42	40	28.44	75	45.72
50.5	61.77	40.5	28.62	75.5	45.87
51	62.81	41	29.15	76	46.32
51.5	63.16	41.5	29.33		
52	64.21	42	29.87		
52.5	64.56	42.5	30.05		
53	65.61	43	30.58		
53.5	65.96	43.5	30.76		
54	67.00	44	31.29		
54.5	67.35	44.5	31.47		
55	68.40	45	32.00		
55.5	68.75	45.5	32.18		
56	69.80	46	32.71		
56.5	70.15	46.5	32.89		
57	71.19	47	33.42		
57.5	71.54	47.5	33.60		
58	72.59	48	34.13		
58.5	72.94	48.5	34.31		
59	73.99	49	34.84		
59.5	74.34	49.5	35.02		
60	75.39	50	35.56		

Worksheet for Women to Calculate Their Percentage of Body Fat

Average hip measurement _____ (used for constant A)

Average abdomen measurement _____ (used for constant B)

Height _____ (used for constant C)

Using the table on pages 338 and 339, look up each of the average measurements and your height in the appropriate column.

Constant A = _____

Constant B = _____

Constant C = _____

To determine your approximate percentage of body fat, add constants A and B. From that total, subtract constant C. The result is your percentage of body fat, as shown below:

(Constant A + Constant B) − Constant C = % Body Fat

CALCULATING BODY-FAT PERCENTAGES FOR MEN

There are four steps you must take to determine your body-fat percentage:

1. While keeping the tape level, measure the circumference of your waist at the umbilicus (i.e., belly button). Measure three times and compute the average.
2. Measure your wrist at the space between your dominant hand and your wrist bone, at the location where your wrist bends.
3. Record these measurements on the worksheet for men.
4. Subtract your wrist measurement from your waist measurement and find the resulting value listed in the table. On the left-hand side of this table, find your weight. Proceed to the right from your weight and down from your waist-minus-wrist measurement. Where these two points intersect, read your body fat percentage.

Worksheet for Men to Calculate Their Percentage of Body Fat

Average waist measurement _____ (inches)

Average wrist measurement _____ (inches)

Subtract the wrist measurement from the waist measurement. Use the table starting on page 342 to find your weight. Then find your "waist-minus-wrist" number. Where the two columns intersect is your approximate percentage of body fat.

Male Percentage Body Fat Calculations

Waist-Wrist (in inches)	22	22.5	23	23.5	24
Weight (in pounds)					
120	4	6	8	10	12
125	4	6	7	9	11
130	3	5	7	9	11
135	3	5	7	8	10
140	3	5	6	8	10
145		4	6	7	9
150		4	6	7	9
155		4	5	6	8
160		4	5	6	8
165		3	5	6	8
170		3	4	6	7
175			4	6	7
180			4	5	7
185			4	5	6
190			4	5	6
195			3	5	6
200			3	4	6
205				4	5
210				4	5
215				4	5
220				4	5
225				3	4
230				3	4
235				3	4
240					4
245					4
250					4
255					3
260					3
265					
270					
275					
280					
285					
290					
295					
300					

24.5	25	25.5	26	26.5	27	27.5
14	16	18	20	21	23	25
13	15	17	19	20	22	24
12	14	16	18	20	21	23
12	13	15	17	19	20	22
11	13	15	16	18	19	21
11	12	14	15	17	19	20
10	12	13	15	16	18	19
10	11	13	14	16	17	19
9	11	12	14	15	17	18
9	10	12	13	15	16	17
9	10	11	13	14	15	17
8	10	11	12	12	15	16
8	9	10	12	13	14	16
8	9	10	11	13	14	15
7	8	10	11	12	13	15
7	8	9	11	12	13	14
7	8	9	10	11	12	14
6	8	9	10	11	12	13
6	7	8	9	11	12	13
6	7	8	9	10	11	12
6	7	8	9	10	11	12
6	7	8	9	10	11	12
5	6	7	8	9	10	11
5	6	7	8	9	10	11
5	6	7	8	9	10	11
5	6	7	8	9	9	10
5	6	6	7	8	9	10
4	5	6	7	8	9	10
4	5	6	7	8	9	10
4	5	6	7	8	8	9
4	5	6	7	7	8	9
4	5	5	6	7	8	9
4	4	5	6	7	8	9
4	4	5	6	7	8	8
3	4	5	6	7	7	8
3	4	5	6	6	7	8
3	4	5	5	6	7	8

Waist-Wrist (in inches)	28	28.5	29	29.5	30	30.5	31
Weight (in pounds)							
120	27	29	31	33	35	37	39
125	26	28	30	32	33	35	37
130	25	27	28	30	32	34	36
135	24	26	27	29	31	32	34
140	23	24	26	28	29	31	33
145	22	23	25	27	28	30	31
150	21	23	24	26	27	29	30
155	20	22	23	25	26	28	29
160	19	21	22	24	25	27	28
165	19	20	22	23	24	26	27
170	18	19	21	22	24	25	26
175	17	19	20	21	23	24	25
180	17	18	19	21	22	23	25
185	16	18	19	20	21	23	24
190	16	17	18	19	21	22	23
195	15	16	18	19	20	21	22
200	15	16	17	18	19	21	22
205	14	15	17	18	19	20	21
210	14	15	16	17	18	19	21
215	13	15	16	17	18	19	20
220	13	14	15	16	17	18	19
225	13	14	15	16	17	18	19
230	12	13	14	15	16	17	18
235	12	13	14	15	16	17	18
240	12	13	14	15	16	17	17
245	11	12	13	14	15	16	17
250	11	12	13	14	15	16	17
255	11	12	13	14	14	15	16
260	10	11	12	13	14	15	16
265	10	11	12	13	14	15	15
270	10	11	12	13	13	14	15
275	10	11	11	12	13	14	15
280	9	10	11	12	13	14	14
285	9	10	11	12	12	13	14
290	9	10	11	11	12	13	14
295	9	10	10	11	12	13	14
300	9	9	10	11	12	12	13

31.5	32	32.5	33	33.5	34	34.5
41	43	45	47	49	50	52
39	41	43	45	46	48	50
37	39	41	43	44	46	48
36	38	39	41	43	44	46
34	36	38	39	41	43	44
33	35	36	38	39	41	43
32	33	35	36	38	40	41
31	32	34	35	37	38	40
30	31	33	34	35	37	38
29	30	31	33	34	36	37
28	29	30	32	33	34	36
27	28	29	31	32	33	35
26	27	28	30	31	32	34
25	26	28	29	30	31	33
24	26	27	28	29	30	32
24	25	26	27	28	30	31
23	24	25	26	28	29	30
22	23	25	26	27	28	29
22	23	24	25	26	27	28
21	22	23	24	25	26	28
20	22	23	24	25	26	27
20	21	22	23	24	25	26
19	20	21	22	23	24	25
19	20	21	22	23	24	25
18	19	20	21	22	23	24
18	19	20	21	22	23	24
18	18	19	20	21	22	23
17	18	19	20	21	22	23
17	18	19	19	20	21	22
16	17	18	19	20	21	22
16	17	18	19	19	20	21
16	16	17	18	19	20	21
15	16	17	18	19	19	20
15	16	17	17	18	19	20
15	15	16	17	18	19	19
14	15	16	17	17	18	19
14	15	16	16	17	18	19

Waist-Wrist (in inches)	35	35.5	36	36.5	37
Weight (in pounds)					
120	54				
125	52	54			
130	50	52	53	55	
135	48	50	51	53	55
140	46	48	49	51	53
145	44	46	47	49	51
150	43	44	46	47	49
155	41	43	44	46	47
160	40	41	43	44	46
165	38	40	41	43	44
170	37	39	40	41	43
175	36	37	39	40	41
180	35	36	37	39	40
185	34	35	36	38	39
190	33	34	35	37	38
195	32	33	34	35	37
200	31	32	33	35	36
205	30	31	32	34	35
210	29	30	32	33	34
215	29	30	31	32	33
220	28	29	30	31	32
225	27	28	29	30	31
230	26	27	28	30	31
235	26	27	28	29	30
240	25	26	27	28	29
245	25	26	27	27	28
250	24	25	26	27	28
255	24	24	25	26	27
260	23	24	25	26	27
265	22	23	24	25	26
270	22	23	24	25	25
275	22	22	23	24	25
280	21	22	23	24	24
285	21	21	22	23	24
290	20	21	22	23	23
295	20	21	21	22	23
300	19	20	21	22	22

37.5	38	38.5	39	39.5	40	40.5
54						
52	54	55				
50	52	53	55			
49	50	52	53	55		
47	48	50	51	53	54	
45	47	48	50	51	52	54
44	45	47	48	49	51	52
43	44	45	47	48	49	51
41	43	44	45	47	48	49
40	41	43	44	45	46	48
39	40	41	43	44	45	46
38	39	40	41	43	44	45
37	38	39	40	41	43	44
36	37	38	39	40	41	43
35	36	37	38	39	40	42
34	35	36	37	38	39	40
33	34	35	36	37	38	39
32	33	34	35	36	37	38
32	33	34	35	36	37	38
31	32	33	34	35	36	37
30	31	32	33	34	35	36
29	30	31	32	33	34	35
29	30	31	31	32	33	34
28	29	30	31	32	33	34
27	28	29	30	31	32	33
27	28	29	29	30	31	32
26	27	28	29	30	31	31
26	27	27	28	29	30	31
25	26	27	28	29	29	30
25	26	26	27	28	29	30
24	25	26	27	27	28	29
24	25	25	26	27	28	28
23	24	25	26	26	27	28

Waist-Wrist (in inches)	41	41.5	42	42.5	43	43.5
Weight (in pounds)						
120						
125						
130						
135						
140						
145						
150						
155						
160						
165	55					
170	54	55				
175	52	53	55			
180	50	52	53	54		
185	49	50	51	53	54	55
190	48	49	50	51	52	54
195	46	47	49	50	51	52
200	45	46	47	48	50	51
205	44	45	46	47	48	49
210	43	44	45	46	47	48
215	42	43	44	45	46	47
220	41	42	43	44	45	46
225	40	41	42	43	44	45
230	39	40	41	42	44	44
235	38	39	40	41	42	43
240	37	38	39	40	41	42
245	36	37	38	39	40	41
250	35	36	37	38	39	40
255	34	35	36	37	38	39
260	34	35	35	36	37	38
265	33	34	35	36	36	37
270	32	33	34	35	36	37
275	32	32	33	34	35	36
280	31	32	33	33	34	35
285	30	31	32	33	34	34
290	30	31	31	32	33	34
295	29	30	31	32	32	33
300	29	29	30	31	32	33

44	44.5	45	45.5	46	46.5	47
55						
53	55					
52	53	54	55			
51	52	53	54	55		
49	50	51	53	54	55	
48	49	50	51	52	53	54
47	48	49	50	51	52	53
46	47	48	49	50	51	52
45	46	47	48	49	50	51
44	45	46	47	48	49	50
43	44	45	46	46	47	48
42	43	44	44	45	46	47
41	42	43	44	44	45	46
40	41	42	43	44	44	45
39	40	41	42	43	43	44
38	39	40	41	42	43	43
37	38	39	40	41	42	43
37	38	38	39	40	41	42
36	37	38	38	39	40	41
35	36	37	38	39	39	40
35	35	36	37	38	39	39
34	35	36	36	37	38	39
33	34	35	36	36	37	38

Waist-Wrist (in inches)	47.5	48	48.5	49	49.5	50
Weight (in pounds)						
120						
125						
130						
135						
140						
145						
150						
155						
160						
165						
170						
175						
180						
185						
190						
195						
200						
205						
210						
215	55					
220	54	55				
225	53	54	55			
230	52	53	54	55		
235	51	51	52	53	54	55
240	49	50	51	52	53	54
245	48	49	50	51	52	53
250	47	48	49	50	51	52
255	46	47	48	49	50	51
260	45	46	47	48	49	50
265	44	45	46	47	48	49
270	43	44	45	46	47	48
275	43	43	44	45	46	47
280	42	43	43	44	45	46
285	41	42	43	43	44	45
290	40	41	42	43	43	44
295	39	40	41	42	43	43
300	39	39	40	41	42	43

Appendix F

References

Introduction

Sears, B. *The Zone*. New York: ReganBooks, 1995.

Chapter 1. What Is Wellness?

Oates, J. A. "The 1982 Nobel prize in physiology or medicine." *Science* 218:765–768 (1982).

Sears, B. *The Zone*. New York: ReganBooks, 1995.

Sears, B. *The Anti-Aging Zone*. New York: ReganBooks, 1999.

Sears, B. *The Omega Rx Zone*. New York: ReganBooks, 2002.

Chapter 2. Why Is Silent Inflammation So Dangerous?

Braunwald, E. "Cardiovascular medicine at the turn of the millennium: triumphs, concerns, and applications." *N Engl J Med* 337:1360–1369 (1997).

McGeer, P. L., M. Shulzer, and E. G. McGeer. "Arthritis and anti-inflammatory agents as possible protective factors for Alzheimer's disease: a review of 17 epidemiological studies." *Neurology* 47:425–432 (1996).

Morris, M. C., D. A. Evans, J. L. Bienias, C. C. Tangney, D. A. Bennett, R. S. Wilson, N. Aggarwal, and J. Schneider. "Consumption of fish and n-3 fatty acids and risk of incident Alzheimer disease." *Arch Neurol* 60:940–966 (2003).

Moghadasian, M. H. "Experimental atherosclerosis. A historical overview." *Life Sci* 70:855–865 (2002).

Olser, W. *Lectures on Angina Pectoris and Allied States*. New York: Appleton, 1897.

Ross, R. "Atherosclerosis is an inflammatory disease." *N Engl J Med* 340:115–126 (1999).

Wolfe, M. M., R. D. Lichtenstein, and G. Singh. "Gastrointestinal toxicity of nonsteroidal anti-inflammatory drugs." *N Engl J Med* 340:1888–1889 (1999).

Yudkin, J. S., C. D. A. Stehouwer, J. J. Emeis, and S. W. Coppack. "C-reactive protein in healthy subjects: associations with obesity, insulin resistance, and endothelial dysfunction—a potential role for cytokines originating from adipose tissue?" *Arterioscler Thromb Vasc Biol* 19:972–978 (1999).

Chapter 3. The Cause and the Cure for Silent Inflammation

Sears, B. *The Zone*. New York: ReganBooks, 1995.
Sears, B. *The Anti-Aging Zone*. New York: ReganBooks, 1999.
Sears, B. *The Omega Rx Zone*. New York: ReganBooks, 2002.

Chapter 4. Testing for Silent Inflammation

Adams, P., S. Lawson, A. Sanigorski, and A. J. Sinclair. "Arachidonic acid to eicosapentaenoic acid ratio in blood correlates positively with clinical symptoms of depression." *Lipids* 31:S157-S161 (1996).
Boizel, R., P. Y. Behhamou, B. Lardy, F. Laporte, T. Foulon, and S. Halimi. "Ratio of triglycerides to HDL cholesterol is an indicator of LDL particle size in patients with type 2 diabetes and normal HDL cholesterol levels." *Diabetes Care* 23:1679–1685 (2000).
Campbell, B., T. Badrick, R. Flatman, and D. Kanowshi. "Limited clinical utility of high-sensitivity plasma C-reactive protein assays." *Ann Clin Biochem* 39:85–88 (2002).
Campbell, B., R. Flatman, T. Badrick, and D. Kanowshi. "Problems with high-sensitivity C-reactive protein." *Clin Chem* 49:201 (2003).
Conquer, J. A., M. C. Tierney, J. Zecevic, W. J. Bettger, and R. H. Fisher. "Fatty acid analysis of blood plasma of patients with Alzheimer's disease, other types of dementia, and cognitive impairment." *Lipids* 35:1305–1312 (2000).
Danesh, J., J. G. Wheeler, G. M. Hirschfield, G. Eiriksdottir, A. Remley, G. D. Lowe, M. B. Pepys, and J. Gudnason. "C-reactive protein and other circulating markers of inflammation in the prediction of coronary heart disease." *N Engl J Med* 350:1387–1397 (2004).
DeLongeril, M., S. Renaud, N. Mamelle, P. Salen, J. L. Martin, I, Monjaud, J. Guidollet, P. Touboul, and J. Delaye. "Mediterranean alpha-linolenic acid rich diet in secondary prevention of coronary heart disease." *Lancet* 343:1454–1459 (1994).
DeLongeril, M., P. Salen, J. L. Martin, I. Monjaud, J. Delaye, and N. Mamelle. "Mediterranean diet, traditional risk factors, and the rate of cardiovascular complications after myocardial infarction: final report of the Lyon Diet Heart Study." *Circulation* 99:779–785 (1999).
Deron, S. J. *C-reactive Protein*. Chicago: Contemporary Books, 2003.
Feng, D., R. P. Tracy, I. Lipinska, J. Murillo, C. McKenna, and G. H. Tofler. "Effect of short-term aspirin use on C-reactive protein." *J Thromb Thrombolysis* 9:37–41 (2000).
Feldman, M., I. Jialal, S. Devaraj, and B. Cryer. "Effects of low-dose aspirin on serum C-reactive protein and thromboxane B2 concentrations: a placebo-controlled study using a highly sensitive C-reactive protein assay." *J Am Coll Cardiol* 37:2036–2041 (2001).
Gaziano, J. M., C. H. Hennekens, C. J. O'Donnell, J. L. Breslow, and J. E. Buring. "Fasting triglycerides, high-density lipoproteins and risk of myocardial infarction." *Circulation* 96:2520–2525 (1997).

Iso, H., S. Sato, A. R. Falsm, T. Shimamoto, A. Terao, R. G. Munger, A. Kitamure, M. Konishi, M. Iida, and Y. Komachi. "Serum fatty acids and fish intake in rual Japanese, urban Japanese, Japanese American and Caucasian American men." *Int J Epidemiol* 18:374–381 (1989).

Jeppesen, J., H. O. Hein, P. Suadicani, and F. Gyntelberg. "Low triglycerides-high high-density lipoprotein cholesterol and risk of ischemic heart disease." *Arch Intern Med* 161:361–366 (2001).

Kagawa, Y., M., Nishizawa, M. Suzuki, T. Miyatake, T. Hamamoto, K. Goto, E. Motonaga, H. Izumikawa, H. Hirata, and A. Ebihara. "Eicosapolyenoic acid of serum lipids of Japanese islanders with low incidence of cardiovascular diseases." *J Nutr Sci Vitaminol* 28:441–453 (1982).

Kluft, C. and M. P. M. de Maat. "Genetics of C-reactive protein." *Arterioscler Thromb Vasc Biol* 23:1956–1959 (2003).

Kromann, N. and A. Green. "Epidemiological studies in Upernavik district, Greenland." *Acta Med Scand* 208:401–406 (1974).

Laidlaw, M. and B. J. Holub. "Effects of supplementation with fish oil-derived n-3 fatty acids and gamma-linolenic acid on circulating plasma lipids and fatty acid profiles in women." *Am J Clin Nutr* 77:37–42 (2003).

Lamarche, B., A. Tchernot, P. Mauriege, B. Cantin, G. R. Gagenais, P. J. Lupien, and J-P. Despres. "Fasting insulin and apolipoprotein B levels and low-density particle size as risk factors for ischemic heart disease." *JAMA* 279:1965–1971 (1998).

Maes, M. "Fatty acid composition in major depression: decreased n-3 fractions in cholesterol esters and increased C20:n6/C20:5n3 ratio in cholesterol ester and phospholipids." *J Affect Dis* 38:35–46 (1996).

Maes, M., A. Christophe, J. Delanghe, C. Altamura, H. Neels, and H. Y. Meltzer. "Lowered omega-3 polyunsaturated fatty acids in serum phospholpids and cholesteryl esters of depressed patients." *Pscyhiatry Res* 85:275–291 (1999).

Nakamura, T., A. Azuma, T. Kuribayashi, H. Sugihara, S. Okuda, and M. Nakagawa. "Serum fatty acid levels, dietary style and coronary heart in three neighbouring areas in Japan." *Br J Nutr* 89:267–272 (2003).

Nordvik, I., K. M. Myhr, H. Nyland, and K. S. Bjerve. "Effect of dietary advice and n-3 supplementation in newly diagnosed MS patients." *Acta Neurol Scand* 102:143–149 (2000).

Pedesen, H. S., G. Mulvad, K. N. Seidelin, G. T. Malcom, and D. A. Doudreau. "N-3 fatty acids as a risk marker for haemorrhagic stroke." *Lancet* 353:812–813 (1999).

Pirro, M., J. Bergeron, G. R. Dagenais, P-M. Bernard, B. Cantin, J-P. Depres, and B. Lamarche. "Age and duration of follow-up as modulators of the risk for ischemic heart disease associated with high plasma C-reactive protein levels in men." *Arch Intern Med* 161:2474–2480 (2001).

Ridker, P. M. "High-sensitivity C-reactive protein." *Circulation* 103:1813–1818 (2001).

Ridker, P. M., M. Cushman, M. J. Stampfer, R. P. Tracy, and C. H. Hennekens. "Inflammation, aspirin, and the risk of cardiovascular disease in apparently healthy men." *N Engl J Med* 336:973–979 (1996).

Ridker, P. M., N. Fifai, M. J. Stampfer, and C. H. Hennekens. "Plasma concentration of interleukin-6 and the risk of future myocardinal infarction among apparently healthy men." *Circulation* 101:1767–1772 (2000).

Ridker, P. M., C. H. Hennekens, J. E. Buring, and N. Rifai. "C-reactive protein and other markers of inflammation in the prediction of cardiovascular disease in women." *New Engl J Med* 42:836–843 (2000).

Ridker, P. M., N. Rifai, M. A. Pfeffer, F. M. Sacks, L. A. Moye, S. Goldman, G. C. Flaker, E. Braunwald. "Inflammation, pravastatin, and the risk of coronary events after myocardial infarction in patients with average cholesterol levels. Cholesterol and Recurrent Events (CARE) Investigators." *Circulation* 98:839–44 (1998).

Rifai, N. and P. M. Ridker. "High-sensitivity C-reactive protein: a novel and promising marker of coronary heart disease." *Clin Chem* 47:403–411 (2001).

Sears, B. *The Omega Rx Zone*. New York: ReganBooks, 2002.

Stevens, L. J. and J. Burgess. "Omega-3 fatty acids in boys with behavior, learning, and health problems." *Physiology Behavior* 59:915–920 (1996).

Stevens, L. J., S. S. Zentall, J. L. Deck, M. L. Abate, B. A. Watkins, S. A. Lipp, and J. R. Burgess. "Essential fatty acid metabolism in boys with attention-deficit hyperactivity disorder." *Am J Clin Nutr* 62:761–768 (1995).

Takeda, T., S. Hoshida, M. Nishino, J. Tanouchi, K. Otsu, and M. Hori. "Relationship between effects of statins, aspirin and angiotensin II modulators on high-sensitive C-reactive protein levels." *Atherosclerosis* 169:155–188 (2003).

Tall, A. R. "C-reactive protein reassessed." *N Engl J Med* 350:1450–1452 (2004).

Upritchard, J. E., W. H. Sutherland, and J. I. Mann. "Effect of supplementation with tomato juice, vitamin E, and vitamin C on LDL oxidation and products of inflammatory activity in type 2 diabetes." *Diabetes Care* 23:733–738 (2000).

Yamada, T., J. P. Strong, T. Ishii, T. Ueno, M. Koyama, H. Wagayama, A. Shimizu, T. Sakai, G. T. Malcom, and M. A. Guzman. "Atherosclerosis and omega-3 fatty acids in the populations of a fishing village and a farming village in Japan." *Atherosclerosis* 153:469–481 (2000).

Yeni-Komshian, H., M. Caratoni, F. Abbasi, and G. M. Reaven. "Relationship between several surrogate estimates of insulin resistance and quantification of insulin-mediated glucose disposal in 490 healthy nondiabetic volunteers." *Diabetes Care* 23:171–175 (2000).

Chapter 5. Your First Line of Defense Against Silent Inflammation: The Zone Diet

Astrup, P. A., D. T., Meinert Larsen, and A. Harper. "Atkins and other low-carbohydrate diets: hoax or an effective tool for weight loss?" *Lancet* 364:897–899 (2004).

Bell, S. J. and B. Sears. "Low glycemic load diets: impact on obesity and chronic diseases." *Crit Rev Food Sci Nutr* 43:357–377 (2003).

Bell, S. J. and B. Sears. "A proposal for a new national diet: a low glycemic load diet with a unique macronutrient composition." *Metabolic Syndrome and Related Disorders* 1:199–200 (2003).

Flegal, K. M., M. D. Carroll, C. L. Ogden, and C. L. Johnson. "Prevalence and trends in obesity among US adults, 1999–2000." *JAMA* 288:1723–1727 (2002).

Foster-Powell, K., S. H. Holt, J. C. Brand-Miller. "International table of glycemic index and glycemic load values: 2002." *Am J Clin Nutr* 76:5–56 (2002).

Jenkins, D. J., T. M. Wolever, R. H. Taylor, H. Barker, H. Fielden, J. M. Baldwin, A. C. Bowling, H. C. Newman, A. L. Jenkins, and D. V. Goff. "Glycemic index of foods: a physiological basis for carbohydrate exchange." *Am J Clin Nutr* 34:362–366 (1981).

Leeds, A. R. "Glycemic index and heart disease." *Am J Clin Nutr* 76:286S-289S (2002).

Liu, S., J. E. Manson, J. E. Buring, M. J. Stampfer, W. C. Willett, and P. M. Ridker. "Relation between a diet with a high glycemic load and plasma concentrations of high-sensitivity C-reactive protein in middle-aged women." *Am J Clin Nutr* 75:492–498 (2002).

Liu, S., J. E. Manson, M. J. Stampfer, M. D. Holmes, F. B. Hu, S. E. Hankinson, and W. C. Willett. "Dietary glycemic load assessed by food-frequency questionnaire in relation to plasma high-density-lipoprotein cholesterol and fasting plasma triacylglycerols in post-menopausal women." *Am J Clin Nutr* 73:560–566 (2001).

Liu, S., W. C. Willett, M. J. Stampfer, F. B. Hu, M. Franz, L. Sampson, C. H. Hennekens, and J. E. Manson. "A prospective study of dietary glycemic load, carbohydrate intake, and risk of coronary heart disease in US women." *Am J Clin Nutr* 71:1455–1461 (2002).

Ludwig, D. S. "The glycemic index: physiological mechanisms relating to obesity, diabetes, and cardiovascular disease." *JAMA* 287:2414–2423 (2002).

Ludwig, D. S., J. A. Majzoub, A. Al-Zahrani, G. E. Dallal, I. Blanco, and S. B. Roberts. "High glycemic index foods, overeating, and obesity." *Pediatrics* 103:E26 (1999).

Mokdad, A. H., E. S. Ford, B. A. Bowman, W. H. Dietz, F. Vinicor, V. S. Bales, and J. S. Marks. "Prevalence of obesity, diabetes, and obesity-related health risk factors, 2001." *JAMA* 289:76–79 (2003).

Mokdad, A. H., E. S. Ford, B. A. Bowman, D. E. Nelson, M. M. Engelgau, F. Vinicor, and J. S. Marks. "Diabetes trends in the U.S." 1990–1998." *Diabetes Care* 23:1278–1283 (2000).

Ogden, C. L., K. M. Flegal, M. D. Carroll, and C. L. Johnson. "Prevalence and trends in over-weight among US children and adolescents, 1999–2000." *JAMA* 288:1728–32 (2002).

Roberts, S. B. "High-glycemic index foods, hunger, and obesity: is there a connection?" *Nutr Rev* 58:163–169 (2000).

Salmeron, J., J. E. Manson, M. J. Stampfer, G. A. Colditz, A. L. Wing, and W. C. Willett. "Dietary fiber, glycemic load, and risk of non-insulin-dependent diabetes mellitus in women." *JAMA* 277:472–477 (1997).

Sears, B. *The Zone.* New York: ReganBooks, 1995.

Sears, B. *Mastering the Zone.* New York, ReganBooks, 1997.

Sears, B. *A Week in the Zone.* New York: ReganBooks, 2000.

Sears, B. and S. J. Bell. "The Zone Diet: an anti-inflammatory, low glycemic-load diet." *Metabolic Syndrome and Related Disorders* 2:24–38 (2004).

Sears, B. and L. Sears. *Zone Meals in Seconds.* New York: ReganBooks, 2002.

Willett, W., J. Manson and S. Liu. "Glycemic index, glycemic load, and risk of type 2 diabetes." *Am J Clin Nutr* 76:274S-280S (2002).

Chapter 6. Turning Your Kitchen into an Anti-Inflammatory Pharmacy

Sears, B. *The Zone.* New York: ReganBooks, 1995.

Sears, B. *Mastering the Zone.* New York, ReganBooks, 1997.

Sears B. *Zone Perfect Meals in Minutes.* New York: ReganBooks, 1998.

Sears B. *Zone Food Blocks.* New York: ReganBooks, 1998.

Sears B. *Top 100 Zone Foods*. New York: ReganBooks, 1999.

Sears, B. *A Week in the Zone*. New York: ReganBooks, 2000.

Sears, B. and L. Sears. *Zone Meals in Seconds*. New York: ReganBooks, 2004.

Chapter 7. Your Ultimate Defense Against Silent Inflammation: High-Dose Fish Oil

Arisawa, K., T. Matsummura, C. Tohyama, H. Saito, M. Hagai, M. Morita, and T. Suzuki. "Fish intake, plasma omega-3 polyunsaturated fatty acids, and polychlorinated dibenzo-p-dioxins/polychlorinated dibenzo-furans and co-planar polychlorinated biphenyls in the blood of the Japanese population." *Int Arch Occup Environ Health* 76:205–215 (2003).

Pedesen, H. S., G. Mulvad, K. N. Seidelin, G. T. Malcom, and D. A. Doudreau. "N-3 fatty acids as a risk marker for haemorrhagic stroke." *Lancet* 353:812–813 (1999).

Sears, B. *The Omega Rx Zone*. New York: ReganBooks, 2002.

Zuijdgeest-van Leeuwen, S. D., P. C. Dagnelie, T. Rietveld, J. W. O. van den Berg, and J. H. P. Wilson. "Incorporation and washout of rally administered n-3 fatty acid ethyl esters in different plasma lipid fracions." *Brit J Nutr* 82:481–488 (1999).

Chapter 8. Additional Supplements to Help Reduce Silent Inflammation

Albert, M. A., R. J. Glynn, and P. M. Ridker. "Alcohol consumption and plasma concentration of C-reactive protein." *Circulation* 107:443–447 (2003).

DeLongeril, M., S. Renaud, N. Mamelle, P. Salen, J. L. Martin, I. Monjaud, J. Guidollet, P. Touboul, and J. Delaye. "Mediterranean alpha-linolenic acid rich diet in secondary prevention of coronary heart disease." *Lancet* 343:1454–1459 (1994).

DeLongeril, M., P. Salen, J. L. Martin, I. Monjaud, J. Delaye, and N. Mamelle. "Mediterranean diet, traditional risk factors, and the rate of cardiovascular complications after myocardial infarction: final report of the Lyon Diet Heart Study." *Circulation* 99:779–785 (1999).

GISSI-Prevenzione Investigators. "Dietary supplementation with n-3 polyunsaturated fatty acids and vitamin E after myocardial infarction: results of the GISSI-Prevenzione trial." *Lancet* 354:447–455 (1999).

Higdon, J. V., S. H. Du, Y. S. Lee, T. Wu, and R. C. Wander. "Supplementation of post-menopausal women with fish oil does not increase overall oxidation of LDL ex vivo compared to dietary oils rich in oleate and linoleate." *J Lipid Res* 42:407–418 (2001).

Horrocks, L. A. and Y. K. Yeo. "Health benefits of docosahexaenoic acid (DHA)." *Pharmacol Res* 40:211–225 (1999).

Jacobs, E. J., C. J. Connell, A. V. Patel, A. Chao, C. Rodriguez, J. Seymour, M. L. McCullough, E. E. Calle, and M. J. Thun. "Vitamin C and vitamin E supplement use and colorectal cancer mortality in a large American Cancer Society cohort." *Cancer Epidemiol Biomarkers Prev* 10:17–23 (2001).

Kangasaho, M., M. Hillbom, M. Kaste, and H. Vapaatalo. "Effects of ethanol intoxication and hangover on plasma levels of thromboxane B2 and 6-keto-prostaglandin F1 alpha and on thromboxane B2 formation by platelets in man." *Thromb Haemost* 48:232- 234 (1982).

Lee, S. H. and I. A. Blair. "Vitamin C–induced decomposition of lipid hydroperoxides to endogenous genotoxins." *Science* 292:2083–2086 (2001).

Leitzmann, M. F., M. J. Stampfer, D. S. Michaud, K. Augustsson, G. C. Colditz, W. C. Willett, and E. L. Giovannucci. "Dietary intake of n-3 and n-6 fatty acids and the risk of prostate cancer." *Am J Clin Nutr* 80:204–216 (2004).

Lonn, E., S. Yusuf, B. Hoogwerf, J. Pogue, Q. Yi, B. Zinman, J. Bosch, G. Dagenais, J. F. Mann, and H. C. Gerstein. "Effects of vitamin E on cardiovascular and microvascular outcomes in high-risk patients with diabetes: results of the HOPE study and MICRO-HOPE substudy." *Diabetes Care* 25:1919–1927 (2002).

Omenn, G. S., G. E. Goodman, M. D. Thornquist, J. Balmes, M. R. Cullen, A. Glass, J. P. Keogh, F. L. Meyskens, B. Valanis, J. H. Williams, S. Barnhart, M. G. Cherniack, C. A. Brodkin, and S. Hammar. "Risk factors for lung cancer and for intervention effects in CARET, the Beta-Carotene and Retinol Efficacy Trial." *J Natl Cancer Inst* 88:1550–1559 (1996).

Stephens, N. G., A. Parsons, P. M. Schofield, F. Kelly, K. Cheeseman, and M. J. Mitchinson. "Randomised controlled trial of vitamin E in patients with coronary disease: Cambridge Heart Antioxidant Study (CHAOS)." *Lancet* 347:781 786 (1996).

Tornwall, M. E., J. Virtamo, P. A. Korhonen, M. J. Virtanen, P. R. Taylor, D. Albanes, and J. K. Huttunen. "Effect of alpha-tocopherol and beta-carotene supplementation on coronary heart disease during the 6-year post-trial follow-up in the ATBC study." *Eur Heart J* 25:1171–1178 (2004).

Chapter 9. Smart Exercise to Help Reduce Silent Inflammation

Calder, P. C. and P. Yaqoob. "Glutamine and the immune system." *Amino Acids* 17:227–241 (1999).

Church, T. S., Y. J. Cheng, C. P. Earnest, C. E. Barlow, L. W. Gibbons, E. L. Priest, and S. N. Blair. "Exercise capacity and body composition as predictors of mortality among men with diabetes." *Diabetes Care* 27:83–88 (2004).

Farrell, S. W., L. Braun, C. E. Barlow, Y. J. Cheng, and S. N. Blair. "The relation of body mass index, cardiorespiratory fitness, and all-cause mortality in women." *Obesity Res* 10:417–423 (2002).

Horner, P. J. and F. H. Gage. "Regenerating the damaged central nervous system." *Nature* 407:963–970

Lee, C. D., S. N. Blair, and A. S. Jackson. "Cardiorespiratory fitness, body composition, and all-cause and cardiovascular disease mortality in men." *Am J Clin Nutr* 69:373–380 (1999).

Neeper, S. A., F. Gomez-Pinilla, J. Choi, and C. W. Cotman. "Physical activity increases mRNA for brain-derived neurotrophic factor and nerve growth factor in rat brain." *Brain Res* 726:49–56 (1996).

Newsholme, P. "Why is L-glutamine metabolism important to cells of the immune system in health, postinjury, surgery or infection?" *J Nutr* S131:2515S-2522S (2001).

Sears, B. *The Omega Rx Zone.* New York: ReganBooks, 2002.

Wojtaszewski, J. R. P., B. F. Hansen, J. Gade, B. Kiena, J. F. Markuna, L. J. Goodyear, and E. A. Richter. "Insulin signaling and insulin sensitivity after exercise in human skeletal muscle." *Diabetes* 49:325–331 (2000).

Chapter 10. Decreasing the Collateral Damage of Silent Inflammation: Cortisol Reduction Strategies

Benson, H. *The Relaxation Response*. New York: William Morrow, 1975.

Carrington, P. *The Book of Mediation*. Boston: Element Books, 1998.

Hamazaki, T., M. Itomura, S. Sawazaki, and Y. Nagao. "Anti-stress effects of DHA." *Biofactors* 13:41–45 (2000).

Homer, H., D. Packan, and R. M. Sapolsky. "Glucocorticoids inhibit glucose transport in cultured hippocampal neurons and glia." *Neuroendocrinology* 52:57–63 (1990).

Kamei, T., Y. Toriumi, H. Kimura, S. Ohno, H. Kumano, and K. Kimura. "Decrease in serum cortisol during yoga exercise is correlated with alpha wave activation." *Percept Mot Skills* 90:1027–1032 (2000).

MacLean, C. R., K. G. Walton, S. R. Wenneberg, D. K. Levitsky, J. P. Mandarino, R. Waziri, S. L. Hillis, and R. H. Schneider. "Effects of the Transcendental Meditation program on adaptive mechanisms: changes in hormone levels and responses to stress after 4 months of practice." *Psychoneuroendocrinology* 22:277–295 (1997).

Maes, M., A. Christophe, E. Bosmans, A. Lin, and H. Neels. "In humans, serum polyunsaturated fatty acid levels predict the response of proinflammatory cytokines to psychologic stress." *Psychiatry* 47:910–920 (2000).

Maier, S. F. and L. R. Watkins. "Cytokines for psychologists: implications of bidirectional immune-to-brain communication for understanding behavior, mood, and cognition." *Psychol Rev* 105:83–107 (1998).

Sears, B. *The Anti-Aging Zone*. New York: ReganBooks, 1999.

Sears, B. *The Omega Rx Zone*. New York: ReganBooks, 2002.

Spiegel, K., R. Leproult, and E. Van Cauter. "Impact of sleep debt on metabolic and endocrine function." *Lancet* 354:1435–1439 (1999).

Spolsky, R. M. *Stress, the Aging Brain, and the Mechanisms of Neuron Death*. Cambridge, MA: MIT Press, 1992.

Spolsky, R. M., D. R. Packan, and W. W. Vale. "Glucocorticoid toxicity in the hippocampus." *Brain Res* 453:367–371 (1988).

Sudsuang, R., V. Chentanez, and K. Veluvan. "Effect of Buddhist meditation on serum cortisol and total protein levels, blood pressure, pulse rate, lung volume and reaction time." *Physiol Behav* 50:543–548 (1991).

Talbott, S. and W. Kramer. *The Cortisol Connection*. Berkeley, CA: Hunter House, 2002.

Vgontzas, A. N., E. Zoumakis, E. O. Bixler, H. M. Lin, H. Follett, A. Kales, and G. P. Chrousos. "Adverse effects of modest sleep restriction on sleepiness, performance, and inflammatory cytokines." *J Clin Endocrinol Metab* 89:2119–2126 (2004).

Wilson, J. L. *Adrenal Fatigue*. Petaluma, CA: Smart Publications, 2001.

Chapter 12. Eicosanoids: The Good, the Bad, and the Neutral

Barham, J. B., M. B. Edens, A. N. Fonteh, M. M. Johnson, L. Easter, and F. H. Chilton. "Addition of eicosapentaenoic acid to gamma-linolenic-acid supplemented diets prevents serum arachidonic acid accumulation in humans." *J Nutr* 130:1925–1931 (2000).

Brenner, R. R. "Nutrition and hormonal factors influencing desaturation of essential fatty acids." *Prog Lipid Res* 20:41–48 (1982).

Burr, G. O. and M. R. Burr. "A new deficiency disease produced by rigid exclusion of fat from the diet." *J Biol Chem* 82:345–367 (1929).

Chapkin, R. S., S. D. Somer, and K. L. Erickson. "Dietary manipulation of macrophage phospholipids classes: selective increase in dihomo gamma linolenic acid." *Lipids* 23:776–770 (1988).

Chavali, S. R. and R. A. Forse. "Decreased production of interleukin-6 and prostaglandin E2 associated with inhibition of delta-5 desaturation of omega 6 fatty acids in mice fed safflower oil diets supplemented with sesamol." *Prostaglandins Leukot Essent Fatty Acids* 61:347–352 (1999).

Cho, H. P., M. Nakamura, and S. D. Clarke. "Cloning, expression, and fatty acid regulation of human delta 5 desaturase." *J Biol Chem* 274:37335–37399 (1999).

Clarke, S. D. "Polyunsaturated fatty acid regulation of gene transcription: a mechanism to improve energy balance and insulin resistance." *Br J Nutr* 83:S59-S66 (2000).

Connor, W. E. "Importance of n-3 fatty acids in health and disease." *Am J Clin Nutr* 71:S171S-S175 (2000).

Conquer, J. A. and B. J. Holub. "Dietary docosahexaenoic acid as a source of eicosapentaenoic acid in vegetarians and omnivores." *Lipids* 32:341–345 (1997).

El Boustani, S., J. E. Gausse, B. Descomps, L. Monnier, F. Mendy, and A. Crastes de Paulet. "Direct in vivo characterization of the delta-5 desaturase activity in humans by deuterium labeling: effect of insulin." *Metabolism* 38:315-3321 (1989).

Ferreria, S. H., S. Moncada, and J. R. Vane. "Indomethacin and aspirin abolish prostaglandin release from the spleen." *Natur New Bio* 231:237–239 (1971).

Garg, M. L., A. B. R. Thomson, and M. T. Clandinin. "Effect of dietary cholesterol and/or omega-3 fatty acids on lipid composition and delta 5-desaturase activity of rat liver microsomes." *J Nutr* 118:661–668 (1998).

Hill, E. G., S. B. Johnson, L. D. Lawson, M. M. Mahfouz, and R. T. Holman. "Perturbation of the metabolism of essential fatty acids by dietary partially hydrogenated vegetable oil." *Proc Natl Acad Sci U S A* 79:953–957 (1982).

Oates, J. A. "The 1982 Nobel prize in physiology or medicine." *Science* 218:765–768 (1982).

Pelikonova, T., M. Kohout, J. Base, Z. Stefka, L. Kovar, L. Kerdova, and J. Valek. "Effect of acute hyperinsulinemia on fatty acid composition of serum lipid in non-insulin dependent diabetics and healthy men." *Clin Chem Acta* 203:329–337 (1991).

Phinney, S. "Potential risk of prolonged gamma-linolenic acid use." *Ann Intern Med* 120:692 (1994).

Robertson, R. P., D. J. Gavarenski, D. Porte, and E. L. Bierman. "Inhibition of in vivo insulin secretion by prostaglandin E1." *J Clin Invest* 54:310–315 (1974).

Sears, B. *The Zone*. New York: ReganBooks, 1995.

Sears, B. *The Anti-Aging Zone*. New York: ReganBooks, 1999.

Sears, B. *The Omega Rx Zone*. New York: ReganBooks, 2002.

Serhan, C. N. "Lipoxins and aspirin-triggered 15-epi-lipoxin biosynthesis: an update and role in anti-inflammation and pro-resolution." *Prostaglandins Other Lipid Mediat* 69:433–455 (2002).

Shimizu, S., K. Akimoto, Y. Shinmen, H. Kawashima, M. Sugano, and H. Yamada. "Sesamin is a potent and specific inhibitor of delta 5 desaturase in polyunsaturated fatty acid biosynthesis." *Lipids* 26:512–516 (1991).

Smith, D. L., A. L. Willis, N. Nguyen, D. Conner, S. Zahedi, and J. Fulks. "Eskimo plasma constituents, dihomo gamma linolenic acid, eicosapentaenoic acid, and docosahexaenoic acid inhibit the release of atherogenic mitogens." *Lipids* 24:70–75 (1989).

Stone, K. J., A. L. Willis, M. Hurt, S. J. Kirtland, P. B. A. Kernof, and G. F. McNichol. "The metabolism of dihomo gamma linolenic acid in man." *Lipids* 14:174–180 (1979).

Von Euler, U. S. "On specific vasodilating and plain muscle stimulating substances from accessory genital glands in men and certain animals (prostaglandins and vesiglandin)." *J Physiol (London)* 88:213–234 (1936).

Willis, A. L. *Handbook of Eicosanoids, Prostaglandins, and Related Lipids*. Boca Raton: CRC Press, 1987.

Yam, D., B. Elitaz, B. Eliraz, and M. Elliot. "Diet and disease: the Israeli paradox: possible dangers of a high omega-6 polyunsaturated fatty acid diet." *Isr J Med Sci* 32:1134–1143 (1996).

Chapter 13. Why Inflammation Hurts, How Inflammation Heals

Babcok, T., W. S. Helton, and N. J. Espat. "Eicosapentaenoic acid: an anti-inflammatory omega-3 fat with potential clinical applications." *Nutrition* 16:1116–1118 (2000).

Bazan, N. G. and R. L. Flower. "Lipid signals in pain control." *Nature* 420:135–138 (2002).

Bechoua, S., M. Dubois, G. Nemoz, P. Chapy, E. Vericel, M. Lagarde, and A. F. Prigent. "Very low dietary intake of n-3 fatty acids affects the immune function of healthy elderly people." *Lipids* 34:S143 (1999).

Bleumink, G. S., J. Feenstra, M. C. M. J. Sturkenboom, and B. H. C. Stricker. "Nonsteroidal anti-inflammatory drugs and heart failure." *Drugs* 63:525–534 (2003).

Blok, W. L., M. B. Katan, and J. W. van der Meer. "Modulation of inflammation and cytokine production by dietary (n-3) fatty acids." *J Nutr* 126:1515–1533 (1996).

Calder, P. C. "n-3 polyunsaturated fatty acids and cytokine production in health and disease." *Ann Nutr Metab* 41:203–234 (1997).

Calder, P. C. "n-3 polyunsaturated fatty acids, inflammation and immunity." *Nutr Res* 21:309–341 (2001).

Calder, P. C. "Dietary modification of inflammation with lipids." *Proc Nutr Soc* 61:345–358 (2002).

Endres, S. "Messengers and mediators: interactions among lipids, eicosanoids, and cytokines." *Am J Clin Nutr* 57:798S–800S (1993).

Endres, S. "n-3 polyunsaturated fatty acids and human cytokine synthesis." *Lipids* 31:S239–242 (1996).

Endres, S., R. Ghorbani, V. E. Kelley, K. Georgilis, G. Lonnemann, J. W. van der Meer, J. G. Cannon, T. S. Rogers, M. S. Klempner, and P. C. Weber. "The effect of dietary supplementation with n-3 polyunsaturated fatty acids on the synthesis of interleukin-1 and tumor necrosis factor by mononuclear cells." *N Engl J Med* 320:265–271 (1989).

Endres, S., R. Lorenz, and K. Loeschke. "Lipid treatment of inflammatory bowel disease." *Curr Opin Clin Nutr Metab Care* 2:117–20 (1999).

Endres, S. and von Schacky, C. "n-3 polyunsaturated fatty acids and human cytokine synthesis." *Curr Opin Lipidol* 7:48–52. (1996).

Hong, S., K. Gronert, P. R. Devchand, R. L. Moussignac, and C. N. Serhan. "Novel docosatrienes and 17S-resolvins generated from docosahexaenoic acid in murine brain, human blood, and glial cells. Autocoids in anti-inflammation." *J Biol Chem* 278:14677–14687 (2003).

Jozsef, L., C. Zouki, N. A. Petasis, C. N. Serhan, and J. G. Filep. "Lipoxin A4 and aspirin-triggered 15-epi-lipoxin A4 inhibit peroxynitriete formation, NF kappa B and AP-1 activation, and IL-8 gene expression in human leukocytes." *Proc Natl Acad Sci U S A* 99:13266–13271 (2002).

Lawrence, T., D. A. Willoughby, and D. W. Gilroy. "Anti-inflammatory lipid mediators and insights into the resolution of inflammation." *Nature Rev Immunol* 2:787–795 (2002).

Levy, B., C. B. Clish, B. Schmidt, K. Gronert, and C. N. Serhan. "Lipid mediator class switching during acute inflammation: signals in resolution." *Nature Immunol* 2:612–619 (2001).

Lo, C. J., K. C. Chiu, M. Fu, R. Lo, and S. Helton. "Fish oil decreases macrophage tumor necrosis factor gene transcription by altering the NF kappaB activity." *J Surg Res* 82:216–221 (1999).

Meydani, S. N. "Effect of n-3 polyunsaturated fatty acid on cytokine production and their biological action." *Nutrition* 12:S8–14 (1996).

Perretti, M., N. Chiang, M. La, I. M. Fierro, S. Marullo, S. J. Getting, E. Solito, and C. N. Serhan. "Endogenous lipid- and peptide derived anti-inflammatory pathways generated with glucocorticoid and aspirin treatment activate the lipoxin A4 receptor." *Nature Med* 9:1296–1302 (2002).

Serhan, C. N. "Lipoxins and aspirin-triggered 15-epi-lipoxin biosynthesis: an update and role in anti-inflammation and pro-resolution." *Prostaglandins Other Lipid Mediat* 69:433–455 (2002).

Serhan, C. N., S. Hong, K. Gronert, S. P. Colgan, P. R. Devchand, G. Mirick, and R. L. Moussignac. "Resolvins: a family of bioactive products of omega-3 fatty acid transformation circuits intiated by aspirin treatment that counter proinflammation signals." *J Exp Med* 196:1025–1037 (2002).

Sperling, R. I. "The effects of dietary n-3 polyunsaturated fatty acids on neutrophils." *Proc Nutr Soc* 57:527–534 (1998).

Tak, P. P., and G. S. Firestein. "NF-kappaB: a key role inflammatory diseases." *J Clin Invest* 107:7–11 (2001).

Teitelbaum, J. E., and W. Allan Walker. "The role of omega-3 fatty acids in intestinal inflammation." *J Nutr Biochem* 12:21–32 (2001).

Tracey, K. J. "The inflammatory reflex." *Nature* 420:853–859 (2002).

Trowbridge, H. O. and R. C. Emling. *Inflammation*. Chicago: Quintessence Publishing, 1997.

Van Dyke, T. E., and C. N. Serhan. "Resolution of inflammation." *J Dental Res* 82:82–90 (2003).

Zurier, R. B. "Eicosanoids and inflammation." In *Prostaglandins in Clinical Practice,* ed. W. D. Watkins, M. B. Peterson, and J. R. Flectcher, pp. 79–96. New York: Raven Press, 1989.

Chapter 14. The Obesity-Diabetes-Silent Inflammation Connection

Allison, D. B., R. Zannolli, M. S. Faith, M. Heo, A. Pietrobelli, T. B. Van Itallie, F. X. Pi-Sunyer, and S. B. Heymsfield. "Weight loss increases and fat loss decreases all-cause mortality rate." *Int J Obes* 23:603–611 (1999).

American Diabetes Association. "Economic costs of diabetes in the U.S. in 2002." *Diabetes Care* 26:917–932 (2003).

Bloomgarden, Z. T. "Cardiovascular disease and diabetes." *Diabetes Care* 26:230–237 (2003).

Bloomgarden, Z. T. "Inflammation and insulin resistance." *Diabetes Care* 26:1922–1926 (2003).

Borkman, M., L. H. Storlien, D. A. Pan, A. B. Jenkins, D. J. Chisholm, and L. V. Campbell. "The relation between insulin sensitivity and the fatty-acid composition of skeletal-muscle phopholipids." *N Engl J Med* 328:911–917 (1993).

Botion, L. M. and A. Green. "Long-term regulation of lipolysis and hormone-sensitive lipase by insulin and glucose." *Diabetes* 48:1691–1697 (1999).

Brandes, J. "Insulin induced overeating in the rat." *Physiol Rev* 18:1095–1102 (1977).

Challem, J., B. Berkson, and M. D. Smith. *Syndrome X.* New York: John Wiley and Sons, 2000.

Coste, T. C., A. Gerbi, P. Vague, G. Pieroni, and D. Raccah. "Neuroprotective effect of docosa-hexaenoic acid–enriched phospholipids in experimental diabetic neuropathy." *Diabetes* 52:2578–2585 (2003).

Cshe, K., G. Winkler, Z. Melczer, and E. Baranyi. "The role of tumor necrosis factor resistance in obesity and insulin resistance." *Diabetologia* 43:525 (2000).

Despres, J-P., I. Lemieux, and D. Prudhomme. "Treatment of obesity: need to focus on high risk abdominally obese patients." *Brit J Med* 322:716–720 (2001).

Drewnowski, A. "Nutrition transition and global dietary trends." *Nutrition* 16:486–487 (2000).

Ebbeling, C. B., M. M. Leidig, K. B. Sinclair, J. P. Hangen, and D. S. Ludwig. "A reduced glycemic load diet in the treatment of adolescent obesity." *Arch Pediatr Adoles Med* 157:773–779 (2003).

Fernandez-Real, J-M., M. Vayreda, C. Richart, C. Gutierrez, M. Broch, J. Vendrell, and W. Ricart. "Circulating interleukin-6 levels, blood pressure, and insulin sensitivity in apparently healthy men and women." *J Clin Endocrinol Metab* 86:1154–1159 (2001).

Festa, A., R. D'Agostino, G. Howard, L. Mykkanen, R. P. Tracy, and S. M. Haffner. "Chronic subclinical inflammation as part of the insulin resistance syndrome." *Circulation* 102:42–47 (2000).

Freeman, D. J., J. Norrie, M. J. Caslake, A. Gaw, I. Ford, G. D. O. Lowe, D. O'Reilly, C. J. Packard, and N. Sattar. "C-reactive protein is an independent predictor of risk for the development of diabetes in the West of Scotland coronary prevention study." *Diabetes* 51:1596–1600 (2002).

Freeth, A., V. Udupi, R. Basile, and A. Green. "Prolonged treatment with prostaglandin E1 increases rate of lipolysis in rat adipocytes." *Life Sci* 73:393–401 (2003).

Friedman, A. N., L. G. Hunsicker, J. Selhub, and A. G. Bostom. "Clinical and nutritional correlates of C-reactive protein in type 2 diabetic nephropathy." *Atherosclerosis* 172:121–125 (2004).

Folsom, A. R., J. Ma, P. G. McGovern, and H. Eckfeldt. "Relationship between plasma phospholipid saturated fatty acids and hyperinsulinemia." *Metabolism* 45:223–228 (1996).

Fontaine, K. R., D. T. Redden, C. Wang, A. O. Westfall, and D. B. Allison. "Years of life lost due to obesity." *JAMA* 289:187–193 (2003).

Ford, E. S., W. H. Giles, and W. H. Dietz. "Prevalence of the metabolic syndrome among US adults." *JAMA* 287:356–359 (2002).

Ford, E. S., W. H. Giles, G. L. Myers, N. Rifai, P. M. Ridker, and D. M. Mannino. "C-reactive protein concentration distribution among US children and young adults." *Clin Chem* 49:1353–1357 (2003).

Fruhbeck, G., J. Gomez-Ambrosi, F. J. Muruzabal, and M. A. Burrell. "The adipocyte: a model for integration of endocrine and metabolic signaling in energy metabolism regulation." *Am J Physiol Endocrinol Metab* 280:E827–E847 (2001).

Gannon, M. C., F. Q. Nuttall, A. Saeed, K. Jordan, and H. Hoover. "An increase in dietary protein improves the blood glucose response in persons with type 2 diabetes." *Am J Clin Nutr* 78:734–741 (2003).

Garg, A. "High-monounsaturated fat diets for patients with diabetes mellitus: a meta analysis." *Am J Clin Nutr* 67:577S–582S (1998).

Gerbi, A., J-M. Maixent, J-L. Ansaldi, M. Pierlovisi, T. Coste, J-F. Pelissier, P. Vague, and D. Raccah. "Fish oil supplementation prevents diabetes-induced nerve conduction velocity and neuroanatomical changes in rats." *J Nutr* 129:207–213 (1999).

Gerbi, A., J-M. Maixent, O. Barbey, I. Jamme, M. Pierlovishi, T. Coste, G. Pieroni, A. Nouvelot, P. Vague, and D. Raccah. "Neuroprotective effect of fish oil in diabetic neuropathy." *Lipids* 34:S93–S94 (1999).

Haemmerle, G., R. Zimmermann, and R. Zechner. "Letting lipids go: hormone-sensitive lipase." *Cur Opin Lipidol* 14:289–297 (2003).

Hasler, G., D. J. Buysse, R. Klaghofer, A. Gamma, V. Ajdacic, D. Eich, W. Rossler, and J. Angst. "The association between short sleep duration and obesity in young adults: a 13-year prospective study." *Sleep* 15:661–666 (2004).

Hauner, H. "Insulin resistance and the metabolic syndrome—a challenge of the new millennium." *Eur J Clin Nutr* 56:S25–S29 (2002).

Herkner, H., N. Klein, C. Joukhadar, E. Lackner, H. Langenberger, M. Frossard, C. Bieglmayer, O. Wagner, M. Roden, and M. Muller. "Transcapillary insulin transfer in human skeletal muscle." *Eur J Clin Invest* 33:141–146 (2003).

Hostens, K., D. Pavlovic, Y. Zambre, Z. Ling, C. van Schravendijk, D. L. Eizirik, and D. G. Pipeleers. "Exposure of human islets to cytokines can result in the disproportionately elevated proinsulin release." *J Clin Invest* 104:67–72 (1999).

Hotamisligil, G. S. "Mechanisms of TNF induced insulin resistance." *Exp Clin Endocrinol Diabetes* 107:119–125 (1999).

Hotamisligil, G. S., P. Arner, J. F. Caro, R. L. Atkinson, and B. M. Spiegelman. "Increase adipose tissue expression of tumor necrosis factor in human obesity and insulin resistance." *J Clin Invest* 95:2409–2415 (1995).

Jansen, M. D. "Cytokine regulation of lipolysis in humans." *J Clin Endocrinol Metab* 88:3003–3004 (2003).

Javisalo, M. J., A. Harmoinen, M. Hakanen, U. Paakunainen, J. Vilkari, J. Hariala, T. Lehtimaki, O. Simell, and O. T. Raitakari. "Elevated C-reactive protein levels and early arterial changes in healthy children." *Arterioscler Thromb Vasc Biol* 22:1323–1328 (2002).

Jensen, T., S. Stender, K. Goldstein, G. Holmer, and T. Deckert. "Partial normalization by dietary cod liver oil of increased microvascular albumin leakage in patients with insulin-dependent diabetes and albuminuria." *N Engl J Med* 321:1572–1577 (1989).

Kahn, B. B. and J. S. Flier. "Obesity and insulin resistance." *J Clin Invest* 106:473–481 (2000).

Katan, M. B., S. M. Grundy, and W. C. Willett. "Should a low-fat, high-carbohydrate diet be recommended for everyone? Beyond low-fat diets." *N Engl J Med* 337:563–567 (1997).

Kern, P. A., S. Ranganathan, C. Li, L. Wood, and G. Ranganathan. "Adipose tissue tumor necrosis factor and interleukin-6 expression in human obesity and insulin resistance." *Am J Physiol Endocrinol Metab* 280:E745–E751 (2001).

Khan, L. K. and B. A. Bowman. "Obesity: a major global public health problem." *Ann Rev Nutr* 19:xii–xvii (1999).

Kim, S. and N. Moustaid-Moussa. "Secretory, endocrine and autocrine/paracrine function of the adipocyte." *J Nutr* 130:3110S–3115S (2000).

Krogh-Madsen, R., P. Plomgaaard, Keller Pernlle, C. Keller, and B. K. Pedersen. "Insulin stimulates interleukin-6 and tumor necrosis factor-alpha gene expression in human subcutaneous adipose tissue." *Am J Physiol Endocrinol Metab* 286:E234–E238 (2004).

Kyselova, P., M. Zourek, Z. Rusavy, L. Trefil, and J. Racek. "Hyperinsulinemia and oxidative stress." *Physiol Res* 51:591–595 (2002).

Lehrke, M. and M. A. Lazar. "Inflamed about obesity." *Nature Med* 10:126–127 (2004).

Luo, J., S. W. Rizkalla, J. Boillot, C. Alamowitch, H. Chaib, F. Bruzzo, N. Desplanque, A. M. Dalix, G. Durand, and G. Slama. "Dietary (n-3) polyunsaturated fatty acids improve adipocyte insulin action and glucose metabolism in insulin-resistant rats: relationship to membrane fatty acids." *J Nutr* 126:1951–1958 (1996).

Marett, A. "Molecular mechanisms of inflammation in obesity-linked insulin resistance." *Int J Obesity* 27:S46–S48 (2003).

Markovic, T. P., A. C. Fleury, L. V. Campbell, L. A. Simons, S. Balasubramanian, D. J. Chisholm, and A. B. Jenkins. "Benefical effect on average lipid levels from energy restriction and fat loss in obese individuals with or without type 2 diabetes." *Diabetes Care* 21:695–700 (1998).

Markovic, T. P., A. B. Jenkins, L. V. Campbell, S. M. Furler, E. W. Kragen, and D. J. Chisholm. "The determinants of glycemic responses to diet restriction and weight loss in obesity and NIDDM." *Diabetes Care* 21:687–694 (1998).

McLaughlin, T., F. Abbasi, C. Lemendola, L. Liang, G. Reaven, P. Schaaf, and P. Reaven. "Differentiation between obesity and insulin resistance in the association with C-reactive protein." *Circulation* 106:2908–2912 (2002).

Mobbs, C. V. "Genetic influences on glucose neurotoxicity, aging and diabetes: a possible role for glucose hysteresis." *Genetica* 91:239–253 (1993).

Mokdad, A. H., E. S. Ford, B. A. Bowman, W. H. Dietz, F. Vinicor, V. S. Bales, and J. S. Marks. "Prevalence of obesity, diabetes, and obesity-related health risk factors, 2001." *JAMA* 289:76–79 (2003).

Mokdad, A. H., E. S. Ford, B. A. Bowman, D. E. Nelson, M. M. Engelgau, F. Vinicor, and J. S. Marks. "Diabetes trends in the U.S." 1990–1998." *Diabetes Care* 23:1278–1283 (2000).

Mokdad, A. H., M. K. Serdula, W. H. Dietz, B. A. Bowman, J. S. Marks, and J. P. Kaplan. "The spread of the obesity epidemic in the United States. 1991–1998." *JAMA* 282:1519–1522 (1999).

Montague, C. T., and S. O'Rahilly. "The perils of portliness: causes and consequences of visceral adiposity." *Diabetes* 49:883–888 (2000).

Montori, V. M., A. Farmer, P. C. Wollan, and S. F. Dinneen. "Fish oil supplementation in type 2 diabetes: a quantitative systematic review." *Diabetes Care* 23:1407–1415. (2000).

Moran, T. H. "Cholecystokinin and satiety." *Nutrition* 16:858–865 (2000).

Mori, T. A., D. Q. Bao, V. Burke, I. B. Puddey, G. F. Watts, L. J. Beilin. "Dietary fish as a major component of a weight-loss diet: effect on serum lipids, glucose, and insulin metabolism in overweight hypertensive subjects." *Am J Clin Nutr* 70:817–825 (1999).

Narayan, K. M. V., J. P. Boyle, T. J. Thompson, S. W. Sorensen, and D. F. Williamson. "Lifetime risk for diabetes mellitus in the United States." *JAMA* 290:1884–1890 (2003).

Nichols, G. A., H. S. Glauber, and J. B. Brown. "Type 2 diabetes: incremental medical care costs during the 8 years preceding diagnosis." *Diabetes Care* 23:1654–1659 (2000).

Nuttall, F. Q., M. C. Gannon, A. Saeed, K. Jordan, and H. Hoover. "The metabolic response of subjects with type 2 diabetes to a high-protein, weight-maintenance diet." *J Clin Endocrinol Metab* 88:3577–3583 (2003).

Park, Y-W., S. Zhu, L. Palaniappan, S. Heshka, M. R. Carethon, and S. Heymsfield. "The metabolic syndrome." *Arch Intern Med* 163:427–436 (2003).

Peraldi, P. and B. Spegelman. "TNF and insulin resistance: summary and future prospects." *Mol Cell Biochem* 182:169–175 (1998).

Pittas, A. G., N. A. Joseph, and A. S. Greenberg. "Adipocytokines and insulin resistance." *J Clin Endocrinol Metab* 89:447–452 (2004).

Pradeepa, R. and V. Mohan. "The changing scenario of the diabetes epidemic: implications for India." *Indian J Med Res* 116:121–132 (2002).

Qi, C. and P. H. Pekala. "Tumor necrosis factor alpha induced insulin resistance in adipocytes." *Proc Soc Exp Biol Med* 223:128–135 (2000).

Raheja, B. S., S. M. Sakidot, R. B. Phatak, and M. B. Rao. "Significance of the N-6/N-3 ratio for insulin action in diabetics." *Ann N Y Acad Sci* 983:258–271 (1993).

Rask-Madsen, C., H. Dominguez, N. Ihlemann, T. Hermann, L. Lober, and C. Torp-Pedersen. "Tumor necrosis factor-alpha inhibits insulin's stimulating effect on glucose uptake and endothelium-dependent vasodilation in humans." *Circulation* 108:1815–1821 (2003).

Reaven, G. M. and A. Laws. *Insulin Resistance. The Metabolic Syndrome X.* Totowa, NJ: Humana Press, 1999.

Rivellese, A., A. Maffettone, C. Iovine, L. Di Marino, G. Annuzzi, M. Mancini, and G. Riccardi. "Long-term effects of fish oil on insulin resistance and plasma lipoprotein in NIDDM patients with hypertriglyceridemia." *Diabetes Care* 19:1207–1213 (1996).

Roberts, S. B. "High glycemic index foods, hunger, and obesity: is there a connection." *Nutr Rev* 58:163–169 (2000).

Rosenbloom, A. L., J. R. Joe, R. S. Young, and W. E. Winter. "Emerging epidemic of type 2 diabetes in youth." *Diabetes Care* 22:345–354 (1999).

Salmeron, J., A. Ascherio, E. B. Rimm, G. A. Colditz, D. Spiegelman, D. J. Jenkins, M. J. Stampfer, A. L. Wing, and W. C. Willett. "Dietary fiber, glycemic load, and risk of NIDDM in men." *Diabetes Care* 20:545–550 (1997).

Salmeron, J., J. E. Manson, and W. C. Willett. "Dietary fiber, glycemic load, and risk of non-insulin dependent diabetes mellitus in women." *JAMA* 277:472–477 (1997).

Samaras, K., and L. V. Campbell. "Increasing incidence of type 2 diabetes in the third millennium." *Diabetes Care* 23:441–442 (2000).

Sears, B. *The Zone*. New York: ReganBooks, 1995.

Sears, B. *The Anti-Aging Zone*. New York: ReganBooks, 1999.

Sears, B. *The Omega Rx Zone*. New York: ReganBooks, 2002.

Seidell, J. C. "Obesity, insulin resistance and diabetes-a worldwide epidemic." *Brit J Nutr* 83:S5–S8 (2000).

Sirtori, C. R., G. Crepaldi, E. Manzato, M. Mancini, A. Rivellese, R. Paolett, F. Pazzucconi, F. Pamparana, and E. Stragliotto. "One-year treatment with ethyl esters of n-3 fatty acids in patients with hypertriglyceridemia and glucose intolerance. Reduced triglyceridemia, total cholesterol and increased HDL-C with glycemic alterations." *Atherosclerosis* 137:419–427 (1998).

Skov, A. R., S. Toubro, B. Renn, L. Holm, and A. Astrup. "Randomized trial on protein vs. carbohydrate in ad libitum fat reduced diet for the treatment of obesity." *Int J Obes* 23:528–536 (1999).

Steinberg, H. O., H. Chaker, R. Learning, A. Johnson, G. Brechtel, and A. D. Baron. "Obesity/insulin resistance is associated with endothelial dysfunction. Implications for the syndrome of insulin resistance." *J Clin Invest* 97:2601–2610 (1996).

Stene, L. C., J. Ulriksen, P. Magnus, and G. Joner. "Use of cod liver oil during pregnancy associated with lower risk of type 1 diabetes in the offspring." *Diabetologia* 42:1093–1098 (2000).

Storlien, L. H., A. B. Jenkins, D. J. Chisholm, W. S. Pascoe, S. Khour, and E. W. Kragen. "Influence of dietary fat composition on development of insulin resistance in rats. Relationship to muscle triglycerides and omega-3 fatty acids in muscle phospholipids." *Diabetes* 40:280–289 (1991).

Storlien, L. H., E. W. Kraegen, D. J. Chisholm, G. L. Ford, D. G. Bruce, and W. S. Pascoe. "Fish oil prevents insulin resistance induced by high-fat feeding in rats." *Science* 237:885–888 (1987).

Unger, R. H. "Glucagon and the insulin-glucagon ratio in diabetes and other catabolic illnesses." *Diabetes* 20:834–838 (1971).

Unger, R. H. and P. J. Lefebvre. *Glucagon: Molecular Physiology, Clinical and Therapeutic Implications*. Oxford: Pergamon Press, 1972.

Vessby, B., S. Tengblad, and H. Lithell. "Insulin sensitivity is related to the fatty acid composition of serum lipids and skeletal muscle phospholipids in 70-year-old men." *Diabetologia* 37:1044–1050 (1994).

Vinik, A. I., T. S. Park, K. B. Stansberry, and G. L. Pittenger. "Diabetic neuropathies." *Diabetologia* 43:957–973 (2000).

Visser, M. "Higher levels of inflammation in obese children." *Nutrition* 17:480–484 (2001).

Visser, M., L. M. Bouter, G. M. McQuillan, M. H. Wener, and T. B. Harris. "Elevated C-reactive protein levels in overweight and obese adults." *JAMA* 282:2131–2315 (1999).

Willett, W. C. "Dietary fat and obesity: an unconvincing relation." *Am J Clin Nutr* 68:1149–1150 (1998).

Willett, W. C. "Is dietary fat a major source of body fat?" *Am J Clin Nutr* 67:556S–562S (1998).

Yudkin, J. S., M. Kumari, S. E. Humphries, and V. Modamed-Ali. "Inflammation, obesity, stress and coronary heart disease: is interleukin-6 the link?" *Atherosclerosis* 148:209–214 (2000).

Yudkin, J. S., C. D. A. Stehouwer, J. J. Emeis, and S. W. Coppack. "C-reactive protein in healthy subjects: associations with obesity, insulin resistance, and endothelial dysfunction— a potential role for cytokines originating from adipose tissue?" *Arterioscler Thromb Vasc Biol* 19:972–978 (1999).

Chapter 15. Why Heart Disease Has Very Little to Do with Cholesterol but Everything to Do with Silent Inflammation

Albert, C. M., H. Campos, M. J. Stampfer, P. M. Ridker, J. E. Manson, W. C. Willett, and J. Ma. "Blood levels of long-chain n-3 fatty acids and risk of sudden death." *N Engl J Med* 346:1113–1118 (2002).

Albert, C. M., C. H. Hennekens, C. I. O'Donnel, U. A. Ajani, V. J. Carey, and W. C. Willett. "Fish consumption and risk of sudden cardiac death." *JAMA* 279:23–28 (1998).

Anderson, J. L., and J. B. Muhlestein. "Restenosis after coronary intervention: narrowing C-reactive protein's prognostic potential?" *Am J Med* 115:147–149 (2003).

Anderson, K. M., W. P. Castelli, and D. Levy. "Cholesterol and mortality: 30 years of follow-up from the Framingham Study." *JAMA* 257:2176–2180 (1987).

Angerer, P. and C. von Schacky. "N-3 polyunsaturated fatty acids and cardiovascular system." *Curr Opin Lipidol* 11:57–63 (2000).

Ascherio, A., C. H. Hennekens, J. E. Buring, C. Master, M. J. Stampfer, and W. C. Willett. "Trans fatty acid intake and risk of myocardial infarction." *Circulation* 89:94–101 (1994).

Ascherio, A., E. B. Rimm, M. J. Stampfer, E. L. Giovannucci, and W. C. Willett. "Dietary intake of marine n-3 fatty acids, fish intake, and risk of coronary heart disease among men." *N Engl J Med* 332:977–982 (1995).

Ascherio, A. and W. C. Willett. "Health effects of trans fatty acids." *Am J Clin Nutr* 66:1006S-1010S (1997).

Austin, M. A. "Plasma triglcyceride and coronary heart disease." *Arterioscler Thromb Vasc Biol* 11:2–14 (1991).

Austin, M. A., J. L. Breslow, C. H. Hennekens, J. E. Buring, W. C. Willett, and R. M. Krauss.

"Low density lipoprotein subclass patterns and risk of myocardinal infarction." *JAMA* 260:1917–1920 (1988).

Bang, H., O. Dyerberg, and A. B. Nielsen. "Plasma lipid and lipoprotein pattern in Greenlandic west-coast Eskimos." *Lancet* i:1143–1145 (1971).

Bao, W., S. R. Srinivasan, and G. S. Berenson. "Persistent elevation of plasma insulin levels is associated with increased cardiovascular risk in children and young adults." *Circulation* 93:54–59 (1996).

Bataile, R., and B. Klein. "C-reactive protein levels as a direct indicator of interleukin-6 levels in humans in vivo." *Arthritis Rheum* 35:982–983 (1992).

Bellamy, C. M., P. M. Schofield, E. B. Faragher, and D. R. Ramsdale. "Can supplementation of diet with omega-3 polyunsaturated fatty acids reduce coronary angioplasty restenosis rate?" *Eur Heart J* 13:1626–1631 (1992).

Bellosta, S., N. Ferri, F. Bernini, R. Paoletti, and A. Corsini. "Non-lipid related effects of statins." *Ann Med* 32:164–176 (2000).

Billman, G. E., J. X. Kang, and A. Leaf. "Prevention of sudden cardiac death by dietary pure omega-3 polyunsaturated fatty acids in dogs." *Circulation* 99:2452–2457 (1999).

Black, H. R. "The coronary artery disease paradox. The role of hyperinsulinemia and insulin resistance and implications for therapy." *J Cardiovascular Pharmacol* 15:26S–38S (1990).

Boizel, R., P. Y. Behhamou, B. Lardy, F. Laporte, T. Foulon, and S. Halimi. "Ratio of triglycerides to HDL cholesterol is an indicator of LDL particle size in patients with type 2 diabetes and normal HDL cholesterol levels." *Diabetes Care* 23:1679–1685 (2000).

Bowles, M. H., D. Klonis, T. G. Plavac, B. Gonzales, D. A. Francisco, R. W. Roberts, G. R. Boxberger, L. R. Poliner, and J. P. Galichia. "EPA in the prevention of restenois post PTCA." *Angiology* 42:187–194 (1991).

Braunwald, E. "Cardiovascular medicine at the turn of the millennium: triumphs, concerns, and applications." *N Engl J Med* 337:1360–1369 (1997).

Burr, M. L. "Lessons from the story of n-3 fatty acids." *Am J Clin Nutr* 71:397S–398S (2000).

Burr, M. L., A. M. Fehily, J. F. Gilbert, S. Rogers, R. M. Holliday, P. M. Sweetnam, P. C. Elwood, and N. M. Deadman. "Effects of changes in fat, fish, and fibre intakes on the death and myocardial reinfarction: diet and reinfarction trial (DART)." *Lancet* ii:757–761 (1989).

Busse, R., and I. Flemining. "Endothelial dysfunction in atherosclerosis." *J Vasc Res* 33:181–194 (1996).

Campbell, B., T. Badrick, R. Flatman, and D. Kanowshi. "Limited clinical utility of high-sensitivity plasma C-reactive protein assays." *Ann Clin Biochem* 39:85–88 (2002).

Campbell, B., R. Flatman, T. Badrick, and D. Kanowshi. "Problems with high-sensitivity C-reactive protein." *Clin Chem* 49:201 (2003).

Carantoni, M., F. Abbasi, F. Warmerdan, M. Klebanov, P. W. Wang, Y. D. Chen, S. Azhar, and G. M. Reaven. "Relationship between insulin resistance and partially oxidized LDL particles in healthy, nondiabetic volunteers." *Arterioscler Thromb Vasc Biol* 18:762–767 (1998).

Chan, D. C., G. F. Watts, T. A. Mori, P. H. R. Barrett, L. J. Beilin, and T. G. Redgrave. "Factorial study of the effects of atorvastatin and fish oil on dyslipidaemia in visceral obesity." *Eur J Clin Invest* 32:429–436 (2002).

Christensen, J. H., M. S. Christensen, J. Dyerberf, and E. B. Scmidt. "Heart rate variability and fatty acid content of blood cell membranes: a dose-response study with n-3 fatty acids." *Am J Clin Nutr* 70.331–337 (1999).

Cleland, S. J., N. Sattar, J. R. Petrie, N. G. Forouhi, H. L. Elliott,and J. M. C. Connell. "Endothelial dysfunction as a possible link between C-reactive protein and cardiovascular disease." *Clin Sci* 98:531–535 (2000).

Coresh, J., P. O. Kwiterovich, and H. H. Smith. "Association of plasma triglyceride concentration and LDL particle diameter, density, and chemico-compostion with premature coronary artery disease." *J Lipid Res* 34:1687–1697 (1993).

Corti, M-C., J. M. Guraink, M. E. Saliva, T. Harris, T. S. Field, R. B. Wallace, L. F. Berkman, T. E. Seeman, R. J. Glynn, C. H. Hennekens, and R. J. Havlik. "HDL cholesterol predicts coronary heart disease mortality in older persons." *JAMA* 274:539–544 (1995).

Cullen, P., S. Lorkowski, H. Schulte, U. Seedorf, and G. Assmann. "Inflammation in atherosclerosis, not yet for a paradigm shift?" *Curr Opin Lipidol* 14:325–328 (2003).

Davidson, J. and D. Rotondo. "Lipid metabolism: inflammatory-immune response in atherosclerosis." *Curr Opin Lipidol* 14:337–339 (2003).

Daviglus, M. L., M. Stamler, A. J. Orencia, A. R. Dyer, K. Liu, P. Greenland, M. K. Walsh, D. Morris, and R. B. Shekelle. "Fish consumption and the 30-year risk of myocardial infarction." *N Engl J Med* 336:1046–1053 (1997).

Davignon, J. and J. S. Cohn. "Triglycerides: a risk factor for coronary heart disease." *Atherosclerosis* 124:S57-S64 (1996).

De Caterina, R., M. I. Cybulsk, S. K. Clinton, M. A. Gimbrone, and P. Libby. "The omega-3 fatty acid docosahexaenoate reduces cytokine-induced expression of proatherogenic and proinflammatory protein in human endothelial cells." *Arterioscler Thromb Vasc Biol* 14:1829–1836 (1994).

De Caterina, R. and A. Zampolli. "n-3 fatty acids: antiatherosclerotic effects." *Lipids* 36:S69–S78 (2001).

Dehmer, G. J., J. J. Popma, E. K. van den Ber, E. J. Eichorn, J. B. Prewitt, W. B. Campbell, L. Jennings, J. T. Willerson, and J. M. Schmitz. "Reduction in the rate of early restenosis after coronary angioplasty by a diet supplemented with n-3 fatty acids." *N Engl J Med* 319:733–740 (1988).

DeLongeril, M., S. Renaud, N. Mamelle, P. Salen, J. L. Martin, I. Monjaud, J. Guidollet, P. Touboul, and J. Delaye. "Mediterranean alpha-linolenic acid rich diet in secondary prevention of coronary heart disease." *Lancet* 343:1454–1459 (1994).

DeLongeril, M., P. Salen, and J. Delaye. "Effect of a Mediterranean type of diet on the rate of cardiovascular complications in patients with coronary artery disease." *J Am Coll Cardiology* 28:1103–1108 (1996).

DeLongeril, M., P. Salen, J. L. Martin, I. Monjaud, J. Delaye, and N. Mamelle. "Mediterranean diet, traditional risk factors, and the rate of cardiovascular complications after myocardial infarction: final report of the Lyon Diet Heart Study." *Circulation* 99:779–785 (1999).

Depres, J-P., B. Lamarche, P. Mauriege, B. Cantin, G. R. Dagenais, S. Moorjani, and P-J. Lupien. "Hyperinsulinemia as an independent risk factor for ischemic heart disease." *N Engl J Med* 334:952–957 (1996).

Depres, J-P., B. Lamarche, P. Mauriege, B. Cantin, P. J. Lupien, and G. R. Dagenais. "Risk factors for ischaemic heart disease: is it time to measure insulin?" *Eur Heart J* 17:1453–1454 (1996).

Diomede, L., D. Albani, M. Sottocorno, M. B. Donati, M. Bianchi, Fruscella, and M. Salmona. "In vivo anti-inflammatory effect statins is mediated by nonsterol mevalonate products." *Arterioscler Thromb Vasc Biol* 21:1327–1332 (2001).

Draznin, B., P. Miles, Y. Kruszynska, J. Olefsky, J. Friedman, I. Golovchenko, R. Stjernholm, K. Wall, M. Reitman, D. Accili, R. Cooksey, D. McClain, and M. Goalstone. "Effects of insulin on the prenylation as a mechanism of potentially detrimental influence of hyperinsulinemia." *Endocrinology* 141:1310–1316 (2000).

Dreon, D. M., H. A. Fernstrom, B. Miller, and R. M. Krauss. "Low-density lipoprotein subclass patterns and lipoprotein response to a reduced-fat diet in men." *FASEB J* 8:121–126 (1994).

Dreon, D. M., H. A. Fernstrom, P. T. Williams, and R. M. Krauss. "A very-low fat is not associated with improved lipoprotein profiles in men with a predominance of large, low-density lipoproteins." *Am J Clin Nutr* 69:411–418 (1999).

Duimetiere, P., E. Eschwege, G. Papoz, J. L. Richard, J. R. Claude, and G. Rosselin. "Relationship of plasma insulin to the incidence of myocardial infraction and coronary heart disease mortality in a middle-aged population." *Diabetologia* 19:205–210 (1980).

Durrington, P. N. "Triglycerides are more important in atherosclerosis than epidemiology has suggested." *Atherosclerosis* 141:S57–S62 (1998).

Dyerberg, J., H. O. Bang, E. Stofferson, S. Moncada, and J. R. Vane. "Eicosapentaenoic acid and prevention of thrombosis and atherosclerosis." *Lancet* ii:117–119 (1978).

Eritsland, J., H. Arnesen, K. Bronseth, N. B. Fjeld, and M. Abdelnoor. "Effect of dietary supplementation with n-3 fatty acids on coronary artery bypass graft patency." *Am J Cardiol* 77:31–36 (1996).

Erkkila, A. T., S. Lehto, Pyorala, and M. I. J. Uusitupa. "n-3 fatty acids and 5-y risks of death and cardiovascular disease events in patients with coronary artery disease." *Am J Clin Nutr* 78:65–71 (2003).

Eschwege, E., J. L. Richard, N. Thibult, P. Ducimetiere, J. M. Warsnot, J. R. Claude, and G. E. Rosselin."Coronary heart disease mortality in relation with diabetes, blood glucose, and plasma insulin levels." *Horm Metab Res Suppl* 15:41–46 (1985).

Ferns, G. A. A. "Differential effects of statins on serum CRP levels." *Atherosclerosis* 169:349–351 (2003).

Fischer, S., P. C. Weber, and J. Dyerberg. "The prostacyclin/thromboxane balance is favourably shifted in Greenland Eskimos." *Prostaglandins* 32:235–241 (1986).

Fontbonne, A., M. A. Charles, N. Thibult, J. L. Richard, J. R. Claude, J. M. Warnet, G. E. Rosselin, and E. Eschwege. "Hyperinsulinemia as a predictor of coronary heart disease mortality in a healthy population. The Paris Prospective Study, 15 year follow-up." *Diabetologia* 34:356–361 (1991).

Ford, E. S. and S. Liu. "Glycemic index and serum high-density lipoprotin cholesterol concentration among US adults." *Arch Intern Med* 161:572–576 (2001).

Foster, D. "Insulin resistance-a secret killer?" *N Engl J Med* 320:733–734 (1989).

Frolkis, J. P., G. L. Pearce, V. Nambi, S. Minor, and D. L. Sprecher. "Statins do not meet expectations for lowering low-density lipoprotein cholesterol levels when used in private practice." *Am J Med* 113:625–629 (2002).

Gaziano, J. M., C. H. Hennekens, C. J. O'Donnell, J. L. Breslow, and J. E. Buring. "Fasting triglycerides, high-density lipoproteins and risk of myocardial infarction." *Circulation* 96:2520–2525 (1997).

Gaziano, J. M., P. J. Skerrett, and J. E. Buring. "Aspirin in the treatment and prevention of cardiovascular disease." *Haemostasis* 30:1–13 (2000).

Gertler, M., H. E. Leetma, E. Saluste, J. L. Rosenberger, and R. G. Guthrie. "Ischemic heart disease, insulin, carbohydrate and lipid inter-relationship." *Circulation* 46:103–111 (1972).

Gillman, M. W., A. Cupples, B. E. Millen, C. Ellison, and P. A. Wolf. "Inverse association of dietary fat with development of ischemic stroke in men." *JAMA* 278:2145–2150 (1997).

Ginsburg, G. S., C. Safran, and R. C. Pasternak. "Frequency of low serum high-density lipoprotein cholesterol levels in hospitalized patients with 'desireable' total cholesterol levels." *Am J Cardiol* 1:187–192 (1991).

Ginsberg, H. N. "Insulin resistance and cardiovascular disease." *J Clin Invest* 106:453–458 (2000).

GISSI-Prevenzione Investigators. "Dietary supplementation with n-3 polyunsaturated fatty acids and vitamin E after myocardial infarction: results of the GISSI-Prevenzione trial." *Lancet* 354:447–455 (1999).

Glueck, C. J., J. E. Lang, T. Tracy, L. Sieve-Smith, and P. Wang. "Contribution of fasting hyperinsulinemia to prediction of atherosclerotic cardiovascular disease status in 293 hyperlipidemic patients." *Metabolism* 48:1437–1444 (1999).

Goto, D., S. Fujii, and A. Kitabatake. "Rho/Rho kinase as a novel theraeutic target in the treatment of cardiovascular diseases." *Drugs of the Future* 28:267–271 (2003).

Gould, K. L. "Very low-fat diets for coronary heart disease: perhaps but which one." *JAMA* 275:1402–1403 (1996).

Grundy, S. M. "Small LDL, atherogenic dyslipidemia, and the metabolic syndrome." *Circulation* 95:1–4 (1997).

Haffner, S. M., L. Mykkanen, M. P. Stern, and R. Valdez, J. A. Heisserman, and R. R. Bowsher. "Relationship of proinsulin and insulin to cardiovascular risk factors in nondiabetic subjects." *Diabetes* 42:1297–1302 (1993).

Harris, T. B., L. Ferrucci, R. P. Tracy, M. C. Corti, S. Wacholder, W. H. Ettinger, H. Heimovitz, H. J. Cohen, and R. Wallace. "Association of elevated interleukin-6 and C-reactive protein levels with mortality in the elderly." *Am J Med* 106:506–512 (1999).

Harris, W. S. "n-3 fatty acids and serum lipoproteins: human studies." *Am J Clin Nutr* 65:1645S–1654S (1997).

Harris, W. S., H. N. Ginsberh, N. Arunakul, N. S. Shachter, S. L. Windsor, M. Adams, L. Berlund, and K. Osmundsen. "Safety and efficacy of Omacor in severe hypertriglyceridemia." *J Cardiovasc Risk* 4:385–392 (1997).

Harris, W. S. "n-3 fatty acids and human lipoprotein metabolism: an update." *Lipids* 34:S257–S258 (1999).

Harris, W. S., and W. L. Isley. "Clinical trial evidence for the cardioprotective effects of omega-3 fatty acids." *Curr Atheroscler Rep* 3:174–179. (2001).

Hegele, R. A. "Premature atherosclerosis associated with monogenic insulin resistance." *Circulation* 103:2225–2229 (2001).

Hirai, A., T. Hamazaki, T. Terano, T. Nishikawa, Y. Tamura, A. Kumagai, and J. Sajiki. "Eicosapentaenoic acid and platelet function in Japanese." *Lancet* ii:1132 (1982).

Hirai, A., T. Terano, Y. Tamura, and S. Yoshida. "Eicosapentaenoic acid and adult disease in Japan." *J Intern Med* 225:69–75 (1989).

Hollenbeck, C. and G. M. Reaven. "Variations in insulin-stimulated glucose uptake in healthy individuals with normal glucose tolerance." *J Clin Endocrinol Metab* 64:1169–1173 (1987).

Horne, B. D., J. B. Muhlestein, J. F. Carlquist, T. L. Bair, T. E. Madsen, N. I. Hart, and J. L. Anderson. "Statin therapy, lipid levels, C-reactive protein and the survival of patients with angiographically severe coronary artery disease." *J Am Coll Cardiol* 36:1774–1780 (2000).

Howard, B. V. "Insulin resistance and lipid metabolism." *Am J Cardiol* 84:28J-32J (1999).

Hrboticky, N., L. Tang, B. Zimmer, I. Lux, and P. C. Weber. "Lovastatin increases arachidonic acid levels and stimulates thromboxane synthesis in human liver and monocytic cell lines." *J Clin Invest* 93:195–203 (1994).

Hu, F. B., E. Cho, K. M. Rexrode, C. M. Albert, and J. E. Manson. "Fish and long-chain omega-3 fatty acid intake and risk of coronary heart disease and total mortality in diabetic women." *Circulation* 107:1852–1857 (2003).

Hu, F. B., J. E. Manson, and W. C. Willett. "Types of dietary fat and risk of coronary heart disease: a critical review." *J Am Coll Nutr* 20:5–19 (2001).

Hu, F. B., M. J. Stampfer, J. E. Manson, E. Rimm, G. A. Colditz, F. E. Speizer, C. H. Hennekens, and W. C. Willett. "Dietary protein and risk of ischemic heart disease in women." *Am J Clin Nutr* 70:221–227 (1999).

Hudgins, L. C., M. Hellerstein, C. Seidman, and J. Hirsch. "Human fatty acid synthesis is stimulated by a eucaloric low fat, high carbohydrate diet." *J Clin Invest* 97:2081–2091 (1996).

Ikeda, U., M. Takahashi, and K. Shimad. "C-reactive protein directly inhibits nitric oxide production by cytokine-stimulate vascular smooth muscle cells." *Cardiovasc Pharmacol* 42:607–611 (2003).

Iso, H., S. Sato, A. R. Falsm, T. Shimamoto, A. Terao, R. G. Munger, A. Kitamure, M. Konishi, M. Iida, and Y. Komachi. "Serum fatty acids and fish intake in rual Japanese, urban Japanese, Japanese American and Caucasian American men." *Int J Epidemiol* 18:374–381 (1989).

Jeppesen, J., H. O. Hein, P. Suadicani, and F. Gyntelberg. "Relation of high TG low HDL cholesterol and LDL cholesterol to the incidence of ischemic heart disease-an 8-year follow-up in the Copenhagen Male Study." *Arterioscler Thromb Vasc Biol* 17:1114–1120 (1997).

Jeppesen, J., H. O. Hein, P. Suadicani, and F. Gyntelberg. "Low triglycerides-high high-density lipoprotein cholesterol and risk of ischemic heart disease." *Arch Intern Med* 161:361–366 (2001).

Job, F. P., J. Wolfertz, R. Meyer, A. Hubinger, F. A. Gries, and H. Kuhn. "Hyperinsulinism in patients with coronary artery disease." *Coronary Artery Disease* 5:487–492 (1994).

Kagawa, Y., M. Nishizawa, M. Suzuki, T. Miyatake, T. Hamamoto, K. Goto, E. Motonaga, H. Izumikawa, H. Hirata, and A. Ebihara. "Eicosapolyenoic acid of serum lipids of Japanese islanders with low incidence of cardiovascular diseases." *J Nutr Sci Vitaminol* 28:441–453 (1982).

Kang, J. X., and A. Leaf. "The cardiac antiarrhythmic effects of polyunsaturated fatty acids." *Lipids* S541–544 (1996).

Kannel, W. B., W. P. Castelli, and T. Gordon. "Cholesterol in the prediction of atherosclerotic disease." *Ann Intern Med* 90:85–91 (1979).

Kano, H., T. Hayashi, D. Sumi, T. Esaki, Y. Asai, N. K. Thakur, M. Jayachandran, and A. Iguchi. "A HMG-CoA reductase inhibitor improved regression of atherosclerosis in the rabbit aorta without affecting serum lipid levels: possible relevance of up-regulation of endothelial NO synthase mRNA." *Biochem Biophys Res Commun* 259:414 419 (1999).

Kaplan, N. "The deadly quartet: upper body obesity, glucose intolerance, hypertriglyceridemia, and hypertension." *Arch Intern Med* 149:1514–1520 (1989).

Karhapaa, P., M. Malkki, and M. Laakso. "Isolated low HDL cholesterol: an insulin-resistant state." *Diabetes* 43:411–417 (1994).

Katan, M. B., S. M. Grundy, and W. C. Willett. "Beyond low-fat diets." *N Engl J Med* 337:563–566 (1997).

Kereiakes, D. J. "The fire that burns within." *Circulation* 107:373–374 (2003).

Kesaniemi, Y. A. "Relevance of the reduction of triglycerides in the prevention of coronary heart disease." *Curr Opin Lipidol* 9:571 574 (1998).

Kiinjo, K., H. Sato, Y. Ohnishi, E. Hisida, Nakaka, Y. Matsumura, H. Takeda, and M. Hori. "Impact of high-sensitivity C-reactive protein on predicting long-term mortality of acute myocardial infarction." *Am J Cardiol* 91:9331–935 (2003).

Kluft, C. and M. P. M. de Maat. "Genetics of C-reactive protein." *Arterioscler Thromb Vasc Biol* 23:1956–1959 (2003).

Knopp, R. H. "Serum lipids after a low-fat diet." *JAMA* 279:1345–1346 (1998).

Knopp, R. H., C. E. Walden, B. M. Retzlaff, B. S. McCann, A. A. Dowdy, J. J. Albers, G. O. Gey, and M. N. Cooper. "Long-term cholesterol-lowering effects of 4 fat-restricted diets in hypercholesterolemic and combined hyperlipidemic men: the dietary alternative study." *JAMA* 278:1509–1515 (1997).

Koh, K. K. "Effects of statins on vascular wall: vasomotor function, inflammation, and plaque stability." *Cardio Res* 1:23–32 (2000).

Kondo, T., K. Ogawa, T. Satake, M. Kitazawa, M. Taki, and S. Sugiyama. "Plasma-free eicosapentaenoic/arachidonic acid ratio: a possible new coronary risk factor." *Clinical Cardiology* 9:413–416 (1986).

Kris-Etherton, P. M., W. S. Harris, and L. J. Appel. "Omega-3 fatty acids and cardiovascular disease: new recommendations frm the American Heart Association." *Arterioscler Thromb Vasc Biol* 23:151–152 (2003).

Kromann, N., and A. Green. "Epidemiological studies in the Upernavik district, Greenland. Incidence of some chronic diseases 1950–1974." *Acta Med Scand* 208:401–406 (1980).

Laino, C. "Trans fatty acids in margarine can increase MI risk." *Circulation* 89:94–101 (1994).

Lakshmanan, M. R., C. M. Nepokroeff, G. C. Ness, R. E. Dugan, and J. W. Porter. "Stimulation by insulin of rat liver beta hydroxy methyl HMGCoA reductase and cholesterol synthesizing activities." *Biochem Biophys Res Commun* 50:704–710 (1973).

Lamarche, B., J-P. Despres, S. Moorjani, B. Cantin, G. R. Dagenais, and P. J. Lupien. "Triglycerides and HDL-cholesterol as risk factors for ischemic heart disease: results from the Quebec Cardiovascular Study." *Atherosclerosis* 119:235–245 (1996).

Lamarche, B., I. Lemieux, and J-P. Despres. "The small, dense LDL phenotype and the risk of coronary heart disease: epidemiology, pathophysiology and therapeutic aspects." *Diabetes Metab* 25:199–211 (1999).

Lamarche, B., L. Rashid, and G. F. Lewis. "HDL metabolism in hypertriglyceridemic states: an overview." *Clin Chim Acta* 286:145–161 (1999).

Lamarche, B., A. Tchernof, G. R. Dagenais, B. Cantin, P. J. Lupien, and J-P. Despres. "Small, dense LDL particles and the risk of ischemic heart disease: prospective results from the Quebec Cardiovascular Study." *Circulation* 95:69–75 (1997).

Lamarche, B., A. Tchernot, P. Mauriege, B. Cantin, G. R. Gagenais, P. J. Lupien, and J-P. Despres. "Fasting insulin and apolipoprotein B levels and low-density particle size as risk factors for ischemic heart disease." *JAMA* 279:1965–1961 (1998).

Laws, A., A. C. King, W. L. Haskell, and G. M. Reaven. "Relation of fasting plasma insulin concentration to high density lipoprotein cholesterol and triglyceride concentration in men." *Arterioscler Thromb Vasc Biol* 11:1636–1642 (1991).

Laws, A. J. and G. M. Reaven. "Evidence for an independent relationship between insulin resistance and fasting HDL-cholesterol, triglyceride and insulin concentrations." *J Intern Med* 231:25–30 (1992).

Laws, A. and G. M. Reaven. "Insulin resistance and risk factors for coronary heart disease." *Clin Endocrinol Metab* 7:1063–1078 (1993).

Leaf, A. "Dietary prevention of coronary heart disease: the Lyon diet heart study." *Circulation* 99:733–735 (1999).

Leaf, A. and J. X. Kang. "Dietary n-3 fatty acids in the prevention of lethal cardiac arrhythmias." *Curr Opin Lipidol* 8:4–6 (1997).

Leaf, A., J. X. Kang, Y-F. Xiao, and G. E. Billman. "n-3 fatty acids in the prevention of cardiac arrhythmias." *Lipids* 34:S187-S189 (1999).

Leaf, A. J. X. Kang, Y-F. Xiao, and G. E. Billman. "Clinical prevention of sudden cardiac death by n-3 polyunsaturated fatty acids and mechanism of prevention of arrhythmias by n-3 fish oils." *Circulation* 107:2646–2652 (2003).

Leaf, A. and P. C. Weber. "Cardiovascular effects of omega-3 fatty acids." *N Engl J Med* 318:549–557 (1988).

Lefer, A. M., R. Scalia, and D. J. Lefer. "Vascular effect of HMG CoA-reductase inhibitors (statins) unrelated to cholesterol lowering: new concepts for cardiovascular disease." *Cardiovascular Res* 49:281–287 (2001).

Lefer, D. J. "Statins as potent anti-inflammatory drugs." *Circulation* 106:2041–2042 (2002).

Libby, P. "Inflammation in atherosclerosis." *Nature* 20:868–874 (2002).

Lichtenstein, A. H. "Trans fatty acids and cardiovascular disease risk." *Curr Opin Lipidol* 11:37–42 (2000).

Lichtenstein, A. H. and L. van Horn. "Very low fat diets." *Circulation* 98:935–939 (1998).

Liu, S., W. C. Willett, M. J. Stampfer, F. B. Hu, M. Franz, L. Sampson, C. H. Hennekens, and J. E. Manson. "A prospective study of dietary glycemic load, carbohydrate intake, and risk of coronary heart disease in US women." *Am J Clin Nutr* 71:1455–1461 (2000).

Lopez, P. M. and R. M. Ortega. "Omega-3 fatty acids in the prevention and control of cardiovascular disease." *Eur J Clin Nutr* 57:S22-S25 (2003).

Lundman, P., M. J. Eriksson, A. Silveia, L-O. Hansson, J. Pernow, C-G. Ericsson, A. Hamsten, and P. Tornvall. "Relation of hypertriglyceridemia to plasma concentrations of biochemical markers of inflammation and endothelial activation." *Am J Cardiol* 91:1128–1131 (2003).

Madsen, T., J. H. Christensen, M. Blom, and E. B. Schmidt. "The effect of dietary N-3 fatty acids on serum concentrations of C-reactive protein." *Br J Nutr* 89:517–522 (2003).

Marcheselli, V. L., S. Hong, W. J. Lukiw, X. H. Tian, K. Gronert, A. Musto, M. Hardy, J. M. Gimenz, N. Chian, C. N. Serhan, and G. Bazan. "Novel docosanoids inhibit brain ischemia-reperfusion-mediate leukocyte infiltration and pro-inflammatory gene expression." *J Biol Chem* 278:43807–43817 (2003).

Marchioli, R., F. Barzi, E. Bomba, and C. Chieffo. "Early protection against sudden death by n-3 polyunsaturated fatty acid after myocardial infarction." *Circulation* 105:1897–1903 (2002).

Marz, W., K. Winkler, M. Nauck, B. Bohm, and B. R. Winkelmann. "Effect of statins on C-reactive protein and interleukin-6." *Am J Cardiol* 92:305–308 (2003).

McLaughlin, T., F. Abbasi, C. Lamendola, H. Yen-Komshian, and G. Reaven. "Carbohydrate-induced hypertriglyceridemia: an insight into the link between plasma insulin and triglyceride concentrations." *J Clin Endocrinol Metab* 85:3085–3088 (2000).

McNamara, J. R., J. L. Jenner, Z. Li, P. W. Wilson, and E. J. Schaefer. "Change in LDL particle size is associated with change in plasma triglyceride concentration." *Arterioscler Thromb Vasc Biol* 12:1284–1290 (1992).

Meagher, E. A., O. P. Barry, J. A. Lawson, J. Rokach, and G. A. FitzGerald. "Effects of vitamin E on lipid peroxidation in healthy persons." *JAMA* 285:1178–1182 (2001).

Modan, M., J. Or, A. Karasik, Y. Drory, Z. Fuchs, A. Lusky, and A. Cherit. "Hyperinsulinemia, sex, and risk of atherosclerotic cardiovascular disease." *Circulation* 84:1165–1175 (1991).

Moghadasian, M. H. "Experimental atherosclerosis. A historical overview." *Life Sci* 70:855–865 (2002).

Nair, S. S. D., J. W. Leitch, J. Faalconer, and M. Garg. "Prevention of cardiac arrhythmia by dietary (n-3) polyunsaturated fatty acids and their mechanism of action." *J Nutr* 127:383–393 (1997).

Nakamura, T., A. Azuma, T. Kuribayashi, H. Sugihara, S. Okuda, and M. Nakagawa. "Serum fatty acid levels, dietary style and coronary heart in three neighboring areas in Japan." *Brit J Nutr* 89:267–272 (2003).

O'Keefe, J. H., and W. S. Harris. "Omega-3 fatty acids: time for clinical implementation?" *Am J Cardiol* 85:1239–1241 (2000).

Okumuar, T., Y. Fujioka, S. Morimoto, S. Tsuboi, M. Masai, T. Tsujino, M. Ohyanagi, and T. Iwasaki. "Eicosapentaenoic acid improves endothelial function in hypertriglyceridemic subjects despite increased lipid oxidizability." *Am J Med Sci* 324:247–253 (2002).

Okuyama, H. "High n-6 to n-3 ratio of dietary fatty acid rather than serum cholesterol as a major risk factor for coronary heart disease." *Eur J Lipid Sci and Tech* 103:418–422 (2001).

Olser, W. *Lectures on Angina Pectoris and Allied States.* New York: Appleton, 1897.

Olszewski, A. J. "Fish oil decreases homocysteine in hyperlipidemic men." *Coronary Artery Dis* 4:53–60 (1993).

Orchard, T. J., D. J. Becker, M. Bates, L. H. Kuller, and A. L. Drash. "Plasma insulin and lipoprotein concentrations: an atherogenic association?" *Am J Epidem* 118:326–337 (1983).

Ornish, D., L. W. Scherwitz, J. H. Billings, K. L. Gould, T. A. Merritt, S. Sparler, W. T. Armstrong, T. A. Ports, R. L. Kirkeeide, C. Hogeboom, and R. J. Brand. "Intensive lifestyle changes for reversal of coronary heart disease." *JAMA* 280:2001–2007 (1998).

Palinski, W. "New evidence for beneficial effects of statins unrelated to lipid lowering." *Arterioscler Thromb Vasc Biol* 21:3–5 (2001).

Papanicolau, D. A. and A. N. Vgontzas. "Interleukin-6: the endocrine cytokine." *J Clin Endocrinol Metab* 85:1331–1332 (2000).

Pentikainen, M. O., K. Oorni, M. Ala-Korpela, and P. T. Kovaen. "Modified LDL-trigger of atherosclerosis and inflammation in the arterial initima." *J Intern Med* 247:359–370 (2000).

Perry, I. J., S. G. Wannamethee, P. H. Whincup, A. G. Shaper, M. K. Walker, and K. G. Alberti. "Serum insulin and incident coronary heart disease in middle-aged British men." *Am J Epidemiol* 144:224–234 (1996).

Pinkey, J. A., C.D. Stenhower, S. W. Coppack, and J. S. Yudkin."Endothelial cell dysfunction: cause of insulin resistance syndrome." *Diabetes* 46:S9–S13 (1997).

Pirro, M., J. Bergeron, G. R. Dagenais, P-M. Bernard, B. Cantin, J-P. Depres, and B. Lamarche. "Age and duration of follow-up as modulators of the risk for ischemic heart disase associated with high plasma C-reactive protein levels in men." *Arch Intern Med* 161:2474–2480 (2001).

Pyorala, K., E. Savolainen, S. Kaukula, and J. Haapakowski. "Plasma insulin as coronary heart disease risk factor." *Acad Med Scand* 701:38–52 (1985).

Pyorala, M., H. Miettinen, P. Halonen, M. Laasko, and K. Pyorala. "Insulin resistance syndrome predicts the risk of coronary heart disease and stroke in healthy middle-aged men." *Arterioscler Thromb Vasc Biol* 20:538–544 (2000).

Rader, D. J. "Inflammatory markers of coronary risk." *N Engl J Med* 343:11790–1182 (2000).

Ravnskov, U. *The Cholesterol Myths*. Washington DC: New Trends Publishing, 2000.

Reaven, G. M. "Role of insulin resistance in human disease." *Diabetes* 37:1595–1607 (1989).

Reaven, G. M. "The role of insulin resistance and hyperinsulinemia in coronary heart disease." *Metabolism* 41:16–19 (1992).

Reaven, G. M., Y. D. Chen, J. Jeppesen, P. Maheux, and R. M. Krauss. "Insulin resistance and hyperinsulinemia in individuals with small, dense low density lipoprotein particles." *J Clin Invest* 92:141–146 (1993).

Ridker, P. M. "High-sensitivity C-reactive protein." *Circulation* 103:1813–1818 (2001).

Ridker, P. M., M. Cushman, M. J. Stampfer, R. P. Tracy, and C. H. Hennekens. "Inflammation, aspirin, and the risk of cardiovascular disease in apparently healthy men." *N Engl J Med* 336:973–979 (1996).

Ridker, P. M., R. J. Glynn, and C. H. Hennekens. "C-reactive protein adds to the predictive value of total and HDL cholesterol in determining risk of first myocardial infarction." *Circulation* 97:2007–2011 (1997).

Ridker, P. M., C. H. Hennekens, J. E. Buring, and N. Rifai. "C-reactive protein and other markers of inflammation in the prediction of cardiovascular disease in women." *New Engl J Med* 42:836–843 (2000).

Rise, P., S. Ghezzi, and C. Galli. "Relative potencies of statins in reducing cholesterol synthesis and enhancing linoleic acid metabolism." *Eur J Pharmcol* 467:73–75 (2003).

Rise, P., F. Pazzucconi, C. R. Sirtori, and C. Galli. "Statins enhance arachidonic acid synthesis in hypercholesterolemic patients." *Nutr Metab Cardiovasc Dis* 11:88–94 (2001).

Rodwell, V. W., J. L. Nordstrom, and Mitschelen. "Regulation of HMG-CoA reductase." *Adv Lipid Res* 14:1–76 (1976).

Rohde, L. E. P., C. H. Hennekens, and P. M. Ridker. "Survey of C-reactive protein and cardiovascular risk factors in apparently healthy men." *Am J Cardiol* 84:1018–1022 (1999).

Rosamond, W. D., L. E. Chambless, A. R. Folsom, L. S. Cooper, D. E. Conwill, L. Legg, Ch-H. Wang, and G. Heiss. "Trends in the incidence of myocardial infarction and in mortality due to coronary heart disease, 1987 to 1994." *N Engl J Med* 339:861–867 (1998).

Ross, R. "The pathogensis of atherosclerosis: a perspective for the 1990s." *Nature* 362:801–809 (1993).

Ross, R. "Atherosclerosis is an inflammatory disease." *N Engl J Med* 340:115–126 (1999).

Rubins, H. B., S. J. Robins, D. Collins, A. Iranmanesh, T. J. Wilt, D. Mann, M. Mayo-Smith, F. H. Fass, M. R. Elam, and G. H. Rutan. "Distribution of lipids in 8,500 men with coronary heart disease." *Am J Cardiol* 75:1196–1201 (1995).

Sacks, F. M., M. A. Pfeffer, L. A. Moye, J. L. Pouleau, J. D. Rutherford, T. G. Cole, L. Brown, J. W. Warnica, J. M. Arnold, C. C. Wun, B. R. Davis, and E. Braunwald. "The effect of pravastatin on coronary events after myocardial infarction in patients with average cholesterol levels." *N Engl J Med* 335:1001–1009 (1996).

Salmeron, J., J. E. Manson, M. J. Stampfer, G. A. Colditz, A. L. Wing, and W. C. Willett. "Dietary fiber, glycemic load, and risk of coronary heart disease in women." *JAMA* 277:472–477 (1997).

Scandinavian Simvastatin Survival Study Group. "Randomized trial of cholesterol lowering in 4444 patients with coronary heart disease: the Scandinavian simvastatin survival study (4S)." *Lancet* 344:1383–1389 (1994).

Sears, B. *The Zone.* New York: ReganBooks, (1995).

Sears, B. *The Anti-Aging Zone.* New York: ReganBooks, (1999).

Sears, B. *The Omega Rx Zone.* New York: ReganBooks, (2002).

Serhan, C. N. and E. Oliw. "Unorthodox routes to prostanoid formation: new twists in cyclooxygenase-initiated pathways." *J Clin Invest* 107:1481–1489 (2001).

Serhan, C. N., C. B. Clish, J. Brannon, S. P. Colgan, N. Chiang, and K. Gronert. "Novel functional sets of lipid-derived mediators with antiinflammatory actions generated from omega-3 fatty acids via cyclooxygenase 2-nonsteroidal antiinflammatory drugs and transcellular processing." *J Exp Med* 192:1197–1204 (2000).

Serhan, C. N., C. B. Clish, J. Brannon, S. P. Colgan, K. Gronert, and N. Chiang. "Antimicroinflammatory lipid signals generated from dietary n-3 fatty acids via cyclooxygenase-2 and transcellular processing: a novel mechanism for NSAID and n-3 PUFA therapeutic actions." *J Physiol Pharmacol* 51:643–654 (2000).

Serhan, C. N., K. Gotlinger, S. Hong, and M. Arita. "Resolvins, docosatrienes, and neuroprotectins, novel omega-3-derived mediators, and their aspirin-triggered endogenous epimers: an overview of their protective roles in catabasis." *Prostaglandins Other Lipid Mediat* 73:155–172 (2004).

Serhan, C. N. "Lipoxins and novel aspirin-triggered 15-epi-lipoxins." *Prostaglandins* 53:107–137 (1997).

Shanoff, H. M., J. A. Little, and A. Csima. "Studies of male survivors of myocardial infarction: xii. Relation of serum lipids and lipoproteins to survival over a 10-year period." *Can Med Assoc J* 103:927–931 (1970).

Sinclair, H. M. "Deficiency of essential fatty acids and atherosclerosis, et cetera." *Lancet* i:381–383 (1956).

Singh, R. B., M. A. Niaz, J. P. Sharma, R. Kumar, V. Rastogi, and M. Moshiri. "Randomized, double-blind, placebo-controlled trial of fish oil and mustard oil in patients with suspected acute myocardial infarction. The Indian Experiment of Infarct Survival-4." *Cardiovasc Drugs Ther* 11:485–491 (1997).

Siscovick, D. S., R. N. Lemaitre, and D. Mozaffarian. "The fish story. A diet-heart hypothesis with clinical implications: n-3 polyunsaturated fatty acids, myocardial vulnerability, and sudden death." *Circulation* 107:2632–2634 (2003).

Solheim, S., H. Arnesen, L. Eikvar, M. Hurlen, and I. Seljeflot. "Influence of aspirin on inflammatory markers in patients after acute myocardial infarction." *Am J Cardiol* 92:843–845 (2003).

Sprecher, D. L. "Triglycerides as a risk factor for coronary artery disease." *Am J Cardiol* 82:49U–56U (1998).

Steering Committee of Physicians Health Study Research Group. "Preliminary Report: findings for aspirin component of the on-going physician health study." *N Engl J Med* 320:262–264 (1988).

Stout, R. "The relationship of abnormal circulating insulin levels to atherosclerosis." *Atherosclerosis* 27:1–13 (1977).

Tchernof, A., B. Lamarche, D. Prud'Homme, A. Nadeau, S. Moorjani, F. Labrie, P. J. Lupien, and J. D. Depres. "The dense LDL phenotype: association with plasma lipoprotein levels, visceral obesity and hyperinsulinemia in men." *Diabetes Care* 19:629–637 (1996).

Thies, F., J. M. C. Garry, P. Yaqoob, K. Kerkasem, J. Williams, C. P. Shearman, P. J. Gallaher, P. C. Calder, and R. F. Grimble. "Association of n-3 polyunsaturated fatty with stability of atherosclerotic plaques." *Lancet* 361:477–485 (2003).

Thompson, P. D. "More on low-fat diets." *New Engl J Med* 338:1623–1624 (1998).

Torjesen, P. A., K. J. Kirkeland, S. A. Andersson, I. Hjermann, I. Holme, and P. Urdal. "Lifestyle chanages may reverse development of the insulin resistance syndrome." *Diabetes Care* 30:26–31 (1997).

Tracy, R. P. "Inflammation in cardiovascular disease." *Arterioscler Thromb Vasc Biol* 22:1514–1515 (2002).

Van der Meer, I. R., P. M. de Maat, A. J. Kiliaan, D. A. M. van der Kuip, A. Hofman, and J. A. M. Witteman. "The value of C-reactive protein in cardiovascular risk prediction." *Arch Intern Med* 163:13231328 (2003).

Villa, B., L. Calabresi, G. Chiesa, P. Rise, C. Galli, and C. R. Sirtori. "Omega-3 fatty acid ethyl esters increase heart rate variability in patients with coronary disease." *Pharmacol Res* 45:475 (2002).

Virchow, R. *Die cellularpathologie in ihrer begrundung auf physiologische und pathologische gewebelehre.* Berlin: Verlag von August Hirschwald, 1858.

Volek, J. S., A. L. Gomez, and W. J. Kraemer. "Fasting lipoprotein and postprandial triacylglycerol responses to a low-carbohydrate diet supplemented with n-3 fatty acids." *J Am Coll Nutr* 19:383–391 (2000).

Von Lente, F. V. "Markers of inflammation as predictors in cardiovascular disease." *Clin Chim Acta* 293:31–52 (2000).

Von Schacky, C. "Omega-3 fatty acids: from Eskimos to clinical cardiology—what took us so long?" *World Rev Nutr Diet* 88:90–99 (2001).

Von Schacky, C. "Prophylaxis of atherosclerosis with marine omega-3 fatty acids." *Ann Intern Med* 107:890–899 (1987).

Von Schacky, C., P. Angerer, W. Kothny, K. Theisen, and H. Mudra. "The effect of dietary omega-3 fatty acids on coronary atherosclerosis: a randomized, double-blind placebo-controlled trial." *Ann Intern Med* 130:554–562 (1999).

Weiner, B. H., I. S. Ockene, P. H. Levine, H. F. Cuenoud, M. Fisher, B. F. Johnson, A. S. Daoud, J. Jarmolych, D. Hosmer, and M. H. Johnson. "Inhibition of atherosclerosis by cod-liver oil in a hyperlipidemic swine model." *N Engl J Med* 315:841–846 (1986).

Westphal, S. A., M. C. Gannon, and F. Q. Nutrall. "Metabolic response to glucose ingested with various amounts of protein." *Am J Clin Nutr* 62:267–272 (1990).

Wierzbicki, A. S., R. Poston, and A. Ferro. "The lipid and non-lipid effects of statins." *Pharmacol and Therapeutics* 99:95–112 (2003).

Willams, P. T. and R. M. Krauss. "Low-fat diets, lipoprotein subclasses, and heart disease risk." *Am J Clin Nutr* 70:949–950 (1999).

Yarnell, J. W. G., P. M. Sweetnam, V. Marks, and J. D. Teale. "Insulin in ischaemic heart disease: are associations explained by triglyceride concentrations? The Caerphilly prospective study." *Br Heart J* 171:293–296 (1994).

Young, B., M. Gleeson, and A. W. Cripps. "C-reactive protein: a critical review." *Pathology* 23:118–124 (1991).

Yudkin, J. S., M. Kumari, S. E. Humphries, and V. Mohamed-Ali. "Inflammation, obesity, stress and coronary heart disease: is interleukin-6 the link?" *Atherosclerosis* 148:209–214 (2000).

Zaman, A. G., G. Helft, S. G. Worthley, and J. J. Badimon. "The role of plaque rupture and thombosis in coronary artery disease." *Artheosclerosis (Ireland)* 149:251–266 (2000).

Zavroni, I., L. Bonini, M. Fantuzzi, E. Dall'Aglio, M. Passeri, and G. M. Reaven. "Hyperinsulinemia, obesity, and syndrome X." *J Intern Med* 235:51–56 (1994).

Zavaroni, I., E. Bonora, M. Pagliara, E. Dall'Aglio, L. Luchetti, G. Buonnanno, P.A. Bonati, M. Bergonzani, L. Gnudi, M. Passeri, and G. Reaven. "Risk factors for coronary artery disease in healthy persons with hyperinsulinemia and normal glucose tolerance." *N Engl J Med* 320:702–706 (1989).

Zhou, Y. R., G. Csako, J. T. Grayston, S.P. Wang, Z. X. Yu, M. Shou, M. Leon, and S. E. Epstein. "Lack of association of restenosis following coronary angioplasty with elevated C-reactive protein levels or seropositivity to Chlamydia pneumoniae." *Am J Cardiol* 84:595–598 (1999).

Zwaka, T. P., V. Hombach, and Torzewski. "C-reactive protein-mediated low density lipoprotein uptake by macrophage: implications for atherosclerosis." *Circulation* 103:2094–2099 (2000).

Chapter 16. Cancer and Silent Inflammation

Ablin, R. J. and M. W. Shaw. "Prostaglandin modulation of prostate tumor growth and metastases." *Anticancer Res* 6:327–388 (1986).

Akre, K., A. M. Ekstrom, L. B. Signorello, L. E. Hansson, and O. Nyren. "Aspirin and risk for gastric cancer." *Br J Cancer* 84:965–968 (2001).

Aktas, H. and J. A. Halperin. "Translational regulation of gene expression by omega-3 fatty acids." *J Nutr* 134:2487S-2491S (2004).

Aronson, W. J., J. A. Glaspy, S. T. Reddy, D. Reese, D. Heber, and D. Bagga. "Modulation of omega-3/omega-6 polyunsaturated ratios with dietary fish oils in men with prostate cancer." *Urology* 58:283–288 (2001).

Attiga, F. A., P. M. Fernandez, A. T. Weeraratna, M. J. Manyak, and S. R. Patierno. "Inhibitors of prostaglandin synthesis inhibit human prostate tumor cell invasiveness and reduce the release of matrix metalloproteinases." *Cancer Res* 60:4629–4637 (2000).

Augustin, L. S. A., L. Dal Maso, C. La Vecchia, M. Papinel, E. Negri, S. Vaccarella, C. W. C. Kendal, D. J. A. Jenkins, and S. Francechi. "Dietary glycemic index and glycemic load, and breast cancer risk." *Ann Ocol* 12:1533–1538 (2001).

Augustsson, K., D. S. Michaud, E. B. Rimm, M. F. Leitzmann, M. J. Stampfer, W. C. Willett, and E. Giovannucci. "A prospective study of intake of fish and marine fatty acids and prostate cancer." *Cancer Epidemiology, Biomarkers and Prevention* 12:64–67 (2003).

Bagga, D., S. Capone, H. J. Wang, D. Heber, M. Lill, L. Chap, and J. A. Glaspy. "Dietary modulation of omega-3/omega-6 polyunsaturated fatty acid ratios in patients with breast cancer." *J Natl Cancer Inst* 6:1123–1131 (1997).

Barber, M. D. "Cancer cachexia and its treatment with fish oil enriched nutritional supplementation." *Nutrition* 217:751–755 (2001).

Barber M. D. and K. C. H. Fearon. "Tolerance and incorporation of a high-dose eicosapentaenoic acid diester emulsion by patients with pancreatic cancer cachexia." *Lipids* 36:347–351 (2001).

Barber, M. D., J. A. Ross, and K. C. H. Fearon. "Changes in nutritional, functional, and inflammatory markers in advanced pancreatic cancer." *Nutr Cancer* 35:106–110 (1999).

Baron, J. A., and R. S. Sandler. "Nonsteroidal anti-inflammatory drugs and cancer prevention." *Ann Rev Med* 51:511–523 (2000).

Baronzio, G. F., F. Galante, A. Gramaglia, A. Barlocco, S. de Grandi, and I. Freitas. "Tumor microcirculation and its significance in therapy: possible role of omega-3 fatty acids as rheological modifiers." *Med Hypotheses* 50:175–82 (1998).

Bartsch, H., J. Nair, and R. W. Owen. "Dietary polyunsaturated fatty acids and cancer of the breast and colorectum: emerging evidence for their role as risk modifiers." *Carcinogenesis* 20:2209–2218 (1999).

Bougnoux, P. "n-3 polyunsaturated fatty acids and cancer." *Curr Opin Clin Nutr Metab Care* 2:121–126. (1999).

Bougnoux, P., E. Germain, V. Chajes, B. Hubert, C. Lhuillery, O. Le Floch, G. Body, and G. Calais. "Cytotoxic drugs efficacy correlates with adipose tissue docosahexaenoic acid level in locally advanced breast carcinoma." *Br J Cancer* 79:1765–1769 (1999).

Bruce, W. R., Wolever T. M. S, and A. Giacca. "Mechanisms linking diet and colorectal cancer: the possible role of insulin resistance." *Nutr Cancer* 37:19–26 (2000).

Bruning, P. F., J. M. G. Bonfrer, P. A. H. van Noodr, A. A. M. Hart, M. de Jong-Bakker, and W. J. Nooijen. "Insulin resistance and breast cancer." *Int J Cancer* 52:511–516 (1992).

Burns, C. P., S. Halabi, G. H. Clamon, V. Hars, B. A. Wagner, R. J. Hohl, E. Lester, J. J. Kirshner, V. Vinciguerra, and E. Paskett. "Phase I clinical study of fish oil fatty acid capsules for patients with cancer cachexia: cancer and leukemia group B study 9473." *Clin Cancer Res* 5:3942–3947 (1999).

Cannizzo Jr., F. and S. A. Broitman. "Postpromotional effects of dietary marine or safflower oils on large bowel or pulmonary implants of CT-26 in mice." *Cancer Res* 49:4289–4294 (1989).

Capuron, L., A. Ravaud, and R. Dantzer. "Early depressive symptoms in cancer patients receiving interleukin 2 and/or interferon alfa-2b therapy." *J Clin Oncol* 18:2143–2151 (2000).

Chapkin, R. S., N. E. Hubbard, D. K. Buckman, and K. L. Erickson. "Linoleic acid metabolism in metastatic and nonmetastatic murine mammary tumor cells." *Cancer Res* 49: 4724–4728 (1989).

Chatenoud, L., C. La Vecchia, S. Franceschi, A. Tavani, D. R. Jacobs, M. T. Parpinel, M. Sosler, and E. Negri. "Refined-cereal intake and risk of selected cancers in Italy." *Am J Clin Nutr* 70:1107–1110 (1999).

Chen, Y. Q., Z. M. Duniec, B. Liu, W. Hagmann, X. Gao, K. Shimoji, L. J. Marnett, C. R. Johnson, and K. V. Honn. "Endogenous 12(S)-HETE production by tumor cells and its role in metastasis." *Cancer Res* 15:1574–1579 (1994).

Chen, Y. Q., B. Liu, D. G. Tang, and K. V. Honn. "Fatty acid modulation of tumor cell-platelet-vessel wall interaction." *Cancer Metastasis Rev* 11:389–409 (1992).

Cho, E., D. Spiegelman, D. J. Hunter, W. Y. Chen, G. A. Colditz, and W. C. Willett. "Premenopausal dietary carbohydrate, glycemic index, and glycemic load, and fiber in relation to risk of breast cancer." *Cancer Epidemiology, Biomarkers and Prevention* 12:1153–1158 (2003).

Claria, J., M. H. Lee, and C. N. Serhan. "Aspirin-triggered lipoxins are generated by human lung adrenocarcinoma cell (A549)-neutrophil interactions and are potent inhibitors of cell proliferation." *Mol Med* 2:583–596 (1996).

Colas, S., L. Paon, F. Denis, M. Prat, P. Louisot, C. Hoinard, O. Le Floch, G. Ogilive, and P. Bougnoux. "Enhanced radiosensitivity of rat autochthonous mammary tumors by dietary docosahexaenoic acid." *Int J Cancer* 109:449–454 (2004).

Connolly, J. M., X. H. Liu, and D. P. Rose. "Dietary linoleic acid-stimulated human breast cancer cell growth and metastasis in nude mice and their suppression by indomethacin, a cyclooxygenase inhibitor." *Nutr Cancer* 25:231–240 (1996).

Copeland, G. P., S. J. Leinster, J. C. Davis, and L. J. Hipkin. "Insulin resistance in patients with colorectal cancer." *Br J Surg* 74:1031–1036 (1987).

Damtew, B. and P. J. Spagnuolo. "Tumor cell-endothelial cell interactions: evidence for roles for lipoxygenase products of arachidonic acid in metastasis." *Prostaglandins Leukot Essent Fatty Acids* 56:295–300 (1997).

DeLongeril, M., P. Salen, J. L. Martin, I. Monjaud, P. Boucher, and N. Mamelle. "Mediterranean dietary pattern in a randomized trial: prolonged survival and possible reduced rate of cancer." *Arch Intern Med* 158:1181–1188 (1998).

Dewailly, E., G. Mulvad, H. S. Pedersen, J. C. Hansen, N. Behrendt, and J. P. H. Hansen. "Inuit are protected against prostate cancer." *Cancer Epidemiology, Biomarkers and Prevention* 12:926–927 (2001).

DuBois, R. N. F. M. Giardiello, and W. E. Smalley. "Nonsteroidal anti-inflammatory drugs, eicosanoids, and colorectal cancer prevention." *Gastroenterol Clin North Am* 25:773–791 (1996).

Dunlop. R. J. and C. W. Campbell. "Cytokines and cancer." *J Pain Symptom Manage* 20:214–232 (2000).

Folsom, A. R., Z. Demissi, and L. Harnack. "Glycemic index, glycemic load, and incidence of endometrial cancer." *Nutr Cancer* 46:119–124 (2003).

Form, D. M. and Auerbach. "PGE2 and angiogenesis." *Exp Biol Med* 172:214–218 (1983).

Ellis, L. M., E. N. Copeland, K. I. Bland, and H. S. Sitren. "Inhibition of tumor growth and metastasis by chronic intravenous infusion of prostaglandin E1." *Ann Surg* 212:45–50 (1990).

Fernandez, E., L. Chatenoud, C. La Vecchia, E. Negri, and S. Franceschi. "Fish consumption and cancer risk." *Am J Clin Nutr* 70:85–90 (1999).

Franceschi, S., L. Dal Maso, L. Augustin, E. Negri, M. Parpinci, P. Boyle, D. J. Jenkins, and C. La Vecchia. "Dietary glycemic load and colorectal cancer risk." *Ann Oncol* 12:173–178 (2001).

Franceschi, S., A. Favero, A. Decari, E. Negri, C. La Vecchia, M. Ferraroni, A. Russo, S. Salvini, D. Amadori, and E. Conti. "Intake of macronutrients and the risk of breast cancer." *Lancet* 347:1351–1356 (1996).

Franceschi, S., A. Favero, M. Parpinel, A. Giacosa, and C. La Vecchia. "Italian study study of colorectal cancer with emphasis on influence of cereals." *Eur J Cancer Prev* 7:S19-S223 (1998).

Franceschi, S., C. La Vecchia, A. Russo, A. Favero, E. Negri, E. Conti, M. Montella, R. Filiberti, D. Amadori, and A. Decarli. "Macronutrient intake and risk of colorectal cancer in Italy." *Int J Cancer* 76:321–324 (1998).

Fulton, A. M. "The role of eicosanoids in tumor metastasis." *Prostaglandins Leukot Essent Fatty Acids* 34:229–237 (1988).

Gago-Dominguez, M., J. E. Castelao, C-L. Sun, D. van den Berg, W-P. Koh, H-P. Lee, and M. C. Yu. "Marine n-3 fatty acid intake, glutathione S-transferease polymorphisms and breast cancer risk in postmenopausal Chinese women in Singapore." *Carcinogenesis* 25:978–982 (2004).

Gao, X., W. Hagmann, A. Zacharek, N. Wu, M. Lee, A. T. Porter, and K. V. Honn. "Eicosanoids, cancer metastasis, and gene regulation: an overview." *Adv Exp Med Biol* 400A:545–55 (1997).

Garcia-Rodriguez, L. A., and C. Huerta-Alvarez. "Reduced risk of colorectal cancer among long-term users of aspirin and nonaspirin nonsterodial anti-inflammatory drugs." *Epidemiology* 12:88–93 (2001).

Germain, E., V. Chajes, S. Cognault, C. Lhuillery, and P. Bougnoux. "Enhancement of doxorubicin cytotoxicity by polyunsaturated fatty acids in the human breast tumor cell line MDA-MB-231: relationship to lipid peroxidation." *Int J Cancer* 75:578–583 (1998).

Germain, E., F. Lavandier, V. Chajes, V. Schubnel, P. Bonnet, C. Lhuillery, and P. Bougnoux. "Dietary n-3 polyunsaturated fatty acids and oxidants increase rat mammary tumor sensitivity to epirubicin without change in cardiac toxicity." *Lipids* 34:S203 (1999).

Ghost, J. and C. E. Myers. "Arachidonic acid stimulates prostate cancer cell growth: critical role of 5-lipooxygenase." *Biochem Biophys Res Commun* 235:418–423 (1997).

Ghost, J. and C. E. Myers. "Arachidonic acid metabolism and cancer of the prostate." *Nutrition* 14:48–57 (1998).

Giardiello, F. M., G. J. Offerhaus, and R. N. DuBois. "The role of nonsteroidal anti-inflammatory drugs in colorectal cancer prevention." *Eur J Cancer* 31A:1071–1076 (1995).

Giovannucci, E. "Insulin and colon cancer." *Cancer Causes and Control* 6:164–179 (1995).

Gogos, C. A., P. Ginopoulos, B. Salsa, E. Apostolidou, N. C. Zoumbos, and F. Kalfarentzos.

"Dietary omega-3 polyunsaturated fatty acids plus vitamin E restore immunodeficiency and prolong survival for severely ill patients with generalized malignancy: a randomized control trial." *Cancer 1998* 82:395–402 (1998).

Hansen-Petrik, M. B., M. F. McEntee, C-H. Chiu, and J. Whelan. "Antagonism of arachidonic acid is linked to the antitumorigenic effect of dietary eicosapentaenoic acid acid in APC mice." *J Nutr* 130:1153–1158 (2000).

Hardman, W. E., C. P. Avula, G. Fernandes, and I. L. Cameron. "Three percent dietary fish oil concentrate increased efficacy of doxorubicin against mda-mb 231 breast cancer xenografts." *Clin Cancer Res* 7:2041–2049 (2001).

Hardman, W. E., M. P. Moyer, and I. L. Cameron. "Dietary fish oil sensitizes A549 lung xenografts to doxorubicin chemotherapy." *Cancer Lett* 151:145–151 (2000).

Honn, K. V., D. G. Tang, X. Gao, I. A. Butovich, B. Liu, J. Timar, and W. Hagmann. "12-lipoxygenases and 12(S)-HETE: role in cancer metastasis." *Cancer Metastasis Rev* 13:365–396 (1994).

Honn, K.V., D. G. Tang, I. M. Grossi, C. Renaud, Z. M. Duniec, C. R. Johnson, and C. A. Diglio. "Enhanced endothelial cell retraction mediated by 12(S)-HETE: a proposed mechanism for the role of platelets in tumor cell metastasis." *Exp Cell Res* 210:1–9 (1994).

Huang, Y.C., J. M. Jessup, and G. L. Blackburn. "N-3 fatty acids decrease colonic epithelial cell proliferation in high-risk bowel mucosa." *Lipids* 31:S313-S316 (1996).

Hubbar, N. E., D. Lim, and K. L. Erickson. "Alternation of murine mammary tumorigenesis by dietary enrichment with n-3 fatty acids in fish oil." *Cancer Lett* 124:1–7 (1998).

Hussey, H. J., and M. H. Tidale. "Inhibition of tumour growth by lipoxygenase inhibitors." *Br J Cancer* 74:683–687 (1996).

Hwang, D., D. Scollard, J. Byrne, and E. Levine. "Expression of cyclooxygenase-1 and cyclooxygenase-2 in human breast cancer." *J Natl Cancer Res* 90:455–460 (1998).

Iniguez, M. A., A. Rodriguez, O. V. Volpert, M. Fresno, and J. M. Redondo. "Cyclooxygenase-2: a therapeutic target in angiogenesis." *Trends in Mol Med* 9:73–78 (2003).

Jiag, W. G., R. P. Bryce, and D. F. Horrobin. "Essential fatty acids: molecular and cellular basis of their anti-cancer action and clinical implications." *Crit Rev Oncol Hematol* 27:179–209 (1998).

Kaizer, L., N. F. Boyd, V. Kriukov, and D. Trichler. "Fish consumption and breast cancer risk." *Nutr Cancer* 12:61–68 (1989).

Karmali, R. "N-3 fatty acids: biochemical actions in cancer." *J Nutr Sci Vitaminol (Tokyo)* Spec No:148–52 (1992).

Karmali, R. A. "Eicosanoids and cancer." *Prog Clin Biol Res* 222:687–697 (1986).

Karmali, R. A. "Historical perspective and potential use of n-3 fatty acids in therapy of cancer cachexia." *Nutrition* 12:S2–S4 (1996).

Karmali, R. A. "N-3 fatty acids and cancer." *J Intern Med* 225:197–200 (1989).

Kinoshita, K., M. Noguchi, M. Earashi, M. Tanaka, and T. Sasaki. "Inhibitory effects of purified eicosapentaenoic acid and docosahexaenoic acid on growth and metastasis of murine transplantable mammary tumor." *In Vivo* 8:371–374 (1994).

Kopp, E. and S. Ghosh. "Inhibition of NF-kappa B by sodium salicylate and aspirin." *Science* 265:956–959 (1994).

Kort, W. J., I. M. Weijma, A. M. Bijma, W. P. van Schalkwijk, A. J. Vergroesen, and D. L. Westbroek. "Omega-3 fatty acids inhibiting the growth of a transplantable rat mammary adeno-carcinoma." *J Natl Cancer Inst* 79:593–599 (1987).

Lane, J., R. E. Mansel, and W. G. Jiang. "Expression of human delta 6-desaturase is associated with aggressiveness of human breast cancer." *Int J Mol Med* 12:253:257 (2003).

Levi, F., C. Pasche, R. Lucchini, L. Chatenoud, D. R. Jacobs, and C. La Vecchia. "Refined and whole grain cereals and the risk of oral, esophageal and laryngeal cancer." *Eur J Clin Nutr* 54:487–489 (2000).

Liu, B., R. J. Maher, Y. A. Hannum, A. T. Porter, and K. V. Honn. "12-HETE enhancement of prostate tumor cell invasion: selective role of PKC alpha." *J Natl Cancer Inst* 86:1145–1151 (1994).

Lloyd, F. P., V. Slivova, T. Valaachovicova, and D. Sliva. "Aspirin inhibits highly invasive prostate cancer cells." *Int J Oncol* 23:1277–1283 (2003).

Lundholm, K., G. Holm, and T. Schersten. "Insulin resistance in patients with cancer." *Cancer Res* 38:4665–4670 (1978).

Marcus, A. J. "Aspirin as prophylaxis against colorectal cancer." *N Engl J Med* 333:656–658 (1995).

Marks, F., K. Muller-Decker, and A. Furstenberger. "A casual relationship between unscheduled eicosanoid signaling and tumor development: cancer chemoprevention by inhibitors of arachidonic acid metabolism." *Toxicology* 153:11–26 (2000).

McCarty, M. F. "Fish oil may impede tumour angiogenesis and invasiveness by down-regulating protein kinase C and modulating eicosanoid production." *Med Hypotheses* 46:107–115 (1996).

McKeown-Eyssen, G. "Epidemiology of colorectal cancer revisted: are serum triglycerides and/or plasma glucose associated with risk?" *Cancer Epidemiol Biomarkers and Prev* 3:687–695 (1994).

Michaud, D. S., S. Liu, E. Giovannucci, W. C. Willett, G. A. Colditz, and C. S. Fuchs. "Dietary sugar, glycemic load, and pancreatic cancer risk in a prospective study." *J Nat Cancer Inst* 94:1293–300 (2002).

Moysich, K. B., C. Mettlin, M. S. Piver, N. Natarajan, R. J. Menezes, and H. Swede. "Regular use of analgesic drugs and ovarian cancer risk." *Cancer Epidemiol Biomarkers Prev* 10:903–906 (2001).

Mukutmoni-Norris, M., N. E. Hubbard, and K. L. Erickson. "Modulation of murine mammary tumor vasculature by dietary n-3 fatty acids in fish oil." *Cancer Lett* 150:101–109 (2000).

Narisawa, T., H. Kusaka, Y. Yamazaki, M. Takahashi, H. Koyama, K. Koyama, Y. Fukaura, and A. Wakizaka. "Relationship between blood plasma prostaglandin E2 and liver and lung metastases in colorectal cancer." *Dis Colon Rectum* 33:840–845 (1990).

Natarajan, R. and J. Nadler. "Role of lipoxygenases in breast cancer." *Front Biosci* 3:E81–88. (1998).

Nie, D., G. G. Hillman, T. Geddes, K. Tang, C. Pierson, D. J. Grignon, and K. V. Honn. "Platelet-type 12-lipoxygenase in a human prostate carcinoma stimulates angiogenesis and tumor growth." *Cancer Res* 58:4047–4051 (1998).

Nie, D., J. Nemeth, Y. Qiao, A. Zacharek, L. Li, K. Hanna, K. Tang, G. G. Hillman, M. L. Cher, D. J. Grignon, and K. V. Honn. "Increased metastatic potential in human prostate carcinoma cells by overexpression of arachidonate 12-lipoxygenase." *Clin Exp Metastasis* 20:657–663 (2003).

Nie, D., K. Tang, K. Szekeres, M. Trikha, and K. V. Honn. "The role of eicosanoids in tumor growth and metastasis." *Ernst Schering Res Found Workshop* 31:201–217 (2000).

Nie, D., K. Tang, K. Szekeres, L. Li, and K. V. Honn. "Eicosanoid regulation of angiogenesis: role of endothelial arachidonate 12-lipoxygenase." *Ann N Y Acad Sci* 905:165–176 (2000).

Noguchi, Y., T. Yoshikawa, D. Marat, C. Doi, T. Makin, K. Fukuzawa, A. Tsuburaya, S. Staoh, T. Ito, and S. Mitsuse. "Insulin resistance in cancer patients is associated with enhanced tumor necrosis factor expression in skeletal muscle." *Biochem Biophys Res Commun* 253:887–892 (1998).

Norrish, A. E., C. M. Skeaff, G. L. Arribas, S. J. Sharpe, and R. T. Jackson. "Prostate cancer risk and consumption of fish oils: a dietary biomarker-based case-control study." *Br J Cancer* 81:1238–1242 (1999).

Ogilvie, G. K., M. J. Fettman, C. H. Mallinckrodt, J. A. Walton, R. A. Hansen, D. J. Davenport, K. L. Gross, K. L. Richardson, Q. Rogers, and M. S. Hand. "Effect of fish oil, arginine, and doxorubicin chemotherapy on remission and survival time for dogs with lymphoma: a double-blind, randomized placebo-controlled study." *Cancer* 88:1916–1928 (2000).

Okuno, K., H. Jinnai, Y. S. Lee, K. Nakamura, T. Hirohata, H. Shigeoka, and M. Yasutomi. "A high level of prostaglandin E2 (PGE2) in the portal vein suppresses liver-associated immunity and promotes liver metastases." *Surg Today* 25:954–958 (1995).

Pham, H., T. Banerjee, G. M. Nalbandian, and V. A. Ziboh. "Activation of peroxisome proliferators-activated receptor gamma by 15S-hydroxyeicosatrienoic acid parallels growth suppression of androgen-dependent prostatic adenocarcinoma cells." *Cancer Lett* 17–23 (2003).

Pratt, V. C., S. Watanable, E. Bruera, J. Mackey, M. R. Clandinin, V. E. Baracos, and C. J. Field. "Plasma and neutrophil fatty acid composition in advanced cancer patients and response to fish oil supplementation." *Br J Cancer* 87:1370–1378 (2002).

Prescott, S. M. and F. A. Fitzpatrick. "Cyclooxygenase-2 and carcinogenesis." *Biochim Biophys Acta* 1470:M69-M78 (2000).

Radisky, D., C. Hagios, and M. J. Bissell. "Tumors are unique organs defined by abnormal signaling and context." *Cancer Biol* 11:87–95 (2001).

Reich, R. and G. R. Martin. "Identification of arachidonic acid pathways required for the invasive and metastatic activity of malignant tumor cells." *Prostaglandins* 51:1–17 (1996).

Rigas, B., I. S. Goldman, and L. Levine. "Altered eicosanoid levels in human colon cancer." *J Lab Clin Med* 122:518–523 (1993).

Rioux, N. and Castonguay. "Inhibitors of lipoxygenase: a new class of cancer chemopreventative inhibitors." *Carcinogenesis* 19:1393–1400 (1998).

Rohdeburg, G. L., A. Bernhard, and O. Krehniel. "Sugar tolerance in cancer." *JAMA* 72:1528 (1919).

Rolland, P. H., M. Martin, and M. Toga. "Prostaglandin in human breast cancer: evidence suggesting the elevated prostaglandin production is a marker of high metastatic potential." *J Nat Cancer Inst* 64:1061–1070 (1980).

Rose, D. P. and J. M. Connolly. "Antiangiogenicity of docosahexaenoic acid and its role in the suppression of breast cancer cell growth in nude mice." *Int J Oncol* 15:1011–1015 (1999).

Rose, D. P. and J. M. Connelly. "Omega-3 fatty acids as cancer chemopreventive agents." *Pharmacol Ther* 83:217–244 (1999).

Rose, D. P. and J. M. Connolly. "Regulation of tumor angiogenesis by dietary fatty acids and eicosanoids." *Nutr Cancer* 37:119–127. (2000).

Rudra, P. K. and H. E. Krokan. "Cell-specific enhancement of doxorubicin toxicity in human tumour cells by docosahexaenoic acid." *Anticancer Res* 21(1A):29–38 (2001).

Sauer, L. A., R. T. Dauchy, and D. E. Blask. "Mechanism for the antitumor and anticachectic effects of n-3 fatty acids." *Cancer Res* 60:5289–5295 (2000).

Sawaoka, H., S. Tsuji, M. Tsuji, E. S. Gunawan, Y. Sasaki, S. Kawano, and M. Hori. "Cyclooxygenase inhibitors suppress angiogenesis and reduce tumor growth in vivo." *Lab Invest* 79:79:1469–1477 (1999).

Schirner, M., R. B. Lichtner, and M. R. Schneider. "The stable prostacyclin analogue Cicaprost inhibits metastasis to lungs and lymph nodes in the 13762NF MTLn3 rat mammary carcinoma." *Clin Exp Metastasis* 12:24–30 (1994).

Schoen, R. E., C. M. Tengen, L. H. Kuller, G. L. Bruke, M. Cushman, R. P. Tracy, A. Dops, and P. J. Savage. "Increased blood glucose and insulin, body size, and incidence of colorectal cancer." *J Natl Cancer Inst* 91:1147–1154 (1999).

Sears, B. *The Zone.* New York: ReganBooks, 1995.

Sears, B. *The Anti-Aging Zone.* New York: ReganBooks, 1999.

Sears, B. *The Omega Rx Zone.* New York: ReganBooks, 2002.

Sheehan, K. M., K. Sherhan, D. P. O'Donoghue, F. MacSweeney, R. M. Conroy, D. J. Fitzgerald, and F. E. Murray. "The relationship between cyclooxygenase-2 expression and colorectal cancer." *JAMA* 282:1254–1257 (1999).

Shiff, S. J. and B. Rigas. "Aspirin for cancer." *Nature Medicine* 5:1348–1349 (1999).

Singh, J., R. Hamid, and B. S. Reddy. "Dietary fat and colon cancer: modulation of cyclooxygenase-2 by types and amount of dietary fat during the post-initiation stage of colon carcinogenesis." *Cancer Res* 57:3465–3470 (1997).

Steele, V. E., C. A. Holmes, E. T. Hawk, L. Kipelovich, R. A. Lubet, J. A. Crowell, C. C. Sigman, and G. J. Kelloff. "Lipoxygenase inhibitors as potential cancer chemopreventives." *Cancer Epidemiol Biomarkers Prevent* 8:467–483 (1999).

Stoll, B. A. "Essential fatty acids, insulin resistance, and breast cancer risk." *Nutrition and Cancer* 31:72–77 (1998).

Stoll, B. A. "Western nutrition and the insulin resistance syndrome: a link to breast cancer." *Eur J Clin Nutr* 53:83–87 (1999).

Takahata, K., M. Tada, K. Yazawa, and T. Tamaki. "Protection from chemotherapy-induced alopecia by docosahexaenoic acid." *Lipids* 34:S105 (1999).

Taketo, M. M. "Cyclooxygenase-2 inhibitors in tumorigenesis (Part II)." *J Natl Cancer Inst* 90:1609–1620 (1998).

Tang, D. G., C. Renaud, S. Stojakovic, C. A. Diglio, A. Porter, and K. V. Honn. "12-HETE is a mitogenic factor for microvascular endothelial cells: its potential role in angiogenesis." *Biochem Biophys Res Comm* 211:462–468 (1995).

Tang, K., and K. V. Honn. "12(S)-HETE in cancer metastasis." *Adv Exp Med Biol* 447:181–191 (1999).

Terry, P., P. Lichtenstein, M. Feychting, A. Ahlbom, and A. Wolk. "Fatty fish consumption and risk of prostate cancer." *Lancet* 357:1764–1766 (2001).

Thun, M. J. "NSAID use and decreased risk of gastrointestinal cancers." *Gastroenterol Clin North Am* 25:333–348 (1996).

Tran, T. T., A. Medline, and W. R. Bruce. "Insulin promotion of colon tumors in rats." *Cancer Epidemiol Biomarkers Prev* 5:1013–1015 (1996).

Tsujii, M., S. Kawano, and R. N. DuBois. "Cyclooxygenase-2 expression in human colon cancer cells increases metastatic potential." *Proc Natl Acad Sci U S A* 94:3336–3340 (1997).

Uefuji, K., T. Ichikura, and H. Mochizuki. "Cyclooxygenase-2 expression is related to prostaglandin biosynthesis and angiogenesis in human gastric cancer." *Clin Cancer Res* 6:135–138 (2000).

Vergote, I. B., P. A. van Dam, G. M. Laekeman, G. H. Keersmaeckers, F. L. Uyttenbroeck, and A. G. Herman. "Prostacyclin/thromboxane ratio in human breast cancer." *Tumour Biol* 12:261–266 (1991).

Welch, H. G., L. M. Schwartz, and S. Woloshin. "Are increasing 5-year survival rates evidence of success against cancer?" *JAMA* 283:2975–2978 (2000).

Wen, B., E. Deutsch, P. Opolon, A. Auperin, V. Frascogna, E. Connault, and J. Bourhis. "n-3 polyunsaturated fatty acids decrease mucosal/epidermal reactions and enhance antitumour effect of ionizing radiation with inhibition of tumour angiogenesis." *Br J Cancer* 89:1102–1107 (2003).

Wigmore, S. J., M. D. Barber, J. A. Ross, M. J. Tisdale, and K. C. Fearon. "Effect of oral eicosapentaenoic acid on weight loss in patients with pancreatic cancer." *Nutr Cancer* 36:177–814 (2000).

Willams, C. S., M. Mann, and R. N. DuBois. "The role of cyclooxygenases in inflammation, cancer, and development." *Oncogene* 18:7980–7916 (1999).

Yam, D. "Insulin-cancer relationships. Possible dietary implications." *Med Hypotheses* 38:111–117 (1992).

Yam, D., A. Peled, and M. Shinitzky. "Suppression of tumor growth and metastasis by dietary fish oil combined with vitamins E and C and cisplatin." *Cancer Chemother Pharmacol* 47:34–40 (2001).

Yokoyama, I., S. Hayashi, T. Kobayashi, M. Negita, M. Yasutomi, K. Uchida, and H. Takagi. "Prevention of experimental hepatic metastasis with thromboxane synthase inhibitor." *Res Exp Med (Berl)* 195:209–215 (1995).

Yoshikawa, T., Y. Noguchi, C. Doi, T. Makino, and K. Noruma. "Insulin resistance in patients with cancer: relationships with tumor site, tumor stage, body-weight loss, acute-phase response, and energy expenditure." *Nutrition* 17:590–593 (2001).

Chapter 17. Brain Drain Due to Silent Inflammation

Adams, P., S. Lawson, A. Sanigorski, and A. J. Sinclair. "Arachidonic acid to eicosapentaenoic acid ratio in blood correlates positively with clinical symptoms of depression." *Lipids* 31:S157–S161 (1996).

Ahmann, P. A., S. J. Waltonen, K. A. Olson, F. W. Theye, A. J. van Erem, and R. J. LePlant. "Placebo-controlled evaluation of Ritalin side effects." *Pediatrics* 91:1101–1106 (1993).

Aisen, P. S. "Anti-inflammatory therapy for Alzheimer's disease." *Neurobiol Aging* 21:447–448 (2000).

Aisen, P. S. "Anti-inflammatory therapy for Alzheimer's disease: implication of the prednisone trial." *Acta Neurol Scand* 176:85–89 (2000).

Akiyama, H., T. Arai, H. Kondo, E. Tanno, C. Haga, and K. Ikeda. "Cell mediators of inflammation in the Alzheimer disease brain." *Alzheimer Disease and Associated Disorders* 14:S47–S53 (2000).

Amen, D. G. *Change Your Brain, Change Your Life*. New York: Random House, 1998.

Amen, D. G. *Healing ADD*. New York: G.P. Putnam, 2001.

Bell, J.G., E. E. MacKinlay, J. R. Dick, D. J. MacDonald, R. M. Boyle, and A. C. Glen. "Essential fatty acids and phospholipase A(2) in autistic spectrum disorders." *Prostaglandins Leukot Essent Fatty Acids* 71:201–204 (2004).

Burdge, G. C., S. M. Wright, J. O. Warner, and A. D. Postle. "Fetal brain and liver phospholipids fatty acid composition in a guinea pig model of fetal alcohol syndrome: effect of maternal supplementation with tuna oil." *J Nutr Biochem* 8:438–444 (1997).

Burgess, J. R., L. Stevens, and L. Peck. "Long-chain polyunsaturated fatty acids in children with attention-deficit hyperactivity disorder." *Am J Clin Nutr* 71:327S-330S (2000).

Bush, G., J. A. Frazier, S. L. Rauch, L. J. Seidman, P. J. Whalen, M. A. Jenike, B. R. Rosen, and J. Biederman. "Anterior cingulated cortex dysfuction in attention deficit/hyperactivity disorder revealed by fMRI and the counting stroop." *Biol Psychiatry* 45:1542–1552 (1999).

Calon, F., G. P. Lim, F. Yang, T. Morihara, B. Teter, O. Ubeda, P. Rostaing, A. Triller, N. Salem, K. H. Ashe, S. A. Frutschy, and G. M. Cole. "Docosahexaenoic acid protects for dendritic pathology in a Alzheimer's disease mouse model." *Neuron* 43:633–645 (2004).

Carrie, I., M. Clement, D. De Javel, H. Frances, and J. M. Bourre. "Learning deficits in the first generation OF1 mice deficient in (n-3) polyunsaturated fatty acids do not result from visual alteration." *Neurosci Lett* 266:69–72 (1999).

Connor, W. E., M. Neuringer, and S. Reisbick. "Essential fatty acids: importance of n-3 fatty acids in the retina and brain." *Nutr Rev* 50:21–29 (1992).

Conquer, J. A., M. C. Tierney, J. Zecevic, W. J. Bettger, and R. H. Fisher. "Fatty acid analysis of blood plasma of patients with Alzheimer's disease, other types of dementia, and cognitive impairment." *Lipids* 35:1305–1312 (2000).

Cooper, N. R., R. N. Kalaria, P. L. McGeer, and J. Rogers. "Key issues in Alzheimer's disease inflammation." *Neurobiology Aging* 21:451–453 (2000).

Delion, S., S. Chalon, D. Guilloteau, J. C. Besnard, and G. Durand. "Alpha-linolenic acid deficiency alters age-related changes of dopaminergic and serotoninergic neurotransmitters in the rat frontal cortex." *J Neurochem* 66:1582–1591 (1996).

Delion, S., S. Chalon, J. Herault, D. Guilloteau, J. C. Besnard, and G. Durand. "Chronic dietary alpha-linolenic acid deficiency alters dopaminergic and serotoninergic neurotransmitters in rats." *J Nutr* 124:2466–2476 (1994).

Ensel, M., H. Milon, and A. Malnoe. "Effect of low intake of n-3 fatty acids during development of brain phospholipid, fatty acid composition and exploratory behavior in rats." *Lipids* 26:203–208 (1991).

Fenton, W. S., J. Hibbeln, and M. Knable. "Essential fatty acids, lipid membrane abnormalities, and the diagnosis and treatment of schizophrenia." *Biol Psychiatry* 47:8–21 (2000).

Fernstrom, J. D. "Effects of dietary polyunsaturated fatty acids on neuronal function." *Lipids* 34:161–169 (1999).

Freychet, P. "Insulin receptors and insulin actions in the nervous system." *Diabetes Metab Res Rev* 16:390–392 (2000).

Gayo, A., L. Mozo, A. Suarez, A. Tunon, C. Lahoz, and C. Gutierrez. "Inteferon beta treatment modulates TNF and interferon gamma spontaneous gene expression in MS." *Neurology* 52:1764–1770 (1999).

Gesch, C. B., S. M. Hammond, S. E. Hampson, A. Eves, and M. J. Crowder. "Influence of supplementary vitamins, minerals and essential fatty acids on the anti-social behavior of young adult prisoners." *Br J Psychiatry* 181:22–28 (2002).

Glueck, C. J., M. Tieger, R. Kunkel, T. Tracy, J. Speirs, P. Streicher, and E. Illig. "Improvement in symptoms of depression and in an index of life stressors accompany treatment of severe hypertriglyceridemia." *Biol Psychiatry* 34:240–252 (1993).

Hallahan, B. and M. R. Garland. "Essential fatty acids and their role in the treatment of impulsivity disorders." *Prostaglandins Leukot Essent Fatty Acids* 71:211–216 (2004).

Hallowell, E. and J. J. Ratey. *Driven to Distraction.* New York: Touchstone Books, 1995.

Hamazaki, T. and S. Hirayama. "The effect of docosahexaenoic acid-containing food administration on symptoms of attention-deficit/hyperactivity disorder—a placebo control double-blind study." *Eur J Clin Nutr* 58:838 (2004).

Hamazaki, T., S. Sawazaki, M. Itomura, E. Asaoka, Y. Nagao, N. Nishimura, K. Yazawa, T. Kuwamori, and M. Kobayashi. "The effect of docosahexaenoic acid on aggression in young adults." *J Clin Invest* 97:1129–1134 (1996).

Hamaszki, T., S. Sawazaki, M. Itomura, Y. Nagao, A. Thienprasert, T. Nagasawa, and S. Watanabe. "Effect of docosahexaenoic acid on hostility." *World Rev Nutr Diet* 88:47–52 (2001).

Hibbeln, J.R. "Fish consumption and major depression." *Lancet* 351:1213 (1998).

Hibbeln, J. R. "Seafood consumption and homicide mortality." *World Rev Nutr Diet* 88:41–46 (2001).

Hibbeln, J. R. and N. Salem. "Dietary polyunsaturated fatty acids and depression: when cholesterol does not satisfy." *Am J Clin Nutr* 62:1–9 (1995).

Hirayama, S., T. Hamazaki, and K. Terasawa. "Effect of docosahexaenoic acid -containing food administration on symptoms of attention-deficit/hyperactivity disorder—a placebo-controlled double-blind study." *Eur J Clin Nutr* 58:467–473 (2004).

Hohlfeld, R. and H. Wiendl. "The ups and downs of multiple sclerosis therapeutics." *Ann Neurol* 49:281–284 (2001).

Holden, R. J., I. S. Pakula, and P. A. Mooney. "The role of brain insulin in the neurophysiology of serious mental disorders: review." *Med Hypothesis* 52:193–200 (1999).

Hoozemans, J. J. M., A. J. M. Rozemuller, I. Janssen, C. J. A. De Groot, R. Veerhuls, and P. Eikelenboom. "Cyclooxygenase expression in microglia and neurons in Alzheimer's disease and control brain." *Acta Neuropathol* 101:2–8 (2001).

Hoozemans, J. J. M., R. Veerhuis, I. Janssen, A. J. M. Rozemuler, and P. Eikelenboom. "Interleukin-1 beta induced cyclooxygenase 2 expression and prostaglandin E2 secretion by human neroblastoma cells: implications for Alzheimer's disease." *Exp Gerontology* 36:559–570 (2001).

Horrobin, D. F. "Essential fatty acids, prostaglandins, and alcoholism: an overview." *Alcohol Clin Exp Res* 11:2–9 (1987).

Hunot, S., and E. C. Hirsch. "Neuroinflammatory processes in Parkinson's disease." *Ann Neurol* 53:S49–S60 (2003).

Ikemoto, A., A. Nitta, S. Furukawa, M. Ohishi, A. Nakamure, Y. Fujii, and H. Okuyama. "Dietary n-3 fatty acid deficiency decreases nerve growth factor content in rat hippocampus." *Neurosci Lett* 285:99–102 (2000).

Kademi, M., E. Wallstrom, M. Andersson, F. Piehl, R. Di Marco, and T. Olsson. "Reduction of both pro- and anti-inflammatory cytokines after 6 months of interferon beta-1a treatment of multiple sclerosis." *J Neurochem* 103:202–210 (2000).

Kalmijn, S., D. Foley, L. White, C. M. Burchfiel, J. D. Curb, H. Petrovitch, G. W. Ross, R. J. Havlik, and L. J. Launer. "Metabolic cardiovascular syndrome and risk of dementia in Japanese-American elderly men." *Arterioscler Thromb Vasc Biol* 20:2255–2260 (2000).

Kawas, C. H. and R. Brookmeyer. "Aging and the public health: effects of dementia." *N Engl J Med* 344:1160–1161 (2001).

Kyle, D. J., E. Schaefer, G. Patton, and A. Beiser. "Low serum docosahexaenoic acid is a significant risk factor for Alzheimer's dementia." *Lipids* 34:S245 (1999).

Lauritzen, I., N. Blondeau, C. Heurteaux, C. Widmann, G. Romey, and M. Lazdunski. "Polyunsaturated fatty acids are potent neuroprotectors." *EMBO J* 19:1784–1793 (2000).

Maes, M. "Fatty acid composition in major depression: decreased n-3 fractions in cholesterol esters and increased C20:n6/C20:5n3 ratio in cholesterol ester and phospholipids." *J Affect Dis* 38:35–46 (1996).

Maes, M., A. Christophe, J. Delanghe, C. Altamura, H. Neels, and H. Y. Meltzer. "Lowered omega-3 polyunsaturated fatty acids in serum phospholpids and cholesteryl esters of depressed patients." *Psychiatry Res* 85:275–291 (1999).

Manev, H., U. Tolga, K. Sugaya, and T. Qu. "Putative role of neuronal 5-lipoxygenase in an aging brain." *FASEB J* 14:1464–1469 (2000).

Marcheselli, V. L., S. Hong, W. J. Lukiw, X. H. Tian, K. Gronert, A. Musto, M. Hardy, J. M. Gimenz, N. Chian, C. N. Serhan, and G. Bazan. "Novel docosanoids inhibit brain ischemia-reperfusion-mediate leukocyte infiltration and pro-inflammatory gene expression." *J Biol Chem* 278:43807–43817 (2003).

McGeer, P. L., E. G. McGeer, and K. Yasojima. "Alzheimer disease and neuroinflammation." *J Neural Transm* 59:53–57 (2000).

McGeer, P. L., M. Shulzer, and E. G. McGeer. "Arthritis and anti-inflammatory agents as possible protective factors for Alzheimer's disease: a review of 17 epidemiological studies." *Neurology* 47:425–432 (1996).

Mills, D. E., K. M. Prkochin, K. A. Harvey, and R. P. Ward. "Dietary fatty acid supplementation alters stress reactivity and performance in man." *J Human Hypertension* 3:111–116 (1989).

Mischoulon, D. and M. Fava. "Docosahexanoic acid and omega-3 fatty acids in depression." *Psychiatr Clin North Am* 23:785–794 (2000).

Miyanga, K., K. Yonemura, T. Takagi, R. Kifune, Y. Kishi, F. Miyakawa, K. Yazawa, and Y. Shirota. "Clinical effects of DHA in demented patients." *J Clin Ther Med* 11:881–901 (1995).

Montine, T. J., K. R. Sidell, B. C. Crews, W. R. Markesbery, L. J. Marnett, L. J. Roberts, and J. D. Morrow. "Elevated CSF prostaglandin E2 levels in patients with probable AD." *Neurology* 53:1495–1498 (1999).

Moriguchi, T., R. S. Greiner, and N. Salem. "Behavioral deficits associated with dietary induction of decreased brain docosahexaenoic acid concentration." *J Neurochem* 75:2563–2573 (2000).

Morris, M. C., D. A. Evans, J. L. Bienias, C. C. Tangney, D. A. Bennett, R. S. Wilson, N. Aggarwal, and J. Schneider. "Consumption of fish and n-3 fatty acids and risk of incident Alzheimer disease." *Arch Neurol* 60:940–966 (2003).

Nagatsu, T., M. Mogi, H. Ichinose, and A. Togari. "Cytokines in Parkinson's disease." *J Neural Transm* 58:143–151 (2000).

Nemets, B., Z. Stahl, and R. H. Belmaker. "Addition of omega-3 fatty acid to maintenance medication treatment for recurrent unipolar depressive disorder." *Am J Psychiatry* 159:477–479 (2002).

Neuroinflammation Working Group. "Inflammation and Alzheimer's disease." *Neurobiology Aging* 21:383–421 (2000).

Nightingale, S., E. Woo, A. D. Smith, J. M. French, M. M. Gale, H. M. Sinclair, D. Bates, and D. A. Shaw. "Red blood cell and adipose tissue fatty acids in active and inactive multiple sclerosis patients." *Acta Neurol Scand* 82:43–50 (1990).

Nordvik, I., K-M. Myhr, H. Nyland, and K. S. Bjerve. "Effect of dietary advice and n-3 supplementation in newly diagnosed MS patients." *Acta Neurol Scand* 102:143–149 (2000).

Pasinetti, G. M., and P. S. Aisen. "Cyclooxygenase-2 expression is increased in frontal cortex of Alzheimer's disease brain." *Neuroscience* 87:319–324 (1997).

Pawlosky, R. J. and N. Salem. "Ethanol exposure causes a decrease in docosahexanenoic acid and an increase in docosapentaenoic acid in feline brain and retina." *Am J Clin Nutr* 61:1284–1289 (1995).

Peet, M. "Essential fatty acid deficiency in erthrocyte membranes from chronic schizophrenic patients and clinical effects of dietary supplementation." *Prostaglandins Leukot Essent Fatty Acids* 55:71–75 (1996).

Peet, M., J. Brind, C. N. Ramchand, S. Shah, and G. K. Vankar. "Two double-blind placebo-controlled pilot studies of eicosapentaenoic acid in the treatment of schizophrenia." *Schizophr Res* 49:243–251 (2001).

Pratico, D. and J. Q. Rojanowski. "Inflammatory hypothesis: novel mechanisms of Alzheimer's neurodegradation and new therapeutic targets?" *Neurobiology Aging* 21:441–445 (2000).

Rasgon, N. and L. Jarvik. "Insulin resistance, affective disorders, and Alzheimer's disease." *J Gerontology* 59A:178–183 (2004).

Reisbick, S., M. Neuringer, R. Hasnain, and W. E. Connor. "Home cage behavior of rhesus monkey with long-term deficiency of omega-3 fatty acids." *Physiol Behav* 55:231–239 (1994).

Remarque, E. J., E. L. E. M. Bollen, A. W. E. Weverling-Rijnsburger, J. C. Laterveer, G. J. Blauw, and R. G. J. Westendorp. "Patients with Alzheimer's disease display a pro-inflammatory phenotype." *Exp Gerontology* 36:171–176 (2001).

Richardson, A. J., C. M. Calvin, C. Clisby, D. R. Schoenheimer, P. Montgomery, J. A. Hall, G. Hebb, E. Westwood, J. B, Talcott, and J. F. Stein. "Fatty acid deficiency signs predict the severity of reading and related difficulties in dyslexic children." *Prostaglandins Leukot Essent Fatty Acids* 63:69–74 (2000).

Richardson, A. J. and B. K. Puri. "A randomized double-blind, placebo-controlled study of the effects of supplementation with highly unsaturated fatty acids on ADHD-related symptoms in children with specific learning difficulties." *Prog Neuropsychopharmacol Biol Psychiatry* 26:233- 239 (2002).

Richardson, A. J. and M. A. Ross. "Fatty acid metabolism in neurodevelopmental disorder: a new perspective on associations between attention-deficit/hyperactivity disorder, dyslexia, dyspraxia and the autistic spectrum." *Prostaglandins Leukot Essent Fatty Acids* 63:1- 9 (2000).

Ross, B. M., I. McKenzie, I. Glen, and C. P. Bennett. "Increased levels of ethane, a non-invasive marker of n- 3 fatty acid oxidation, in breath of children with attention deficit hyperactivity disorder." *Nutr Neurosci* 6:277–281 (2003).

Sachdev, P. "Attention deficit hyperactivity disorder in adults." *Psychological Med* 29:507–514 (1999).

Sears, B. *The Zone*. New York: ReganBooks, 1995.

Sears, B. *The Anti-Aging Zone*. New York: ReganBooks, 1999.

Sears, B. *The Omega Rx Zone*. New York: ReganBooks, 2002.

Sonderberg, M., C. Edlund, K. Kristensson, and G. Dallner. "Fatty acid composition of brain phospholipids in aging and Alzheimer's disease." *Lipids* 26:421–423 (1991).

Stein, J. "The neurobiology of reading difficulties." *Prostaglandins Leukot Essent Fatty Acids* 63:109–116 (2000).

Stevens, L. J. and J. Burgess. "Omega-3 fatty acids in boys with behavior, learning, and health problems." *Physiology Behavior* 59:915–920 (1996).

Stevens, L. J., S. S. Zentall, J. L. Deck, M. L. Abate, B. A. Watkins, S. A. Lipp, and J. R. Burgess. "Essential fatty acid metabolism in boys with attention-deficit hyperactivity disorder." *Am J Clin Nutr* 62:761–768 (1995).

Stevens, L., W. Zhang, L. Peck, T. Kuczek, N. Grevstad, A. Mahon, S. S. Zentall, L. E. Arnold, and J. R. Burgess. "EFA supplementation in children with inattention, hyperactivity, and other disruptive behaviors." *Lipids* 38:1007–1021 (2003).

Stewart, W. F., C. Kawas, M. Corrada, and E. J. Metter. "Risk of Alzhemier's disease and duration of NSAID use." *Neurology* 48:626–632 (1997).

Stoll, A. L., E. Sverus, M. P. Freeman, S. Rueter, H. A. Zhoyan, E. Diamond, K. K. Cress, and L. B. Marangell. "Omega-3 fatty acids in bipolar depression: a preliminary double-blind, placebo-controlled trial." *Arch Gen Psychiatry* 56:407–412 (1999).

Stordy, B. J. "Benefit of docosahexaenoic acid supplements to dark adaption in dyslexics." *Lancet* 346:385 (1995).

Su, K. P., S. Y. Huang, C. C. Chiu, and W. W. Shen. "Omega-3 fatty acids in major depressive disorder." *Eur Neuropsychopharmacology* 13:267–271 (2003).

Tanskanen, A. "Fish consumption, depression, and suicidality in a general population." *Arch Gen Psychiatry* 58:512–513 (2001).

Taylor, K. E. and A. J. Richardson. "Visual function, fatty acids and dyslexia." *Prostglandins Leukot Essent Fatty Acids* 63:89–93 (2000).

Terano, T., S. Fujishiro, T. Ban, K. Ymamoto, T. Tanaka, Y. Noguchi, Y. Tamura, K. Yazawa, and T. Hirayama. "Docosahexaenoic acid supplementation improves moderately severe dementia from thrombotic cerebrovascular diseases." *Lipids* 34:S345-S346 (1999).

Teunissen, C. E., M. P. J. van Boxtel, H. Bosma, E. Bosmans, J. Delanghe, De Bruijin, A. Wauters, M. Maes, J. Jolles, H. W. M. Steinbusch, and J. de Vente. "Inflammatory markers in relation to cognition in a healthy aging population." *J Neuroimmunity* 134:142–150 (2003).

Tully, A., H. M. Roche, R. Doyle, C. Fallon, I. Bruce, B. Lawlor, D. Coakley, and M. J. Gibney. "Low serum cholesteryl ester-docosahexaenoic acid levels in Alzheimer's disease." *Br J Nutr* 89:483–489 (2003).

Uauy, R., P. Peirano, D. Hoffman, P. Mena, D. Birch, and E. Birch. "Role of essential fatty acids in the function of the developing nervous system." *Lipids* 31:S167-S176 (1996).

Venters, H. D., R. Dantzer, and K. W. Kelly. "A new concept in neurodegeneration: TNF is a silencer of survival signals." *Trends in Neuroscience* 23:175–180 (2000).

Virkkunen, M. E., D. F. Horrobin, K. Douglas, K. Jenkins, and M. S. Manku. "Plasma phospholipids essential fatty acids and prostaglandin in alcoholic, habitually violent, and impulsive offenders." *Biol Psychiatry* 22:1087–1096 (1987).

Vitkovic, L., J. Bockaert, and C. Jacque. "Inflammatory cytokines: neuromodulators in normal brain?" *J Neurochem* 74:457–471 (2000).

Yehuda, S., S. Rabinovitz, R. L. Carasso, and D. I. Mostofsky. "Essential fatty acid preparation improves Alzheimer's patients quality of life." *Int J Neurosci* 87:141–149 (1996).

Yehuda, S., S. Rabinovitz, and D. I. Mostofsky. "Essential fatty acids are mediators of brain biochemistry and cognitive functions." *J Neurosci Res* 56:565–570 (1999).

Zametkin, A. J., and M. Ernst. "Problems in the management of attention-deficit-hyperactivity disorder." *N Engl J Med* 340:40–46 (1999).

Zametkin, A. J., T. E. Nordahl, A. C. King, W. E. Semple, J. Rumsey, S. Hamburger, and R. M. Cohen. "Cerebral glucose metabolism in adults with hyperactivity of childhood onset." *N Engl J Med* 323:1361–1366 (1990).

Zimmer, L., S. Hembert, G. Durand, P. Breton, D. Guillotau, J. C. Besnard, and S. Chalon. "Chronic n-3 polyunsaturated fatty acid diet-deficiency acts on dopamine metabolism in the rat frontal cortex." *Neurosci Letter* 240:177–181 (1998).

Zimmer, L., S. Vancassel, S. Cantagrel, P. Breton, S. Delamanche, D. Guilloteau, G. Durand, and S. Chalon. "The dopamine mesocorticolimbic pathway is affected by deficiency in n-3 polyunsaturated fatty acids." *Am J Clin Nutr* 75:662–667 (2002).

Chapter 18. Screaming Pain

Adam, O., C. Beringer, T. Kless, C. Lemmen, A. Adam, M. Wiseman, P. Adam, R. Klimmek, and W. Forth. "Anti-inflammatory effects of a low arachidonic acid diet and fish oil in patients with rheumatoid arthritis." *Rheumatol Int* 23:27–36 (2003).

Ariza-Ariza, R., M. Mestanza-Peralta, and M. H. Cardiel. "Omega-3 fatty acids in rheumatoid arthritis: an overview." *Semin Arthritis Rheum* 27:366–370 (1998).

Babcok, T., W. S. Helton, and N. J. Espat. "Eicosapentaenoic acid: an anti-inflammatory omega-3 fat with potential clinical applications." *Nutrition* 16:1116–1118 (2000).

Belluzzi, A., S. Boschi, C. Brignola, A. Munarini, G. Cariani, and F. Miglio. "Polyunsaturated fatty acids and inflammatory bowel disease." *Am J Clin Nutr* 71:339S-42S (2000).

Belluzzi, A., C. Brignola, M. Campieri, A. Pera, S. Boschi, and M. Miglioli. "Effect of an enteric-coated fish-oil preparation on relapses in Crohn's disease." *N Engl J Med* 354:1557–1560 (1996).

Blok, W. L., M. B. Katan, and J. W. van der Meer. "Modulation of inflammation and cytokine production by dietary (n-3) fatty acids." *J Nutr* 126:1515–1533 (1996).

Calder, P. C. "n-3 polyunsaturated fatty acids and cytokine production in health and disease." *Ann Nutr Metab* 41:203–234 (1997).

Calder, P. C. "n-3 polyunsaturated fatty acids, inflammation and immunity." *Nutr Res* 21:309–341 (2001).

Chandrasekar, B., and G. Fernandes. "Decreased pro-inflammatory cytokines and increased antioxidant enzyme gene expression by omega-3 lipids in murine lupus nephritis." *Biochem Biophys Res Commun* 200(2):893–898 (1994).

Clark, W. F., A. Parbtani, C. D. Naylor, C. M. Levinton, N. Muirhead, E. Spanner, M. W. Huff, D. J. Philbrick, and B. J. Holub. "Fish oil in lupus nephritis: clinical findings and methodological implications." *Kidney Int* 44:75–86 (1993).

Cleland, L. G., J. K. French, W. H. Betts, G. A. Murphy, and M. J. Elliot. "Clinical and biochemical effects of dietary fish oil supplements in rheumatoid arthritis." *J Rheumatol* 15:1471–1475 (1988).

Das, U. N. "Beneficial effects of eicosapentaenoic and docosahexaenoic acids in the management of systemic erthematosus and its relationship to the cytokine network." *Prostaglandins Leukot Essent Fatty Acids* 51:207–213 (1994).

Donadio, J. V., J. P. Grande, E. J. Bergstralh, R. A. Dart, T. S. Larson, and D. C. Spencer. "The long-term outcome of patients with IgA nephropathy treated with fish oil in a controlled trial." *J Am Soc Nephrol* 10:1772–1777 (1999).

Endres, S. "Messengers and mediators: interactions among lipids, eicosanoids, and cytokines." *Am J Clin Nutr* 57:798S–800S (1993).

Endres, S. "n-3 polyunsaturated fatty acids and human cytokine synthesis." *Lipids* 31 S239–S242 (1996).

Endres, S., R. Ghorbani, V. E. Kelley, K. Georgilis, G. Lonnemann, J. W. van der Meer, J. G. Cannon, T. S. Rogers, M.S. Klempner, and P.C. Weber. "The effect of dietary supplementation with n-3 polyunsaturated fatty acids on the synthesis of interleukin-1 and tumor necrosis factor by mononuclear cells." *N Engl J Med* 320:265–271 (1989).

Endres, S., R. Lorenz, and K. Loeschke."Lipid treatment of inflammatory bowel disease." *Curr Opin Clin Nutr Metab Care* 2:117–120 (1999).

Endres, S., B. Sinha, and T. Eisenhut. "Omega 3 fatty acids in the regulation of cytokine synthesis." *World Rev Nutr Diet* 76:89–94 (1994).

Endres, S., and C. von Schacky. "n-3 polyunsaturated fatty acids and human cytokine synthesis." *Curr Opin Lipidol* 7:48–52 (1996).

Fox, D. A. "Cytokine blockade as a new strategy to treat rheumatoid arthritis. Inhibition of tumor necrosis factor." *Arch Intern Med* 160:437–444 (2000).

Geusens, P., C. Wouters, J. Nijs, Y. Jiang, and J. Dequeker. "Long-term effect of omega-3 fatty acid supplementation in active rheumatoid arthritis. A 12-month, double-blind, controlled study." *Arthritis Rheum* 37:824–829 (1994).

Kilkens, T. O. C., A. Honig, M. Maes, R. Lousberg, and R. J. Brummer. "Fatty acid profile and affective dysregulation in irritable bowel syndrome." *Lipids* 39:425–431 (2004).

Kremer, J. M. "N-3 fatty acid supplements in rheumatoid arthritis." *Am J Clin Nutr* 71:349S–351S. (2000).

Kremer, J. M., D. A. Lawrence, G. F. Petrillo, L. L. Litts, P. M. Mullaly, R. I. Rynes, R. P. Stocker, N. Parhami, N. S. Greenstein, and B. R. Fuchs. "Effects of high-dose fish oil on rheumatoid arthritis after stopping nonsteroidal antiinflammatory drugs. Clinical and immune correlates." *Arthritis Rheum* 38:1107–1114 (1995).

Lo, C. J., K. C. Chiu, M. Fu, R. Lo, and S. Helton. "Fish oil decreases macrophage tumor necrosis factor gene transcription by altering the NF kappaB activity." *J Surg Res* 82:216–221 (1999).

Meydani, S. N. "Effect of n-3 polyunsaturated fatty acid on cytokine production and their biological action." *Nutrition* 12:S8–14 (1996).

Ozgocmen, S., S. A. Catal, O. Ardicoglu, and A. Kamanli. "Effect of omega-3 fatty acids in the management of fibromyalgia syndrome." *Int J Clin Pharmacol Ther* 38:362–363 (2000).

Pisetsky, D. S. "Tumor necrosis factor blockers in rheumatoid arthritis." *N Engl J Med* 342:810–811 (2000).

Prickett, J. D., D. R. Robinson, and A. D. Steinberg. "Dietary enrichment with polyunsaturated acid eicosapentaenoic acid prevents proteinuria and prolongs survival in NZBxNZW F1 mice." *J Clin Invest* 68:556–559 (1981).

Robinson, D. R., L. L. Xu, S. Tateno, M. Guo, and R. B. Colvin. "Suppression of autoimmune disease by dietary n-3 fatty acids." *J Lipid Res* 34:1435–1444 (1993).

Ross, E. "The role of marine oils in the treatment of ulcerative colitis." *Nutr Rev* 51:47–49 (1993).

Shapiro, H. "Could n-3 polyunsaturated fatty acids reduce pathological pain direct actions on the nervous system." *Prostaglandins Leukot Essent Fatty Acids* 68:219–224 (2003).

Simopoulos, A. P. "Omega-3 fatty acids in inflammation and autoimmune diseases." *J Am Coll Nutr* 21:495–505 (2002).

Sperling, R. I. "The effects of dietary n-3 polyunsaturated fatty acids on neutrophils." *Proc Nutr Soc* 57:527–534 (1998).

Teitelbaum, J. E. and W. Allan Walker. "The role of omega 3 fatty acids in intestinal inflammation." *J Nutr Biochem* 12:21–32 (2001).

Wolfe, F., K. Ross, J. Anderson, I. J. Russel, and L. Hebert. "The prevalence and characteristics of fibromyalgia in the general population." *Arthritis Rheum* 38:19–28 (1995).

Zaloga, G. P. and P. Parik. "Lipid modulation and systemic inflammation." *Crit Care Clin* 17:201–217.

Zurier, R. B. "Prostaglandins, immune responses and murine lupus." *Arth Rheum* 25:804–809 (1982).

Zurier, R. B. "Lipids and lupus." In *Lupus: Molecular and Cellular Pathogenesis*, ed. G. M. Kammer and G. C. Tsokos, pp. 599–611, Totowan, N.J.: Humana Press, 1998.

Chapter 19. Who Is to Blame for the Epidemic of Silent Inflammation?

Darman, N., A. Briend, and A. Drewnowski. "Energy-dense diets are associated with lower diet costs." *Public Health Nutrition* 7:21–27 (2004).

Drewnowski, A. "Energy density, palatability and satiation: implications for weight control." *Nutr Rev* 56:347–353 (1998).

Drewnowski, A. "Fat and sugar: an economic analysis." *J Nutr* 133:838S-840S (2003).

Drewnowski, A. "The role of energy density." *Lipids* 38:109–115 (2003).

Nestle, M. *Food Politics. How the Food Industry Influences Nutrition and Health.* Berkeley, CA: University of California Press, 2002.

Nestle, M. "The ironic politics of obesity." *Science* 299:781 (2003).

Nielsen, S. J., and B. M. Popkin. "Patterns and trends in food portion sizes, 1977–1998." *JAMA* 289:450–453 (2003).

Popkin, B. M. and S. J. Nielsen. "The sweetening of the world's diet." *Obesity Res* 11:1325–1331 (2003).

Chapter 20. Avoiding the Coming Collapse of the Health Care System

Noakes, M., P. R. Foster, J. B. Keogh, and P. M. Clifton. "Meal replacements are as effective as structured weight-loss diets for treating obesity in adults with features of metabolic syndrome." *J Nutr* 134:1894–1899 (2004).

Willet, W. C. *Eat, Drink and Be Healthy. The Harvard Medical School Guide to Healthy Eating.* New York: Fireside, 2001.

Yao, M. and S. B. Roberts. "Dietary energy density and weight regulation." *Nutr Rev* 59:247–258 (2001).

Index

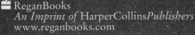